Praise for

Clean

"An objective, if still impassioned, examination of the research on prevention and treatment . . . Sheff is a skilled journalist on an urgent mission . . . His forbearance and clearheadedness could serve as an example for America as it confronts its drug problem. He has performed a vital service by compiling sensible advice on a subject for which sensible advice is in short supply." — *New York Times Book Review*

"Providing a wealth of information and practical advice, *Clean* is the best book on drug abuse and addiction to appear in years . . . *Clean* busts a mountain of myths . . . [An] extraordinarily valuable book." — *Psychology Today*

"[A] guide for those just entering the terrain [David] Sheff knows so well . . . Cardiac patients stop to rest halfway up a flight of stairs not because they want to, but because they have to. Similarly, addicts lie and steal, over and over again, not because they want to but because they must. Wrapping the mind around this formulation requires an enormous act of will, and it is Sheff's foremost achievement that his arguments are likely to influence even the angriest and most judgmental reader . . . *Clean* is a reference work and a manifesto." — *New York Times*

"David Sheff knows addiction as no parent would ever want. Through it all, he's tapped into a unique ability to convey the pain, wisdom, and love that he's experienced through many turbulent years with his son Nic. As a journalist, father, and clear-eyed chronicler of addiction, Sheff is without peer." — **Sanjay Gupta, M.D., chief medical correspondent, CNN**

"Sheff offers new, sustainable solutions to a problem that has reached epidemic levels in this country ... Fascinating ... [*Clean*] offers new models, strategies, and alternative therapies for abuse interventions and promising reform ... Intelligent and thought-provoking."

— *Kirkus Reviews*

"Indisputably important."

— *Library Journal*

"Gripping and vibrant."

— *Publishers Weekly*

"*Clean* will change not only how you look at drug abuse, but also what you think should be done about it. This book is essential reading on one of our most important social problems."

— Eric Schlosser, author of *Fast Food Nation* and *Reefer Madness*

"How do we prevent kids from using drugs, and how do we effectively treat addiction? *Clean* cuts through the technical jargon and marketing nonsense to summarize our best knowledge on these topics ... A major contribution to our understanding of this disease and how to fight it."

— Richard A. Rawson, Ph.D., professor and associate director, Integrated Substance Abuse Programs, Geffen School of Medicine, UCLA

"*Clean* is an important exposé of a failed system; by replacing it, we will save countless lives, help people get clean and stay clean, and help the United States end its catastrophic war on drugs."

— Sir Richard Branson, founder and chairman, Virgin Group, and member of the Global Commission on Drug Policy

Clean

Overcoming Addiction and Ending America's Greatest Tragedy

DAVID SHEFF

An Eamon Dolan Book
Mariner Books
HOUGHTON MIFFLIN HARCOURT
Boston   New York

First Mariner Books edition 2014

Copyright © 2013 by David Sheff

www.hmhco.com

Library of Congress Cataloging-in-Publication Data
Sheff, David.
Clean : overcoming addiction and ending America's greatest tragedy / David Sheff.
pages cm
"An Eamon Dolan book."
Includes bibliographical references and index.
ISBN 978-0-547-84865-5   ISBN 978-0-544-11232-2 (pbk.)
1. Substance abuse — United States. 2. Addicts — Rehabilitation —
United States. 3. Substance abuse — Physiological aspects. I. Title.
RC564.S497 2013
362.29 — dc23
2013000387

Book design by Melissa Lotfy

Printed in the United States of America
DOC 10 9 8 7 6 5 4 3 2

To those afflicted with addiction, to their loved ones,
to those we've lost to this disease,
and to those working to prevent addiction and treat the addicted

And to Karen Barbour

Contents

Author's Note

Over the years I researched *Clean,* many people afflicted with addiction and many of their family members bravely shared their stories. Some spoke under the condition that I use only their first names or pseudonyms and change details that would identify them or their loved ones. Named or not, I'm deeply grateful to them all for their willingness to speak to me and their desire to help others in their straits. Similarly, I report on visits to inpatient and outpatient treatment programs, sober-living residences, and other facilities that, in some cases, allowed me onto the premises only under the condition that neither they nor their patients be identified.

Preface

THE VIEW THAT DRUG use is a moral choice is pervasive, pernicious, and wrong. So are the corresponding beliefs about the addicted — that they're weak, selfish, and dissolute; if they weren't, when their excessive drug taking and drinking began to harm them, they'd stop. The reality is far different. Using drugs or not isn't about willpower or character. Most problematic drug use is related to stress, trauma, genetic predisposition, mild or serious mental illness, use at an early age, or some combination of those. Even in their relentless destruction and self-destruction, the addicted aren't bad people. They're gravely ill, afflicted with a chronic, progressive, and often terminal disease.

People also believe that addicts can't be treated; at best, they can muster their willpower and manage their compulsion for a short time. But while it's true that addicts who seek treatment are seldom cured, their disease is treatable when we reject the pseudoscience, moralizing, and scare tactics that characterize the current system. The disease of addiction can be prevented, and when we treat it the way we treat other diseases, those in its thrall can be freed to live long, full, healthy lives.

The mission of *Clean* is to describe the scope of America's drug problem and explain how and why we've failed in our efforts to combat it. I show why we must waste no time in rejecting the existing paradigm that got us into this catastrophic mess. I provide scientific evidence that will change the way we think about drugs and addiction. Finally, and most important, I present the hopeful news that we can now effectively pre-

vent drug use and treat addiction. When we do, we do more than help
those with drug problems and their families. We also start to remedy
America's single greatest problem, one that affects almost every other
problem you can name — the quality and availability of health care, the
national and international economic crisis, poverty, spousal and child
abuse, suicide, U.S. competitiveness in the world economy, property
crime, violence, shattered families, decimated neighborhoods, and
many others.

As a young child, my firstborn son, Nic, was happy and excited about everything, kind and sincere and funny. Parents like me monitor external
barometers to tell us how our kids are doing, and according to those, as
Nic grew older, he did well. He had friends; he was a good student, an
athlete (on the varsity swim and water polo teams), and a lauded student
journalist. Most important, he seemed so joyful. But, beginning when
he was twelve years old, he was also using drugs, initially smoking pot.

A decade later, I still look back and ask, How did it start? How does
it start for any of our children, our husbands or wives, partners, parents,
siblings, friends — for anyone who becomes addicted? Nic says he tried
drugs because he was curious, and everyone seemed to be using, "at
least, everyone who was cool." When he tried them, he felt fantastic. He
used more and then more. He graduated from high school, but he also
graduated to other drugs. He began college but didn't last long there. Instead, he became homeless, sleeping in cars, abandoned buildings, and
city parks. He lied to his family and stole from us. He took pills (psychedelics, ecstasy, uppers, downers), used cocaine, and — inconceivably to
me — began shooting heroin, crack, and crystal meth.

I wrote about the years our family lived through his addiction in the
book *Beautiful Boy*. Readers of it and of Nic's own books — a pair of
memoirs, *Tweak: Growing Up on Methamphetamines* and *We All Fall
Down* — know many of the gory details. Over the course of a hellish
half a dozen years, Nic dealt drugs, was beaten up, and was wanted by
the police. Once, a doctor informed him that he would probably have
to amputate Nic's arm because it had become infected after Nic shot
heroin and crystal meth. (Miraculously, the doctor was able to save it.)
There were many times when Nic nearly died. I'd think, *This cannot be
happening to my son. Not to Nic.* I thought he'd be protected by his intel-

ligence, his education, us — his family. Nic didn't look like the addicts I'd see on the streets. I'd walk by those hollow-eyed, trembling wraiths and avert my gaze. I thought it was impossible that Nic would become one of them, but he did.

The experts say that addiction is a family disease. For a long time, I didn't understand what that meant. When Nic became addicted, I thought he was the one with the problem. He was the one who needed help. But my son's addiction wasn't destroying only him. It was destroying our family. It was destroying me. I couldn't function. I couldn't work, couldn't take care of the rest of my family. Nic repeatedly disappeared — a day and a night, two days, a week — and I'd be out of my mind with worry. I couldn't sleep. I did what parents who don't know where their children are do. I called the police, the hospital emergency rooms. One time, when I called the local sheriff's office looking for Nic, an officer asked, "Mr. Sheff, have you tried the morgue?"

I was in a state of unrelenting, immobilizing panic. As I described it in *Beautiful Boy*, I became addicted to Nic's addiction. How could I not? My son was mainlining drugs — as I wrote, "shooting poison into his arms, arms that not that long ago threw baseballs and built Lego castles, arms that wrapped around my neck when I carried his sleepy body in from the car at night."

For the sake of Jasper and Daisy, our younger children, my wife, Karen, and I carried on as normally as possible. They were not only confused and intensely worried about their big brother but also traumatized by their parents' distress. When Jasper watched Nic being arrested, he was inconsolable. Back when she was in grade school, Daisy wrote about her childhood for a homework assignment. "I was born into a latticework of lovely oceans and hunched shadowed vampires tangled together in an inseparable knot. Most of what I remember about being little is marvelous, with my two wise brothers carrying me upon their shoulders." But then "everything sort of flipped over. Nic was tired and slinking and then he was gone. My strong pillar parents crumbled."

During those hellish years, I tried everything I could to help Nic. I brought him to therapists and counselors and Twelve Step meetings and checked him into residential treatments, halfway houses, outpatient programs, and more, but his addiction worsened. In family groups and at the Al-Anon meetings I attended, I heard other parents with stories similar to mine. In most cases, nothing had helped their children either. Even worse, when treatment failed, their kids were blamed — they were too weak, weren't committed enough to staying sober, didn't pray hard enough. I also learned that despite how bad it was for us, we were among the lucky ones. Nic survived; many people's loved ones didn't.

Eventually I learned that only a minority of those who are addicted are successfully treated. How bad is the current addiction-treatment system? Tom McLellan, a preeminent addiction researcher, knows as much about addiction as anyone in the world. Yet despite that, his two sons became addicts. "I was the addiction expert," says McLellan, founder of the Treatment Research Institute and former deputy director of the Office of National Drug Control Policy in the Obama administration. "But I didn't know what to do. I asked my colleagues — they're experts — and *they* didn't know what to do." Groping his way through the dark, desperate to help his sons, McLellan did all he could. He had access to the best care possible, but it wasn't good enough. One son is now in recovery, but his younger son died of an overdose of benzodiazepines and alcohol.

Why are we so inept at preventing drug use and keeping early use from progressing to abuse? Why can't we treat most of those who become addicted? A decade ago, I set out to find answers to these questions. More important, I wanted to find a better way to prevent our children — all people, but kids are the most vulnerable — from using and help the addicted get and stay clean.

I learned as much as I could about the physiology and psychology of addiction, its prevention, and its treatment from researchers who have devoted their lives to these subjects. I took into account their opinions and consensus (when there was a consensus) and research that came to conflicting conclusions. I interviewed clinicians and watched them work. I visited emergency rooms and doctors' and therapists' offices. I toured inpatient and outpatient rehabs and sat in on a wide variety of treatment sessions led by therapists of countless stripes. I also attended Twelve Step meetings — AA, NA, Al-Anon, and others. I went to dangerous neighborhoods defined by drugs, destroyed by them. I went to meetings where parents agonized about the drugs flooding into their towns, and to drug-prevention assemblies in school cafeterias. When I left one assembly, I turned a corner and ran into a dozen kids smoking weed under a stairwell.

Sometimes I gleaned the greatest wisdom from addicts themselves. I interviewed many, observed them, commiserated with them. I met with them after they relapsed. I met with them in the middle of relapse. I met addicts who had been clean for days, or months, or years. Some were on the streets — vagrants, derelicts — and some in prison. Some carried on full lives — working, parenting, and in every other way functioning despite their dependence on heroin or crack. I also got to know their families — traumatized parents, children, spouses, and siblings.

The combination of research, expert opinion, and personal stories resulted in volumes of interview transcripts, notes, and articles from medical journals and the lay press; cardboard boxes and gigabytes full of them. I analyzed them over months and then years, slowly distilling them, identifying what had gone wrong. But although the system was, and is, indisputably broken, I found, hidden in corners, little-known but effective prevention and treatment programs. I found psychologists, psychiatrists, and therapists who are implementing lifesaving treatments. And I found researchers who are advancing the understanding of drug use and addiction and, based on their findings, developing and putting into practice prevention and treatment strategies that dramatically improve the chances that children will grow up drug-free and that addicts will be successfully treated.

Clean is a synthesis of what I learned, presented in a way that I hope will prove useful to all of those who are concerned about America's drug problem and want to do something about it. Moreover, I believe the approach put forth in this book will be a revelation for those afflicted with addiction and for their families. It will be particularly revelatory for those who've been told that there's only one way to get and stay clean, and for the many, many people who haven't been helped by the current treatment system and who were told that it was their own fault.

Addicted Nation

Almost 80 percent of America's children under eighteen have used alcohol, and half have smoked marijuana or tried other drugs. No one who tries drugs thinks he'll become addicted. True, some people can smoke pot or take a drink once, and that's it — they stop or use moderately. For others, however, drug use steers life inexorably toward tragedy. It's a cliché to say that addiction is an equal opportunity affliction, but it's worth repeating. Your education, safe neighborhood, good income, strong family — whatever you think will protect you — guarantees nothing.

The devastation begins with the more than twenty million people who are currently addicted to drugs (throughout this book, when I speak of drugs, I include alcohol, one of the many addictive substances). Many of them suffer a lifetime of physical and mental anguish and many die young. Indeed, drugs now kill more people than any other non-natural cause. The Centers for Disease Control and Prevention (CDC) has tracked a doubling of drug-related deaths since the early 1980s. Every day drugs kill over 365 Americans, more than any other preventable health problem. Approximately 135,000 deaths a year in the United States are directly attributed to drugs, but that doesn't take into account the more than 100,000 additional fatalities that are caused by drugs but counted as suicides, homicides, automobile and other accidents, heart attacks, pulmonary disorders, strokes and cerebral hemorrhages, hepatitis and other infections, HIV/AIDS, liver disease, kidney disease, septicemia, and on and on.

Approximately one in twelve Americans over the age of twelve is addicted to drugs. In addition to the deaths it causes, substance abuse leads to more illnesses than any other preventable health condition. Addiction is more prevalent than cancer, stroke, HIV/AIDS, or Alzheimer's disease. Drug abuse and addiction overwhelm America's health-care system; hospitals regularly treat drug overdoses as well as automobile accidents, illnesses, and other life-threatening crises caused by drugs. Indeed, drugs are linked to more ER visits and hospital admissions than any other single cause — 4.6 million of them in 2009, the most recent figure available. That was an 81 percent increase over 2004.

Drugs are also the number one cause of crime. People who are either high or seeking money for drugs are involved in more than half of all burglaries. More than half of America's federal prison inmates today are in on drug convictions. In 2010, 85 percent of the U.S. prison population were incarcerated for crimes committed while under the influence of alcohol or other drugs; crimes committed to get money to buy drugs;

or crimes involving alcohol or drug law violations. Almost 80 percent of kids in the juvenile justice system are there because of problems related to their substance abuse. Drugs are involved in from one-half to three-quarters of all incidences of violence, including child abuse, spousal abuse, homicides, rape, and close to 100 percent of date rapes. Drugs are at the center of myriad other social problems. It's estimated that at least 60 percent of homeless people suffer addiction, which often occurs along with mental illnesses. Drugs have broken up an incalculable number of families and devastated neighborhoods everywhere.

The total overall cost of drug abuse in the United States exceeds $400 billion a year, mostly in health-care and crime-related costs and lost productivity. Looming in the future are the incalculable costs of a generation of kids growing up high. There's much handwringing about America's future competitiveness in light of the educational disparities between the United States and other nations, but we've ignored the fact that American teenagers use drugs at a higher rate than teens in any other country in the world. In this competition, the contest isn't even close.

The Anguish of Addiction

The statistics describe only the scope of the problem, not the suffering, which is immeasurable. Over the past decade, I've felt the anguish and seen it in the hundreds of people I've met who were in agony because of their own or their loved ones' addictions. I can often tell before they say a word. Their faces show me the hell they've endured. Some can barely get out a syllable before they break down in tears. As best they can, they tell their stories. I've also heard from thousands by mail and e-mail, and more write every day. In a typical week, a mother described her son as "the latest sacrificial lamb"; drunk and stoned, he was killed in a head-on collision. Another mother wrote, "We knew K. smoked a little marijuana, but that was the extent of it as far as we knew. The coroner said there was marijuana, cocaine and heroin in her system. She went from the most loving child to someone I didn't recognize, and then I lost her."

"My 19 year old daughter died last month," her father wrote. "I loved her with every ounce of me. The world lost an angel. My life is shattered."

"My precious son died of a drug overdose eight months ago," wrote Kathleen Kelly, a professor at Colorado State University. "He was 24 years old. He got addicted to Oxy and when he couldn't afford it anymore he went to a less expensive opiate — heroin. . . . He hated being an addict." Kathleen sent photographs of her son, Austin. In one, he was pictured with two friends. All three boys in the photograph are dead of overdoses. "First Ben, then Jackson, and now Austin."

Not all of the letters are from parents whose children have not survived. One man described the vigil that many parents know too well. "It's only a matter of time. I can barely breathe as I write this. Every time the phone rings my heart stops. 'This is it,' I know. 'This is the call. He's dead.'" A mother said, "My daughter started with abusing inhalants, then marijuana, and has confessed to taking pills — Adderall, Valium, and ones I haven't heard of. She is 14 years old. My husband and I placed her into a treatment center. . . . She came home and was okay for two months, then she didn't come home one night when she was supposed to be here. We got a call from the hospital. She had overdosed and is in a coma. I'm writing from her room in the hospital. I look up at her blank face. Her chances are 50-50."

A father wrote about his "beautiful, intelligent, talented, and charismatic" son, who was, he said, "on his third attempt at staying clean. He tricked us, snuck out, and scored, and we don't know where he is. Is he alive or dead? All I can do is worry. My son's addiction has destroyed my marriage and estranged me from the rest of my family. I live, pretty much, in isolation. All I want is my son back."

Children write too. One letter began, "I was my parents' beautiful girl. I've taken pills since I was 15. I tried to kill myself by taking twenty Valium, but it didn't work. You'd think that would get me to stop [using], but not me."

Another woman wrote of her addicted husband: "He's not the man I married. He won't even stop for our three- and seven-year-old children. He's a good man, a good husband and father. But he goes on benders and we don't see him. I know he tried crack at least once. He's been in rehab three times. They say to throw him out and close the door, but he is the father of my children."

A letter from a thirty-seven-year-old woman addicted to heroin, written in tiny, shaky script on tissue paper, came in the mail: "If not for the curse of addiction," she wrote, "I would not have a heart locked up tight in my chest, afraid of opening it for anyone. My children have been taken from me, to be raised by someone else, and I have to live with that agony every day of my life. I suffer through the knowledge that I caused them immense pain, and caused them to be fearful of trusting and loving and that I took from them the one thing that all children deserve, a feeling of security and knowing that no matter what is happening in the world, there is one place of safety and that is their home." She concluded, "I am so sorry for the things I have done, and I live with so much regret — sometimes so much that I feel like I can't face another day."

These letters communicate an infinitesimal fraction of the suffering that millions endure every day. If this were a problem that couldn't be solved, I'd be devastated but resigned. Instead, I'm filled with rage, because the suffering and death can be prevented. How? It begins with an understanding of the precepts that underpin *Clean*.

1. Most drug use isn't about drugs; it's about life.

Our prevention and treatment efforts have failed mostly because they've focused on dealing with drugs themselves, but drug abuse is almost always the result of kids starting to use early, genetics, and other problems — stress, trauma, mental illness, or some combination of these factors. The new paradigm is rooted in recognizing that drugs are a symptom, not a cause, and whatever problems underlie them must be (and can be) addressed. Until they are, our prevention and treatment systems will continue to fail most people.

2. Addiction is a disease.

No one chooses leukemia, heart disease, or depression. Abusing drugs, however, appears to many to be a choice, and a reckless and selfish one. It's not. The new approach is based on the fact — a fact I'll prove categorically — that addiction is a disease. Serious illness is always frightening, but it's a relief to understand that it's not a person's fault if she is addicted. Perhaps more to the point, blaming the afflicted for their condition has led to decades of flawed treatment and policy. But the evidence clearly proves that addicts aren't morally bereft or weak-willed. They're ill.

3. This disease is preventable.

Given the scale of illicit drug use and abuse, the ineffectiveness of decades of anti-drug campaigns, and the failure of a war on drugs that has cost more than $1 trillion, most people assume that it's impossible to prevent drug abuse. Parents, schools, communities, and the nation itself have initiated campaigns to stop drug use, but they've failed. However, we now know that prevention initiatives failed not because it's impossible to stop people from using and abusing drugs, but because our efforts were misguided.

4. This disease is treatable.

Most people, including most addicts, assume that addiction can't be treated. On their own or with help, sometimes by relying on the traditional Twelve Step program, some people have learned to manage their addiction and stop using. But many more haven't. Many of those who had successfully stopped using relapsed, often repeatedly. Some early research indicated that addicts could never fully recover because drugs caused permanent brain damage. We've since learned that traditional treatments often failed not because of intractable brain damage, but because they were inadequate. (In fact, some were useless, and some were harmful.) However, a host of recent findings about how addiction works have led to the development of effective treatments, and more are coming. Adding to this promising news is evidence that most brains damaged by drugs can recover. Sufferers of addiction can be restored to health.

5. As with any other illness, the prevention strategies
   and treatments most likely to work aren't based on
   tradition, wishful thinking, or faith, but science.

To date, prevention strategies have failed because they've relied on scare tactics and best guesses of what might work. When these efforts fail and drug use begins and escalates, desperate people who need treatment often wind up in the hands of charlatans, rip-off artists, or well-intentioned but incompetent practitioners. Once we understand that addiction is a disease and that it's preventable and treatable, our course becomes clearer, because we have a model to follow. Just as there are proven prevention strategies that lower incidences of some cancers, diabetes, and heart disease, there are effective approaches to stop people from using drugs and nip early use in the bud, before it advances to full-blown addiction. And just as patients with other serious illnesses pursue the most effective treatments developed by science and tested in clinical trials, so too can addicts and their families.

6. Drug abusers and addicts can do more than get
   off drugs; they can achieve mental health.

As it's defined by the National Academy of Sciences, mental health "is more than the absence of disorder." Usually those with addiction, particularly those who've used drugs since they were teenagers, live their lives in pain and confusion. Drugs impeded their emotional growth at the very time when they would have been learning to navigate the world, to develop close relationships, and to mature in other ways. With sobriety comes the opportunity of transformation and a fulfilling life.

These precepts may seem pretty straightforward, but like everything else related to addiction, each is complicated by nuance and variation. Yes, most drug use isn't about drugs, but it's often impossible to get to the root causes of addiction when a person's using. Drugs mask and exacerbate other problems, so treatment must focus on stopping drug use even as it addresses whatever underlies or accompanies it. Yes, addiction is a disease, but it has characteristics that distinguish it from most other illnesses. Yes, it's preventable, but given the myriad and complex reasons people use drugs, preventing use and abuse is a daunting challenge. Yes, it's treatable, but for now there's no cure. Yes, the treatments most likely to work are those based on science, but it's not an exact science. "This is the place where science meets people," says Steve Shoptaw, psychologist in the department of family medicine at UCLA. Drug use, addiction, and mental illness are as complicated as people are. There are as many permutations as there are people, so there's no one-size-fits-all solution. And yes, the lives of those with addiction can transform, but it can take time, and forward progress can be interrupted by setbacks. Still, healing is almost always possible.

Nothing makes it easy to prevent drug use or treat addiction, but the new paradigm presented in *Clean* makes it easier because it helps people understand what they're up against; shows them how to navigate bewildering, treacherous waters; and guides them in planning the best possible course of action. When people follow this new path, they can avoid wasting effort and precious time. Ultimately, this model can take people through the most confusing, complicated, and devastating times that many will ever face. Confusion and despair can make way for clarity and hope. Addicts can lead full lives free from the pain that plagued them and the disease that controlled them.

I

America on Drugs

1

This Is Your Brain on Drugs

DRUG USE BEGINS INNOCENTLY enough. A child is handed a joint and takes a puff. He's given a beer and has a sip. Some don't like it and they stop. Many of them continue to use occasionally, and some use frequently. Some become addicted. So many of the stories about addiction begin the same way: "He was a good boy"; "She was a joy, moral and smart and funny and . . ." Of her son, Kevin, Jacqueline Periman says, "He was my beautiful golden-haired angel child."

The earliest pictures of Kevin were taken in the hospital on the first day of his life: His mother, striking with long brown hair parted on the side, gazing into the blue of her son's eyes. In a photo that takes my breath away, his head rests on his mother's bare shoulder. Mother and child look serene, at peace.

Jacqueline grew up in West LA near Beverly Hills. She had two much older — older by nearly twenty years — brothers. "I was kind of 'oops.'" Looking back, she says that her childhood was surreal. In her home, it was considered normal for either of her brothers to be passed out drunk or stoned at the dinner table. Her mother mostly didn't notice; she was devoted to the care of her husband, Jacqueline's father, who was dying of Alzheimer's disease.

"We weren't really raised," Jacqueline recalls.

There were fights when one brother accused the other of stealing their father's medication. Paramedics came and went. When Jacqueline called 911, the dispatcher would ask, "Which brother is it now?"

Alzheimer's killed Jacqueline's father and, later, her mother. When she was a teenager, one of her brothers was admitted to UCLA Medical Center after an accident. A doctor told her that he didn't think he would make it. "I thought, *Let's get it over with.*" Her brother survived that time, but not for much longer. Six years later, he committed suicide. Soon after, her other brother died of cancer. Both brothers were high most of their lives.

Jacqueline earned a degree in anthropology at UCLA, where she fell in love with and married a fellow student. Her husband got his pilot's license and a job at a regional airline and then with TWA and American. The couple moved to St. Louis, where she worked at the St. Louis University Hospital as a medical assistant in the ob-gyn department.

They had two children: Kevin, born in 1988, and Jill, born three years later. Jacqueline and her husband divorced in 1996, when the children were eight and five.

Given her brothers' addictions, Jacqueline worried about drugs and talked to her children about them. Kevin had asthma and so she was particularly appalled when she smelled marijuana on him when he came home one evening after playing with friends. He was twelve. "What are you thinking?"

He said what kids say: "I just wanted to try it." And she believed him. When she caught him drinking a beer, he told her the same thing, and she believed him again. She thought, *Kids experiment.*

Kevin read a lot and loved Legos and science; in the evenings, he'd stand mesmerized in the backyard looking through a telescope he'd built himself. He charted the planets and their moons. But then he became an adolescent and all that stopped. He seemed tired all the time. He was surly, and sometimes Jacqueline thought he might be depressed. She brought him to see a psychiatrist, who diagnosed him with ADD and noted that Kevin might also have bipolar disorder. He prescribed Depakote.

Kevin became "different, he drifted away from me," Jacqueline says. He was thirteen when she discovered that he had taken pills from her medicine cabinet. When she confronted him, he again said he was curious. She said: "You have no idea how dangerous this is. You should have asked me if you were curious."

Before they divorced, Kevin's parents had moved to a neighborhood in Chesterfield, Missouri, because it was reputed to have a good school district. Kevin attended Parkway Central High. She began hearing rumors from other parents that she found absurd: that her son had become the "cocaine king" of Chesterfield County. She confronted him. Kevin was adamant in his denial. "You know I'd never do anything like that."

At home, a watch disappeared. A silver bracelet. Both were family heirlooms.

In their upper-class neighborhood late one night, there was gunfire, and Jacqueline ran for her children in their beds, threw them onto the floor, and held them down. It took a while for her to realize that it was their house being shot at. All the basement windows were blasted out.

The next day the police came and arrested Kevin. They found a cache of drugs. He was charged with possession and dealing. He was also charged with burglary. He'd broken into a car and stolen weapons — a crossbow and a sniper rifle.

Kevin was released pending trial. One night, he slipped out, and when he came home he was "sort of crazy — paranoid, anxious." Jacqueline learned he'd taken methamphetamine. "It was already terrible by then, but everything got worse." Once, he held his mother hostage in her room for hours, pacing. She tried to leave and he knocked her down. Finally he became calmer, and she wept and said he had to go into a hospital, but he said no, he knew he was messing up, and he'd stop. She searched his room and found spoons, needles, plastic bags with yellowish powder in them, cut-up 7-Up cans, and pens without cartridges. Soda cans and pens can be used as makeshift pipes for smoking marijuana, crack, and other drugs.

Kevin's court date came. A judge sentenced him to nine months in jail for three felonies, including dealing and the theft of the rifle and crossbow. He served the time. After that, Jacqueline says, "Everyone felt he should get out of Missouri, away from his drug-using friends, and we sent him to LA to be with his grandparents." She thought that maybe things would be okay. But his grandfather, a psychiatrist, discovered that someone had been stealing prescription pads, and there were missing checks.

Jacqueline pleaded with Kevin: This has to stop. Remember your uncles. You have good grades. You can go to college.

His grandparents couldn't handle him and sent him back. She met him at the airport and was horrified. He was wired, grinding his teeth, emaciated. "What could I do? I didn't know." She brought him home. "I just tried to figure it out, talked to people, asked for help. Even at the hospital where I worked, no one knew what to tell me. He'd go out. Was I supposed to sit on him twenty-four-seven? I couldn't. I'd tell people, try to get help."

He turned eighteen, which meant that she had even fewer options, because at that age in most states, children can longer be forced by their parents to go into treatment — they have to sign themselves in. One day, she found more drugs. Baggies. Small crystal rocks — probably cocaine or meth. Suboxone. She went to him and begged him to check into the hospital, but he refused. He locked himself in the bathroom. She called to him but he didn't answer. She waited twenty minutes. A half an hour. An hour. "I worried that he could die, so I called 911."

Cops arrived. The shower was on but they heard cabinets closing. The police told Kevin to come out. When he didn't, they told him to back away from the door because they were going to kick it in. They did. Kevin was on the floor stuffing drugs — cocaine — and paraphernalia into a cabinet. They took him away.

Jacqueline went to work, and that afternoon she was paged and told that her son was downstairs. He'd just been arrested. How could he be downstairs? He'd apparently called her ex-husband, who bailed him out. She went downstairs as hospital security guards were escorting him out of the building.

Jacqueline says, "I'm bawling. He's out there, 'I wanna come home! Mom!' Screaming for me. 'Mom!'"

She shook her head no, and he left.

Soon Kevin was back in jail, but he was released when his father paid his bail again. Jacqueline helped him get into a youth hostel. She'd meet him for breakfast at a restaurant. He had a job, made some money, and began seeing a girl. He seemed happy, Jacqueline says. "And that's what we want for our kids." Shortly after he turned twenty-one, he moved with his girlfriend to LA. He and Jacqueline talked on the phone and texted for a while, but when Kevin stopped returning her calls and texts, she knew. A week went by, two. A text appeared on her phone: *I love you, Mom.*

 She left messages on his phone and sent texts. In every message and text, she told him that she loved him.

Kevin was in LA for four months before he was arrested again. He spent six months in jail, and then a drug court sent him to an inpatient rehab program. He called from there, sounding better. At the rehab, patients who did well were integrated into the surrounding community. Over the months, Kevin gained privileges — worked part-time, enrolled at Santa Monica College. He was discharged in the spring.

Jacqueline sent her son notes of encouragement. She sent notes from the family dog, Gryffindor, named after Harry Potter's house at Hogwarts; Kevin had loved the J. K. Rowling books. But again she stopped hearing from him. When she did, she knew it was getting worse, he was going "down down down." He smoked pot, drank, used cocaine, bath salts (a so-called designer drug related to amphetamine), mushrooms, heroin, and, mostly, methamphetamine. Sometimes he would call — when he was stuck at a gas station, for instance — begging her to wire him money, which she refused to do.

She did send his grandparents money to buy him a cell phone for Christmas after his had been lost or stolen. She thought of it as a lifeline to him. She kept sending him messages. *I love you.* Again and again: *I love you.*

No response.

On the eleventh of February, 2012, the door of a nondescript apartment building in Los Angeles opened and a boy stumbled out into the empty gray street. He collapsed into a nearby bush.

A day later, Kevin's grandmother received a telephone call. Some boy said he was a friend of Kevin. "I want to offer my condolences," he said. "I'm sorry Kevin died."

"What are you talking about?" His grandmother didn't understand.

The boy said, "You didn't know?"

She called Kevin's father, who called Jacqueline.

She heard her ex-husband's voice and knew.

• • •

There was a memorial service. There was an autopsy, and a toxicology report confirmed a long list of drugs in his body.

Jacqueline wrote me and said, "I am trying to get some solace, some meaning from this crazy world. My life is shattered. I loved him with every ounce of me, I know he loved me too. The drugs won in the end."

Another note: "I am on my way to LA for Kevin's funeral. It has been 2 weeks today, and I still do not want to believe what has happened. I had a star named after him."

A week later: "I have to do the hardest thing tomorrow, bury my son's ashes. I am not ready to say goodbye."

Later: "It is six weeks since he passed away. I still can't believe he is truly gone. I have found a cemetery near my house that I go to on Sundays and just sit, sometimes write, and wonder why my son. My entire core aches. I keep looking for something that will connect me to him, but I can't find it."

Another: "Today is 9 weeks. It's really bad. I am having a really hard time with the question of what happens to a person when he dies. I am driving myself crazy."

Sometimes Jacqueline writes to Kevin. "Love you sweet boy, always and forever. I was numb this morning, then I could not stop crying. I love you so much. I can't stop the tears. I wish I had a sweatshirt of yours that I could curl up in. Your blanket, anything."

Later she writes me: "For the first time I saw a young man that looked liked Kevin. He was crossing the street in front of me. He had the same hair as Kevin, I could tell it was that same texture too, and that reddish color his hair got after he had been in the sun for a while. I lost it, I had tears streaming down my face. I wanted to follow this boy and scream Kevin, where is my Kevin."

Wired to Seek Pleasure

Every parent—every spouse, child, or sibling—anyone who experiences the addiction of a loved one is baffled by the transformation of a person he thought he knew into someone unrecognizable, someone unfathomably and unrelentingly destructive and self-destructive. The change defies all logic, but it's explained by the impact of drugs on the human brain and the fact that not all brains react the same way.

A healthy adult brain has a hundred billion neurons that connect at a quadrillion synapses. The neurons continually release chemical pulses that travel between receptors, delivering messages. These signals cause every automatic and intentional action, and they're essential to thought, emotion, and sensation. The incomprehensibly complex system is vital to our ability to function, to survive.

The neurological system is one of precarious equilibrium. Pulses flow continuously, carrying information and instructions, triggering and monitoring responses, and moderating one another. The balance has been fine-tuned over the course of human evolution to work pretty well, at least in most of us, most of the time.

The pulses come in the form of chemicals, neurotransmitters that interact with different receptors in different ways. Each has myriad functions, but they all specialize. One neurotransmitter, norepinephrine, floods the brain when there's imminent danger, igniting the fight-or-flight response that helped our ancestors when, for example, they ran into a saber-toothed tiger. GABA and glycine — called inhibitory neurotransmitters — regulate impulses. Serotonin courses through the neurological system to aid memory storage and retrieval and moderate emotions, moods, and sleep. Dopamine is associated with movement, but its main job is to reward useful behaviors so we'll repeat them. Dopamine flows in response to sights, sounds, tastes, or even thoughts related to essential behaviors like eating and sex, giving us the reinforcing reward of pleasure. That is, humans feel pleasure when dopamine flows, which reinforces whatever behavior caused the pleasure in the first place.

It turns out that pleasure isn't merely a fringe benefit. Like everything else inside us — the fight-or-flight response, for example — pleasure has an evolutionary purpose. Because we respond so positively to pleasure, we want more. The go system, as some scientists call it, is turned on — go as in *Go for it, get more*. Pleasure-seeking was critical to the survival of the species. Berries tasted good, so the action of seeking berries was reinforced. Sex felt good, so humans wanted more. Food and sex were, of course, necessary for sustenance and procreation.

Primordial pleasure-seeking was necessary, but unrestrained, it would have caused trouble. It wasn't conducive to people living together in groups, which required compromise and restraint — the sharing of berries, for example. The go system needed to be corralled. Enter the stop system, which regulates visceral responses.

Scientists seem to like saber-toothed-tiger analogies. One explained that the stop system — the inhibitory system based in the prefrontal cortex of the brain — is an innate mechanism that developed to help ensure our species' survival. Its job is to check the go system, because it's dangerous to respond precipitately to, for example, a charging saber-toothed tiger. Cave people had to think through their options and do so quickly: Running might be a fatal mistake. Fighting might be futile. Maybe they should climb a tree.

The stop system also puts the brakes on unbridled hedonism. *Cool it. You can't have sex with that woman. She's taken. It will cause a counterproductive altercation. Moderation. If you eat too much of that, you'll get sick.* To use a Freudian analogy, the go system is the id, the hunger for pleasure — what Freud described as "the original animality of our nature" and "a cauldron full of seething excitations." The stop system is the superego, the higher self, rationality that keeps the id in check. It's more complicated than that, of course, but the go and stop systems are linked. They talk to each other all the time.

In most people, these interactions serve their purpose well until drugs are added to the mix. Psychoactive drugs artificially stimulate and overstimulate dopamine flow, turning the go system way, way up. (Drugs affect other neurotransmitters as well, but dopamine is central to addiction.) The result is a powerful reward — intense pleasure that can be, as a researcher described it, like "a hundred orgasms at once." The go system's on full blast, with dopamine flooding the receptors. *These aren't just good berries, they're the best goddamn berries I've ever tasted in my life. I want more and more and more.* Restraint? Moderation? The stop system has been rendered useless.

Drugs change the brain. That's the point of them. Prescribed psychoactive drugs alter the chemistry in such a way that, in theory, at least, they correct or compensate for the abnormal; they dull pain, alleviate depression, lessen anxiety, heighten sensation, allow sleep, and otherwise treat mood and psychological disorders. Drugs used illicitly alter the chemistry too, but they aren't finely targeted or moderate in their effects. They change the natural chemical balance, and people feel less or more, depending on the person and the drug or drugs taken. Yes, they often feel better. Sometimes they feel fantastic. The pleasure comes in different varieties. Sometimes people feel energized. They may feel supremely confident. They can feel intense sensuality. Sometimes they feel dreamy, sedated — blissfully stoned. In an online forum, a user wrote that being high on heroin "is as if you are kissing the creator."

When drugs bombard the system, another survival mechanism kicks in. Human bodies mend, or at least try to, to return to homeostasis. That is, the body wants to restore its equilibrium, and so it works to neutralize or adapt to whatever disrupts it, including invasive substances. People take a drug, feel the euphoria, and because of the positive reinforcement, they do it again. Eventually the drug alters the reward system and no longer causes the same euphoria, but meanwhile, the brain has adapted to its presence. "Take it away and the organism goes into a state of dysphoria and withdrawal," explains Ulrike Heberlein, scientific program director at the Howard Hughes Medical Institute's Janelia Farm Research Campus. "Because the brain has adapted to the presence of the drug, people don't get high any longer, but not only don't they get high, they don't feel normal. There's an all-consuming need to feel normal" — which by then means having more of the drug. "A switch is turned on," says Richard Rawson, the associate director of the Integrated Substance Abuse Programs at UCLA. "Once it's activated it cannot be deactivated." That first puff of pot or sip of alcohol or pill has led to addiction.

2

This Is Our Nation on Drugs

FOR DECADES PARENTS, SCHOOLS, and communities have tried to stop children from using drugs. There have been myriad national and local drug-prevention campaigns. But clearly these efforts have failed. The proof? Every day, an average of 8,120 people age twelve and over try drugs for the first time, and 12,800 try alcohol — more than 20,000 people. That's more than seven million people a year. Lifetime marijuana use among teenagers is up 21 percent since 2008. Daily marijuana use among high-school seniors is at its highest level in thirty years. Nearly a quarter of those over twelve years old — sixty million people — binge drink. More than 40 percent of college students do. (Binge drinking is defined as having five or more drinks at a time.) Across all ages and most demographics, abuse of prescription pills is America's fastest-growing drug problem, with skyrocketing mortality rates attributed to them. Between 2000 and 2009, poisoning deaths among teens increased 91 percent, with most of those being caused by overdoses of prescription painkillers. More people died from overdoses of prescription pills than from cocaine and heroin combined.

Most drug use begins when people are young — from twelve to eighteen years old. The median age of initial drug use is fourteen, and 90 percent of those who become addicted begin using before the age of eighteen. Joanna Jacobus, postdoctoral fellow at the Department of Psychiatry at the University of California, San Diego, explains one reason teenagers are so susceptible to using and abusing drugs, and why it's especially dangerous for them. The posterior subcortical region of the brain—where the go system resides, the "more primitive brain structures," Jacobus says—develops early. The prefrontal cortex—the site of the stop system, center of abstract thinking, decision-making, and judgment—takes longer to mature. "Because it's developing more slowly, [it] isn't ready to do its job inhibiting the reward system," Jacobus says. "There's a discrepancy between the development of adolescents' reward systems and impulse control systems, so the reward system is overactive." Joseph Frascella, the director of the Division of Clinical Neuroscience and Behavioral Research at the National Institute on Drug Abuse (NIDA), says, "Kids have a double whammy. The go system rages, the foot's on the gas pedal, and the stop system has a hard time keeping up."

It's actually a triple whammy when kids begin using drugs. Their brain chemistry makes them more susceptible to using, and drugs impede the maturation of the prefrontal cortex, further slowing the development of the brain's braking system. Teenagers are known for impulsivity and reckless behavior. It turns out that they're wired that way. Add drugs to the mix, and their impulsivity and recklessness remain unregulated for longer.

Given teenagers' particular vulnerability, it's logical that most prevention efforts have targeted them. But in spite of the years and the hundreds of millions of dollars spent on education and prevention, teenagers' attitudes about drugs are now *more* positive than they used to be. The Partnership Attitude Tracking Study (PATS), conducted by the Partnership at Drugfree.org, a nonprofit organization devoted to prevention of drug abuse, showed "a growing belief [among teens] in the benefits and acceptability of drug use and drinking." The study reported on a precipitous drop in the number of teenagers who say they don't want to hang around drug users and an increase in teenagers who agree that "being high feels good" and "friends usually get high at parties"—the latter was reported by 75 percent of kids. The study showed that almost half of teens (45 percent) reported they didn't see a "great risk" in heavy daily drinking, and only a third strongly disapproved of their peers getting drunk. Many of their parents appear resigned to such widespread use. Almost 40 percent expect that their children will try illegal drugs, and a majority say they're unable to stop them.

These attitudes tell only part of the story. From researchers, physicians, and therapists who work with adolescents, I repeatedly heard that kids are using more and stronger drugs at earlier ages. Children who enter treatment have what Jim Steinhagen, executive director of youth and young adult services at the renowned addiction-treatment center Hazelden, described as "markedly higher levels of acuity" than ever before. "Most kids we used to see had problems with marijuana and drinking and some may have used ecstasy or pills," he says. "Now there's a steady stream of poly-drug users whose addictions have progressed to levels normally associated with people who've used for decades." Steinhagen concludes, "We used to get kids who were beginning to spin out and we could help arrest their use before too much damage was done. Now we're seeing lots of kids who are full-fledged junkies, addicted to pills, or tweakers."

We've Failed at Prevention

When I was a teenager, my mother once said to me, after watching reports about drugs on the evening news, "You'd never try those drugs, I know that." But I was stoned throughout high school. My parents didn't pay much attention to the specter of drugs even as I went raging forward. It's not their fault. They had no idea what I was doing and didn't know what warning signs to look for. The school tried to scare us, in its ham-fisted way, with mandatory drug-education assemblies. In the auditorium, former football stars described their drug use and its hellish results. These assemblies and similar drug-prevention tactics — there were yearly visits from local police officers too — had no effect on my friends and me, other than inducing derisive laughter. Sitting in these assemblies, we were stoned half the time.

Countless students have endured visits by police, athletes, local TV personalities, and other celebrities in anti-drug campaigns like the ones at my high school. The other main attempt at prevention came in the form of advertising and sloganeering. In 1982, Nancy Reagan, the wife of President Ronald Reagan, spearheaded the memorable Just Say No anti-drug crusade. Before and since, there have been multiple public service campaigns involving TV, radio, and print ads. It's hard to imagine that anyone thought the ubiquitous ads from the 1980s — most memorably, an egg sizzling in a frying pan with the ominous voice-over, "This is your brain on drugs" — would work. One ridiculous ad had a cartoon boy saying, "I smoke pot to impress the ladies." A nearby child responds, "Try football." In a more recent spot aimed at prescription-drug abuse, a dealer complains that he's losing business because kids are finding drugs for free in their parents' medicine cabinets. (It makes raiding the medicine cabinet sound like a more responsible — and convenient — option.)

We've Failed at Treatment

Most prevention efforts have failed, and so too has what passes for a treatment system. Ninety percent of people who need help never receive it. Indeed, people with addiction are more likely to wind up in prison than in rehab. Those who do get treatment enter a broken system that's almost impossible to navigate. When addicts must decide what to do, they're usually in crisis and terrified, consumed by worry, and immobilized, and yet in this compromised state, they must make one of the most complex and important decisions of their lives.

The fortunate ones consult specialists, but even then, reliable professionals are difficult to identify, and they often offer contradictory advice. People seek the advice of school counselors, teachers, psychologists, social workers, psychiatrists, directors of drug-treatment programs, physicians, clergymen, friends, and friends of friends. Many go online, but the web is a repository of misinformation and lies, and it's almost impossible to differentiate between objective information and disguised advertisements for treatment programs.

Often, the more information people get, the more bewildered they become. Parents or spouses of addicts are sometimes told that they must kick their loved ones out of the house. Some say that nothing short of letting an addict hit bottom will help, even though hitting bottom can mean dying. Some people recommend Outward Bound. Others push wilderness programs that are similar to Outward Bound but also include sweat lodges or days and nights spent alone in a forest or desert. Treatment programs can last anywhere from a week to a year or longer. Some programs dispense medication, while others forbid it.

Of course, many people recommend rehab, but what *is* rehab, exactly?

There's no standard definition; it's a generic word for a wide variety of treatments, including some that are outrageous. Some rehabs employ threats and harsh and humiliating punishments. I've been told about programs that require rule-breaking patients to scrub grout on the bathroom floor with a toothbrush and cut the lawn with scissors. Some rehabs are run by self-anointed "experts" with no training or credentials, unless you count their own recoveries from addiction to heroin or crack or some other drug. In many states, anyone can open a rehab. There are online guides such as "How to Open a Drug-Rehabilitation Center." There are faith-based programs, and some operated by cults. Even most of the mainstream programs offer a random mix of Twelve Step meetings, lectures, "processing groups," other group therapy, required chores, and drug testing. Most programs offer, and some require, prayer. Some add yoga; acupuncture; juice cleanses; and art, equine, agriculture, and vitamin therapy. Program directors criticize one another. At some rehabs, admitting personnel attack the veracity of other programs' cited success rates while inflating their own numbers.

People in need become increasingly disillusioned, skeptical of every claim, and distrustful of every promise, because most available addiction treatments are a haphazard collection of cobbled-together, often useless, and sometimes harmful recovery programs based not on medical science but on tradition, wild guesses, wishful thinking, and pseudoscience, some of which borders on voodoo. (I've heard of a program that claims to treat addiction by exorcism and past-life reintegration.)

Many rehabs are for-profit businesses — it's a multibillion-dollar industry. *For profit* doesn't necessarily equate with poor treatment, but for addiction-treatment programs, as for other health-care institutions, the bottom line can influence staffing decisions; highly trained physicians and therapists are expensive. Also, the bottom line may cause a rehab to admit patients who aren't appropriate for it. Some rehabs are mills, churning patients through. Some charge tens of thousands of dollars a month, and if a patient doesn't do as he's told, he's booted out — and there are no refunds. There are testimonials galore, but many are fabricated. I met an employee of a prominent rehab center (he asked me to keep his and the center's name confidential; he doesn't want to lose his job) who reported, "One of my responsibilities here is to write testimonials for our brochure and website. I was given a list of words to use: 'transformation,' 'love,' 'miracle,' 'light,' 'astonishing,' 'wonder,' and 'gratitude.'" Some testimonials are probably genuine, heartfelt words from people who have had dramatic, life-changing, and lifesaving transformations, but it's impossible to know which is which. Given the free-for-all environment, the lack of regulation, the lack of accepted treatment protocols, and some individuals' greed and willingness to exploit the desperately ill and their families, it's no wonder the treatment statistics are so disheartening. A majority of patients who enter treatment never complete it. Among those who do, 40 to 86 percent (the percentage depends on the methodology used and population studied) relapse within the first year (the higher number applies to those with co-occurring psychological disorders). An often-quoted statistic is that 30 percent of addicts remain sober for a year, but even that figure may be high. "The therapeutic community claims a thirty percent success rate, but they only count people who complete the program," according to Joseph A. Califano Jr., the founder of the National Center on Addiction and Substance Abuse (CASA) and a former U.S. secretary of Health, Education, and Welfare. "Seventy to eighty percent drop out in three to six months." In some cases, there are modest measures of success, honestly reported. Father John Hardin, chair of the board of trustees of San Francisco's St. Anthony's, a social services foundation with an addiction-recovery program, says, "Success for us is that a person hasn't died."

Good Kids, Bad Kids

Because the addiction-treatment system is so ineffective, people assume addicts can't get well — that they're hopeless. Because of the failure of prevention strategies, people assume that no matter what anyone does, kids are going to use. But both prevention and treatment fail for the same reason: the stigma of addiction that is based on the widely held but archaic view that good people don't use drugs; bad people do.

It's a logical conclusion.

You wake up on Monday morning and decide to leave early for work so you can get a head start on your day. Or you wake up to a screaming alarm, shut it off, and choose to sleep in. Or you wake up and drive across town to a friend's house to score a quarter ounce of weed and a gram of cocaine.

We choose. Volition and free will define us and distinguish us as human beings. I choose, therefore I am.

Some people choose drugs, even though their drug use hurts their loved ones and themselves. For some, the descent is rapid and obvious, but sometimes it's gradual, barely perceptible. Former First Lady Betty Ford, an alcoholic and prescription-pill addict who cofounded the renowned treatment center that bears her name, said, "My makeup wasn't smeared, I wasn't disheveled, I behaved politely, and I never finished off a bottle, so how could I be alcoholic?" Eventually the façade crumbles, though. Whether slowly or swiftly, subtly or blatantly, a person changes, and a life unravels.

As our children grow up, we tell them that good kids abstain, bad ones use. Yet, as I've reported, 80 percent of America's children will at least try alcohol or other drugs. Do we really believe that most of our children are bad? Though drug users are sometimes celebrated in popular culture, most Americans view addicts as — in the words of respondents to a survey conducted by Hazelden — "stupid," "weak," "selfish," "uncaring," "losers," "undisciplined," and "pitiful." In a *USA Today*/HBO poll, most respondents identified "lack of willpower" as the main problem facing addicts. "Addiction seems to involve a total abdication of reason, a messy tangle of emotions and a lack of will," Peg O'Connor wrote in the *New York Times*. Addiction is seen as a character flaw and a moral weakness. People in the Hazelden study also described addicts as "sinners."

Addicts are harshly judged, and for good reason. Many of them are incorrigible liars. Their deceit can be shocking. We beg them to stop; we scream at them. We give them ultimatums, kick them out, and lock them up, but they don't stop using. They hide their relapses, sometimes with brilliant subterfuge. They become ill, depressed, and remorseful, and still they don't stop. It's understandable that we stigmatize people who, in spite of warnings, pleas, and threats, choose to get high. In a puritanical society, succumbing to the desire for pleasure over everything else is a sin and an affront. We're offended when drug users don't follow the rules that apply to everyone else. Whether they're working or in school, their performance usually suffers; they drop out, get kicked out, or get fired. They take, and we all pay the costs of their selfishness when they become ill and visit emergency rooms and hospitals; we pay billions of dollars a year for their health care. We despise addicts because they're in our faces and they embarrass and disgust us.

When they're on drugs, otherwise gentle people become violent and dangerous. Users shrug off their antisocial behavior; they think it's no big deal to steal a few dollars — or more — from a parent's wallet or take prescription drugs from a friend's medicine cabinet. Rationalizations continue as their actions — and their crimes — become more appalling.

We Celebrate Using

One segment of society judges drug users harshly and tries to inculcate children with anti-drug messages, but another lionizes them. In some peer groups, particularly those of adolescents and young adults, using isn't stigmatized. Abstaining is. Stoners are frequently the hip kids, and they often belittle and make fun of those who say no — the losers and nerds, the "good" kids.

There have always been these opposing factions in human culture, one group demonizing drugs and one group glamorizing them. The viewpoint of the latter has been reinforced in music, movies, books, and television, and by artists we admire. Many of the most revered writers of every age were drinkers and drug users, and you'd be hard-pressed to name a jazz, rock-and-roll, or hip-hop great who abstained.

In a 2008 study, researchers from the University of Pittsburgh School of Medicine counted the references to drugs, alcohol, and tobacco in a representative sample of popular songs. One-third of the songs portrayed substance use. De facto advertisements for drug use appear in countless TV shows and movies that depict stoners as charming and funny. A study cosponsored by the U.S. Department of Health and Human Services showed that drug use in movies is often associated with "wealth or luxury." Citing the University of Pittsburgh study, the *New York Times* noted, "The average adolescent is exposed to approximately 84 references to illicit substance use per day and 591 references per week, or 30,732 references per year. . . . Studies have long shown that media messages have a pronounced impact on childhood risk behaviors." A study of sixteen thousand teenagers in six European countries found that the more drinking kids saw in movies, the more likely they were to binge drink.

Many stars seem proudly wasted, and their fans seek to emulate them. In 2007, a tabloid newspaper ran a photograph of the actress Lindsay Lohan high and passed out in the passenger seat of a car. In the picture, she wore a hooded American Apparel sweatshirt. Within a week, the company sold out of those hoodies. A typical consumer, "Andy," posted his review of the product online: "i saw lindsay lohan passed out in this hoodie, so i went out and bought [it] :)." A popular Facebook page, Charlie Sheen Is My Role Model, is not ironic. In a roast of Charlie Sheen, Priceline pitchman William Shatner advised him to "book your next rehab stay through Priceline.com." Seth MacFarlane introduced the night's honoree as "a man with a big heart, because it's been dangerously enlarged by cocaine use." Everyone laughed. They all made fun of Sheen, and yet there they were, feting him. At the time of his public flameout, a survey found that while a majority of adults had an unfavorable opinion of Sheen, 86 percent of twelve- to eighteen-year-olds admired him.

Agent of the Devil, Elixir of the Gods — a History of Ambivalence

These polarized attitudes toward drugs are hardly new. In fact, the earliest records of drug use — and humans have used drugs for at least ten thousand years — are positive depictions, mostly in rituals and medicine. In archaeological records, drugs and alcohol are often portrayed as central to celebrations, including religious rites, though the darker side was known too. In ancient Rome, for example, drunkenness was normal in celebrations, but it was also denounced as "nothing but voluntary madness." The Bible encourages wine drinking, but in moderation. The "sin" of drunkenness is one of the "works of the flesh," along with adultery, fornication, uncleanness, lasciviousness, idolatry, witchcraft, seditions, heresies, and murder. The Bible warns that "they which do such things shall not inherit the kingdom of God." Some religions, including Islam and Mormonism, forbid drinking altogether. In *The New Yorker,* Malcolm Gladwell wrote, "Muslims and Mormons and many kinds of fundamentalist Christians do not drink because they consider alcohol an invitation to weakness and sin."

Over the course of the past millennium, there have been accounts of alcoholics — dipsomaniacs, lushes, winos — and other abusers who were banished, tortured, put in stocks, imprisoned, or locked in asylums. More recently, in the early twentieth century, the temperance movement sought to ban alcohol. Carry Nation, the famous anti-alcohol crusader, railed against anyone who served alcohol as being a "destroyer of men's souls." Nation claimed that she'd had a vision in which God instructed her to abolish drunkenness, and she devoted herself to the mission. She hurled stones at saloons and, wielding a hatchet, ransacked them. The temperance movement she advocated gained enough support to result in the establishment of Prohibition in 1920; at the time, in the minds of some, "alcohol seemed to exacerbate almost all the evils of a disorderly society," as historian David Musto wrote. Prohibition was ultimately repealed, of course; that failed experiment changed little, and little has changed since then. We still either loathe or venerate drinkers. For every media portrayal of a despicable drunk, there are a dozen depicting charming ones.

Of course, the polarized attitudes weren't limited to alcohol. Opium was originally used as a treatment for disease, but it became associated with paganism and hedonism. A variant of opium, morphine — the name derives from Morpheus, the Greek god of dreams — was used as a painkiller, but it was widely abused, and in the late 1800s, users were vilified, banished, or shunned. There weren't many positive depictions of heroin, another opium derivative originally used as a sedative and painkiller, but Sigmund Freud and Arthur Conan Doyle sang the praises of cocaine, Freud calling it "the magical drug" with its "exhilaration and euphoria." In his Sherlock Holmes books, Doyle described cocaine as "so transcendentally stimulating and clarifying to the mind that its secondary action is a matter of small moment." However, the drug "enslaved its users," causing them to become incapable of functioning. Paul Vallely, in his history of the drug, wrote, "In 1903, the *American Journal of Pharmacy* described cocaine-users as 'bohemians, gamblers, high- and low-class prostitutes, night porters, bell boys, burglars, racketeers, pimps, and casual labourers.'" There was no notable romanticizing of the newer forms of cocaine, freebase and crack. In a 1986 *Newsweek* cover story, psychologist Dr. Arnold Washton branded crack "the most addictive drug known to man." *U.S. News and World Report* called the crack epidemic "a situation experts compare to medieval plagues."

Mixed messages about marijuana have been more consistent. Cannabis was used during the pre-Christian period throughout the Middle East and Africa in ceremonies. It was the drug of beatniks, jazz musicians, rock stars, and, more recently, at least two presidents (though one didn't inhale). But it's also been called the "assassin of youth," and in the 1936 movie *Tell Your Children,* later renamed *Reefer Madness,* the message was that marijuana caused users to commit rape and go insane. Now more than ever, opinion is divided: marijuana is celebrated by some (who claim it's harmless, natural, and even medicinal) and condemned by others (who decry it as addictive and a gateway drug).

Drugs are good. Drugs are bad. No wonder kids are confused.

Good Kids or Popular Kids

Given popular culture's depiction of drugs and alcohol, it's no surprise that many non-using teenagers believe that their peers who smoke pot, drink, or use other drugs are the ones having the most fun. And they're not just imagining a "correlation between popularity and consumption," according to a study by Canadian researcher Jean-Sébastien Fallu of the University of Montreal's School of Psycho-Education. This study found that the more popular a child and his friends were, the more drugs they used. Fallu concluded that teens will do drugs to remain well liked and in order to keep (not necessarily advance, but to maintain) their social status. On their Facebook walls, kids post pictures of themselves wasted, with forties, bongs, and lines of cocaine. A 2011 CASA survey reported that 40 percent of American teens have seen pictures on social-networking sites of their peers "getting drunk, passed out, or using drugs."

Half of them saw the pictures when they were thirteen or younger, and more than 90 percent saw such pictures by the time they turned fifteen.

"The media function as a kind of 'super-peer,'" wrote Victor C. Strasburger in a review of research in *Current Problems in Pediatric Adolescent Health Care*. "Clearly the message that children and adolescents continue to get is that smoking is cool and drinking alcohol is normative behavior. Content analyses show how frequently drug use is portrayed in mainstream media, and teens cannot help but get the feeling that . . . everyone is doing it except for them."

In this parallel narrative, kids learn that the warnings they've heard from authority figures are only a small part of the story. Drugs can be fun, and using them gets kids admission to a club that many desperately want to join. Children must decide whether to be good kids, or popular ones. It can feel as if there's no middle ground.

The Cost of Hypocrisy

Whether kids look on drugs as cool or shameful (or both), their view is distorted and confused. We tell them to say no, not to succumb to peer pressure. However, it's normal for children growing up in a drug-obsessed culture to be curious about drugs. But since they're told drugs are bad, having an interest in them, no matter how normal, is taboo. The drugs-are-bad view in a culture that promotes drugs is partly responsible for our failure to prevent use, because it alienates the very people — teenagers — we want to influence. Those curious about drugs are unlikely to confide in anyone who might be able to help them navigate the minefield they're in. Their honesty may be met with panic, threats, punishments, and draconian prohibitions (against seeing their friends, for example). We tell our children to talk to us, but we often unwittingly motivate them to lie or keep silent. As a result, kids often nod when they're warned about drugs, and they're unlikely to admit if they're tempted. Their fantasies and fears go underground. They conduct their experiments in secret. Countless parents told me that they would have sworn that their children never used drugs until an arrest or overdose revealed that they had been smoking pot, drinking, using cocaine, OxyContin, speed, or other drugs, often for months and sometimes for years.

The stigma doesn't affect only adolescents; it affects every user, particularly as they begin to abuse drugs or become addicted to them. According to a national survey called the Face of Recovery, a quarter of people in recovery reported they had been denied a job or promotion or had had trouble getting insurance, and four in ten said they experienced shame or social embarrassment while in recovery for addiction. Drug abuse is seen as a character flaw, so it's no wonder that both adults, and children keep their worsening problems hidden.

The stigma also affects public policy and treatment. Effective prevention campaigns haven't been adequately funded, and researchers have had a hard time getting money to investigate new treatment options, because legislators and government agencies are unlikely to focus on people they perceive as making selfish choices. Add to this that addicts usually aren't in any position to advocate for themselves, and their families are often too ashamed to take on what appears to be a problem caused by their loved ones' moral deficiencies. As a result, there's little money for research into addiction, which reduces the potential for finding effective treatment options. And addiction is perceived as carrying a relatively poor prognosis, which reinforces the stigma — addicts, unwilling to help themselves and unable to be helped, are seen as hopeless.

The stigma also explains why most insurance plans don't adequately cover addiction treatments (in spite of a bill passed in Congress to make them do so): insurance covers treatments for illnesses, not for bad behavior. The result of all this is that by the time addicts seek treatment — if they do — they're usually in crisis, which makes the illness far more difficult and expensive to treat. In addition, they're likely to be belligerent, angry, and depressed, even violent, so doctors, nurses, counselors, and social workers can be understandably reluctant to treat them. Even doctors contribute to the stigma, blaming patients for their problem and their resistance to treatment. "There's no one in the medical community that likes addicts," says John Mendelson, senior scientist at the Addiction and Pharmacology Research Laboratory at the California Pacific Medical Center Research Institute. "Doctors hate the patients, nurses hate the patients." Some practitioners admit they'd rather spend their energy caring for, as one nurse put it, "appreciative patients rather than antagonistic ones who'll likely be back in the ER in a week or month or two."

This stigma associated with drug use — the belief that bad kids use, good kids don't, and those with full-blown addiction are weak, degenerate, and pathetic — has contributed to the escalation of use and has hampered treatment more than any single other factor.

II

Why We Use

3

Everybody Does It

ADULTS ASSUME THAT KIDS try drugs because they want to fit in, to
be cool. (A Partnership Attitude Tracking Study that focused on parents
confirmed this.) Indeed, that's one reason. "I was a freshman in high
school and a trio of junior girls asked me if I wanted 'to go outside' with
them before class," wrote Seth Mnookin, an award-winning journalist
and recovering heroin addict, on Salon.com. "I had never smoked pot,
and was even vaguely afraid of trying it; as a child, I used to be terrified
of reports that perverted psychopaths dressed as clowns were feeding
kids LSD out of ice-cream trucks. But the girls were cute and I was curious."

Peer pressure is indeed a powerful force that can lead to drug use,
but it's more complicated than kids' desire to fit in. In a research project,
Laurence Steinberg, a Temple University psychology professor, demonstrated what some people had already suspected — that teenagers are
almost a different species than the rest of us, particularly in social situations. Steinberg and his colleagues had groups of teenagers, college students, and adults play a driving video game to see if members of these
groups played differently when their friends were watching them. When
their friends were present, college students and adults didn't take more
risks, but teenagers did. They ran 40 percent more yellow lights and had
60 percent more crashes. Steinberg scanned his subjects' brains while
they played, and he found that in teenagers, brain regions associated
with rewards were much more active when their friends were watching
them play. As Steinberg told the New York Times, "The presence of peers

activated the reward circuitry in the brain of adolescents that it didn't do in the case of adults. . . . We think we've uncovered one very plausible explanation for why adolescents do a lot of stupid things with their friends that they wouldn't do when they are by themselves."

The Pleasure Principle

In the Partnership Study, parents said that they felt their kids' drug use was partly due to peer pressure, but they also believed it had something to do with their selfish pursuit of pleasure. That is, they thought kids tried drugs to fit in with their peers, but a primary reason they kept using was that they liked the feeling — they wanted to be stoned.

Though some people do have negative reactions to first-time use — they become ill, paranoid, or disoriented — most feel great, possibly better than they've ever felt in their lives. Marijuana makes many people feel calm — sleepily mellow — and it can heighten their senses. Psychedelics can heighten the senses even more, and distort them. Heroin can cause indescribable bliss. Ecstasy? The name speaks for itself. Tranquilizers? They offer tranquillity. The highs can be long-lasting, because some drugs not only spark a flood of neurotransmitters but also interrupt the system that recycles them, which means they're floating around freely, causing continuous stimulation. Whereas normal pleasure quickly peaks and dissipates, drug-fueled euphoria can go on and on.

Everyone wants to feel good, but the lag in the development of the prefrontal cortex is responsible for why adolescents' brains respond so strongly to that feeling. I explained that the prefrontal cortex — again, the stop system — develops later than the rest of the brain. So kids aren't desirous of pleasure just because they're selfishly hedonistic but because their go systems are unrestrained. Again: dopamine pours forth, it's not being moderated, and the feeling is intense.

The pleasure-seeking brain regions are also associated with impulsivity, which is another of the myriad reasons kids use. Curiosity and impulsivity are, it turns out, another hallmark of adolescence, an essential trait that helps an individual step into a new stage of life. "Adolescent humans are supposed to taste and to experiment," Shoptaw says.

Toddlers and teenagers have that in common. Curiosity drives them both to experiment and push boundaries in order to enter into a new phase of life. Sometimes their explorations are dangerous. A toddler may touch a hot stove. A teenager may try drugs.

Growing Up

Teenagers' biology explains why they're drawn to drugs, but there are also psychological forces at play — powerful ones that are developmentally appropriate. Adolescents are supposed to begin to separate from their parents, and these days drugs can seem to be a way for them to express and feel their independence. Young children are generally horrified by the idea of drinking coffee, smoking cigarettes, drinking alcohol, or using drugs. Nonetheless, many of them will go on to smoke and use drugs, and most will drink alcohol and coffee. Kids may adopt behaviors (and tastes) that are associated with adults to prove (to others, to themselves) that they're no longer children. A child who was once committed to staying away from drugs may sense that they help him individuate; using them helps him stand up to his parents, who prohibit drugs, and connects him with his peers, including older kids who don't appear to be under their parents' control. Richard K., a nineteen-year-old University of Michigan student in rehab, told a therapy group, "Getting high was a way to say, 'Fuck you.' My parents tried to control me, but they couldn't stop me from getting wasted."

It's exciting to grow up, to separate, to become an adult, but it's also at least a little bit terrifying. Most kids sublimate the apprehension, but it's present, and drugs can help lessen it.

Stress

So teenagers are wired to seek pleasure and are poorly wired to inhibit impulses. Add to that their tendency toward experimentation, their natural curiosity, and their susceptibility to peer pressure. And add to that their sometimes awkward need to grow up, and you begin to understand why many adolescents begin and continue using. And there's still more — another potent force that pushes them.

I reported that in the Drugfree survey, parents said that they believed their children used drugs to feel good and to fit in with their peers. In the survey, 60 percent of kids did admit that they used because drinking (the survey focused on alcohol) was fun. But teenagers' primary motivations to use were to "forget their troubles" (32 percent); deal with problems at home (24 percent); and cope with school pressure (20 percent). Their parents were clueless. In the study, only 7 percent of parents connected drug use with teenagers' stress. Most parents assumed that the number one reason kids used drugs was that "drugs are fun." When kids listed their reasons for using, however, "drugs are fun" came in fifteenth on a list of sixteen. "A lot of young people today aren't using to rebel or because of peer pressure," says Steve Pasierb, the Partnership at Drugfree.org president. "They'll say, 'I'm stressed out. I'm driven on Monday through Friday. On Saturday and Sunday I'm going to get wrecked. To get blasted.' They talk about drugs like in old days people talked about the martini after work — 'I need a drink,' 'a chance for me to chill, to manage the stress I deal with the rest of the time.'"

All stages of life have their stresses, but adolescence is particularly fraught with them because of the external pressures kids face and the fact that their brains are not yet developed enough to handle those pressures effectively. Some stress comes in the form of the day-to-day ennui and time-honored pressures that are especially pronounced during adolescence — many teenagers feel defeated, confused, anxious, alienated, or weird. They may feel inadequate and insecure — about friendships, their appearance, and sex. Kids face bullying and cyber-bullying. Some parents seem to be trying to create the best kids money can buy — but the kids are totally stressed out taking AP and honors classes; SAT prep courses; and ballet, acting, guitar, and tae kwon do lessons. They're on the soccer, lacrosse, and swim teams, and they're logging hours of community service. And it's much worse for many other children: those without parents or competent caretakers, kids who aren't being raised at all; those barely in school; and the many coping with abuse, poverty, and bleak and dangerous neighborhoods.

Drugs make a paradoxical promise: they will help us feel more, and help us feel less. And they deliver. They can provide an escape from whatever we want to escape. For people who haven't found a way to live comfortably in the real world, they offer an alternative world. Drugs can make social situations easier. Drugs can keep sadness at bay. For shy people on drugs, social awkwardness can vanish. For the inhibited, drugs can provide newfound confidence. Drugs and alcohol have long and accurately been described as social lubricants, easing the way for people to interact. For the lonely, drugs can provide a social group — other users — with whom they can connect when they're high. When you're on drugs, languor and isolation and doubts can be replaced, at least for a while, by euphoria, a sense of peace, confidence, and connection — everything a teenager craves.

While it's true that drugs can cause impotence and other problems related to sex, many users learn to associate drugs with sex and rely on them to help lift their inhibitions. As *Science Daily* reported, a study conducted across Europe found that "individuals were significantly more likely to have had sex under sixteen years if they had used alcohol, marijuana, cocaine or ecstasy before that age. Girls in particular were as much as four times as likely to have had sex under the age of sixteen if they drank alcohol or used cannabis." Also, combine the dopamine rush of drugs with natural stimulation, and the result can be even more intense. Teenagers in a group I visited admitted that "normal" sex could be awkward and embarrassing, whereas on drugs it was natural and intense.

It's not only kids who use drugs to treat physical, emotional, or serious psychological problems. Adults do too. Drugs can relieve physical pain. The depressed can become energized. The anxious can be calmed. Drugs can make life seem easier to navigate. For some people, drugs may make life *possible* to navigate. "When you're an addict, you can go without feeling anything except drunk or stoned or hungry," wrote Chuck Palahniuk in the novel *Choke*. "Still, when you compare this to other feelings, to sadness, anger, fear, worry, despair, and depression, well, an addiction no longer looks so bad. It looks like a very viable option."

A year or two ago I sat in a restaurant with a renowned writer who after a half an hour or so pushed away her glass of wine and asked the waiter for vodka. She drank down one glass and asked for another, which she used to wash down a couple of Valiums. She saw me staring. "It keeps the rats from gnawing," she said. People in pain are desperate for relief. Far more of them turn to drugs than to therapy. Why? Many have no access to therapy, and drugs are a quicker fix. The bonus of drugs is that people get to feel high, and the pleasure is in sharp contrast to the pain they feel. For a sublime moment or two, the rats stop gnawing.

High-Risk Kids

Luke Gsell grew up in a modest single-story tract home in the rural community of Petaluma in Northern California with his parents and younger sister. He and his sister attended a Christian grade school. "As kindergartners, we had to have our hands folded, feet on the floor," he says. "We weren't allowed to move. There was a fear-of-God atmosphere. 'You're a sinner.'"

Luke was an athlete — he played soccer, Little League, and then football — but he became less interested in sports when he started drinking and smoking pot. The first time, he was at a friend's house at a sleepover. His friend asked Luke if he wanted to try some alcohol.

His parents had warned him. "There's alcoholism and addiction in the family," they said. "You have to be careful." He had aunts and uncles in recovery, and one of his grandparents too. "So I knew that it kind of ran in the family, but, you know, I was a kid. None of that really stuck, and I said, 'Yeah, sure, let's do that.' I was super-excited."

The boys took liquor out of a cabinet and filled a tall glass. "My friend took a sip and spit it out. He didn't like it. I took a sip and couldn't stop. I just chugged the whole thing. It hit my lips and it was like I was the coolest kid. Nothing really bothered me anymore. I remember being drunk and just not caring at all. I spent the night throwing up in the toilet and I blacked out. Even with that, I remembered that feeling that it gave me. I wanted more."

Luke says that he'd been embarrassed by his family's social status — they were poorer than most kids' families at his school — "and anyway, I'd always had low self-esteem, really felt out of place. When I tried drinking, it was like, *Oh, all that's gone.*"

Luke was twelve.

Luke smoked pot. He drank whenever he could get alcohol. His parents caught him smoking once, but they shrugged it off. Theirs was a typical parents' response: "Oh, he's experimenting," they said. Rumors were going around at school, Luke says, but no one ever caught him using. Or carrying or dealing, which he was also doing.

One night Luke went with a girl to see a rap group in a local club. His date gave him a hit of ecstasy. "And that really became my drug of choice," he says. "That and alcohol." He would go on to try cocaine and meth and pills, but "ecstasy was the one."

Luke began high school at Sonoma Academy, an independent college-prep school set on thirty-four bucolic acres in Santa Rosa, California. It didn't have a football team, so as a freshman he joined the basketball team. The school held a retreat for new freshmen. "I was high all during that," Luke said.

On scholarship at the elite school, Luke felt even more out of place than he had at the religious schools he'd attended. The income disparity between his and the other students' families was more extreme. He was reluctant to have his friends come over to his small home after visiting their mansions.

Using and dealing gave him cachet. "Everyone knew me. I was like the party kid, but only my really close friends knew the extent of what I was using." Luke sold weed to all his freshman friends, "just ripping them off because they had never bought any, didn't know the ropes. I remember I had an attitude like, If you're not like me, if you don't party, I don't want anything to do with you, and I was mean to all those kids, you know? I hung out with a lot of seniors. Smoke in the morning, smoke at lunch, smoke after school. I'd take ecstasy in the morning."

Luke had long hair, wore the same hat backward every day, with a hood over it. "I was kind of pissed off and, *Unless you're buying from me or you're going to get high with me, don't talk to me.*"

In mid-December, Luke sold dope to some freshmen, and their parents caught them. "They immediately ratted me out." He was escorted from class to the office of the dean of students as someone went to search his locker. He'd hidden ecstasy tablets in the battery compartment of his cell phone, and weed in a deodorant can, and he was sure they'd find it. "I'm just sitting there with my head of school, and she had the expulsion sheet out, ready to sign it when they found the drugs." They didn't find them, though, and Luke was sent back to class. There were ongoing rumors, but "they never could pin anything on me."

When his parents heard that Luke had been accused of selling drugs, they grounded him, just as Christmas break began. "I didn't care at all," he says. "I had a bunch of weed and just smoked all break."

It was stressful at home. After years of struggling, his parents were divorcing. Luke recalls yelling and tension. Neither had enough money to move out, though, "so they literally split the house in half — Dad's half, Mom's half," he says. He coped with the tension by getting high every day. "If I didn't have anything, I'd take gasoline out of the lawnmower and huff that."

I asked him what it was like to huff gasoline. "You go kind of deaf," he says, "and you just hear like a *yowwowwow* sound. I learned later that that's your brain cells popping."

I've enumerated many reasons adolescents are drawn to use, but there are others that make some adolescents (and some adults) especially susceptible to abuse and addiction: one or more risk factors related to biology, psychology, and environment. Researchers have identified a long list of these risk factors, and Luke was dealt a handful of them: His relatives were addicts. His parents divorced. His childhood was chaotic and traumatic. Other risks for future drug use include genetics, poverty, learning disorders, behavioral disorders, and mental illness. Also, the younger kids are when they start using, the more likely it is that they'll become addicted.

It's important to note that not all people who have substance-abuse risk factors become addicted, of course. Also, a risk factor for one person may not be an issue for another. That is, having risk factors doesn't guarantee that an individual will use or become addicted, but drugs are more dangerous for him if he does start using. It's another fact that proves most drug use isn't about drugs but about coping with life, and some people have more to cope with than others.

Poverty

People living below the poverty line are 50 percent more likely to use and 100 percent more likely to abuse or be addicted than those with incomes 200 percent over the poverty line, according to a RAND Drug

Policy Research Center analysis of existing studies. Americans living below the federal poverty level are nearly twice as likely as middle- and upper-income Americans to name drug use as the number one cause of poverty. Drugs exist in all places, rich and poor, but there may be fewer alternatives to the drug culture in some areas. Indeed, some neighborhoods and communities are awash in drugs — they're available on every street corner. In some locales, they're the norm. "While several researchers have identified a strong, positive correlation between illegal drug use and poverty, the economic literature is unclear about the extent to which suffering from an illicit drug disorder causes poverty," reports to Beau Kilmer, codirector of the RAND Drug Policy Research Center. "Indeed, some individuals may use illegal substances as a way of coping with poverty and their surroundings."

Trauma

A 2012 study conducted by researchers at the National Institute on Alcohol Abuse and Alcoholism found a high rate of childhood trauma in adult alcoholics in residential treatment. The report explained that it was already known that a history of physical, sexual, or emotional abuse in childhood was a risk factor for later drug use, but the study showed that there was more of a connection than had been thought. Overall, of the alcoholics studied, more than 55 percent had a history of childhood trauma. The prevalence of emotional abuse was about 21 percent; physical abuse, about 31 percent; sexual abuse, about 24 percent; emotional neglect, about 20 percent; and physical neglect, about 20 percent. The sources of trauma are sometimes obvious, such as being in combat. SAMHSA has tracked much higher than average rates of drug use and addiction among veterans. Trauma can result from a single event, or it can occur over the course of years or a lifetime. Trauma can be growing up in a climate of turmoil. A death or serious illness in the family can traumatize people. So can losing one's job. Not all children of divorce are traumatized, but many are. "Addiction is always an attempt to soothe severe emotional suffering which is often rooted in childhood emotional loss or trauma," according to Gabor Maté, an addiction expert who for many years worked as a staff physician at the Portland Hotel, a residence for street people in downtown Vancouver. "Such loss or trauma is imprinted when the child's ability to cope is overwhelmed by adversity — physical, sexual or emotional abuse, extreme parental stress as in a rancorous divorce, violence in the family, and so on. Whether the addiction is to alcohol or heroin or anything else, it is an attempt to change one's mind state from negative to positive in the short term. Adverse early experiences not only induce the pain the addict is wanting to escape, they also shape developing brain circuits in ways that predispose to addiction."

Single-Parent Families and Divorce

As the *New York Times* reported, a study conducted among 4,097 high-school students in Connecticut showed that "teenagers in single-parent households were more likely to report marijuana use than those in two-parent homes." Children of divorce are at high risk for drug use for a number of reasons. The main one is that divorce can be a psychic earthquake for children; the bedrock cracks beneath them. "Divorce can be deceptive — legally it is a single event but psychologically it is a chain, sometimes a never ending chain, of events, relocations and radically shifting relationships strung through time, a process that forever changes the lives of people involved," wrote psychologist Judith Wallerstein. In a study she conducted, 25 percent of children of divorce used drugs and alcohol before age fourteen, compared with 9 percent of a control group. The National Longitudinal Study of Adolescent Health found that teens with divorced parents were four times more likely to use drugs than teens with non-divorced parents.

Dysfunction in Families

Research shows that a strong family bond is a protective factor for addiction; that is, it decreases the likelihood that someone will abuse drugs. However, some families make children's drug abuse more likely. It obviously increases risk when there's abuse, neglect, or violence, or when there's drug use in the home. In fact, one of the greatest risk factors for a child is growing up in a family in which one or both parents abuse alcohol or use drugs. If one parent is a heavy drinker, the child's chances of becoming a heavy drinker increase two to three times. Children of heavy drinkers have been found to "drink more frequently, more heavily, and more often alone" than children of parents without alcohol problems. (Similar rates for cigarette smoking occur with children of smokers.) A study undertaken by the American Academy of Child and Adolescent Psychiatry found that children of alcoholics were four times more likely than other kids to become alcoholics. Kids who have seen their parents drunk are five times more likely than kids who haven't to get drunk one or more times a month.

There are at least 7.5 million children in the United States — 10.5 percent of the population — living with an alcoholic parent. This doesn't take into account kids who live with parents who are addicted to other drugs. Some children of alcoholics and addicts come to loathe drugs and are able to avoid them. But in spite of their intentions or resolve, kids may find that parents who use and stress related to parents' drug use can be forces too powerful to withstand. Beyond their modeling their parents' behavior, children may take drugs to escape from or in reaction to a parent's or relative's addiction. Research at the University of Gothenburg in Sweden has shown that children of alcoholics are more likely than children of nonalcoholics to respond to stress by drinking.

Family dysfunction can be subtler than parents' drug use. Even with the best of intentions, some loving family members can cause stress, and some cause trauma. It's not that these family members directly cause drug use, but they can contribute to a psychological climate in which drug use is more likely and addiction can flourish. A parent's love can only help a child, but dysfunction in families may include manipulation and guilt-inducing behavior disguised as love. In some families, children are systematically devalued, and their self-esteem battered. Drugs can help assuage feelings of worthlessness and insecurity.

A Family's Addiction Cycle and Genetics

Children of addicts aren't influenced only by their parents' drug use. There's a good chance that they've inherited what some scientists call "the addiction gene" — actually a constellation of genes that interact

among themselves and with the environment to increase the likelihood
of addiction. The genetic component of addiction can't be overempha-
sized. "Genes are the blueprint for a host of traits, from the basic archi-
tecture of a brain cell to the behavioral styles that largely define who we
are," according to health scientist Ruben Baler of the National Institute
on Drug Abuse's Science Policy Branch. "They impact how long a drug
will remain active in a users' bloodstream, how many dopamine receptors will be displayed on the surface of a neuron, the proper balance of
mood-controlling chemicals in the brain, and they also influence basic
temperament and personality traits, such as stress sensitivity, impulsivity, and risk taking. Also, because of genetic factors, some people will
be more sensitive to peer influence." It's estimated that 8 to 10 percent
of people have a genetic predisposition to addiction. According to National Institute on Drug Abuse (NIDA) director Nora Volkow, studies
of twins have indicated that genes account for about 50 percent of the
risk for addiction. (The other 50 percent includes use at an early age,
stress, anxiety, environment, mental illness, and more.) For now, it's impossible to know if any particular individual's genetic makeup makes
him more vulnerable to addiction, but people with a family history of
addiction are at higher risk than the general population. And though
many people have family trees abounding with addicts and alcoholics, they're sometimes hidden. "My father's brother's rages, depression,
and absences were explained away as eccentricity," a woman told me.
"We were finally told the truth when he died in a car crash. He was addicted to prescription pills and cocaine and was high when he died."
She said, "We had no idea." Until her mother died and the family found
hidden bourbon bottles throughout her home, a friend of mine didn't
know that her mother was an alcoholic. Dr. Shoptaw calls the addiction
genes "the sleeping monster." Smoking a single joint or drinking one
beer can wake it up. But as with other risk factors, genetic predisposition just increases the chances of getting the disease; it doesn't guarantee
it. It's not unlike other complex diseases: a person's DNA can predict
only the odds of a disease becoming a clinical reality. And conversely, as
Baler says, "Some people have a genetic predisposition to addiction, but
anyone can become an addict under the right — that is, *wrong* — set of
circumstances."

Learning Disabilities

Other kinds of neurological wiring can sharply increase the risk of addiction too. About 20 percent of school-age children in the United States — about eleven million — have learning disabilities, and these have been shown to increase the risk of drug abuse. This may possibly be related to the fact that those with learning disabilities are more likely to struggle in school, engage in disruptive behavior, and be frustrated in their relationships with others, and these difficulties, too, can lead to drug use. "Academic failure and peer rejection are common risk factors associated with substance abuse, so is the lower self esteem that accompanies social difficulty and academic failure," concludes a CASA study. "A lot of the kids who appear not to care or to be lazy, the one in the back of the class either fooling around or checked out, have decided that seeming like they don't care about school is better than looking stupid," says Kyle Redford, education editor for the Yale Center for Dyslexia and Creativity. "Drugs help them not care, or pretend not to care, and help them flee from their confusion and frustration."

Behavioral Disorders, Mental Illnesses

Learning disabilities often accompany other disorders. A child with a learning disability is twice as likely as a child without one to suffer attention disorders, and those with ADD and ADHD have a high incidence of substance abuse. ADHD itself is associated with an early onset of substance abuse and a greater difficulty of treating it. An analysis of several studies suggests that kids with ADHD are one and a half times more likely to use marijuana and twice as likely to use cocaine as kids without ADHD. Those with certain mental illnesses — a long list, including obsessive-compulsive disorder, depression, bipolar disorder, anxiety disorders, and schizophrenia — are highly susceptible to abuse and addiction. A SAMHSA study found that people who experienced mental-health problems were more than three times as likely as others to have drug problems. Dr. Volkow said that six out of ten addicts have at least one co-occurring mental disorder.

Anxiety disorders are the most common mental illnesses — 18 percent of Americans are affected by them — and 10 percent are affected by depression. In 2010, an estimated two million kids between twelve and seventeen had had a major depressive episode during the previous year — that's 8 percent. Numerous studies have found that depression and anxiety are closely linked with drug use. According to the Anxiety and Depression Association of America, about 20 percent of those with an anxiety or mood disorder also have a substance-abuse disorder.

I've visited many rehabs and heard patients talk about the chronic depression or anxiety that eased when they got high — they said they were self-medicating. Some of them abused their prescription medications — antidepressants, anti-anxiety medications, mood stabilizers, or sleeping pills. People with anxiety disorders, a class of disorders that include panic, social anxiety, and generalized anxiety disorder, described the relief they got from marijuana, alcohol, downers, benzodiazepines (like Valium), and opioids (like OxyContin). Various drugs, including marijuana and alcohol, can "treat" depression — at least temporarily, before it floods back in (alcohol is itself a depressant). Some meth addicts with bipolar disorder or depression have reported that when they tried the drug, they didn't feel high; they felt normal. "It was a revelation to get a glimpse of what I imagined other people felt, a lack of pain and depression and anxiety," a girl in a recovery group said. My son Nic, who ultimately was diagnosed with bipolar disorder and depression, told me that when he first tried methamphetamine he thought, *If only I'd been breastfed on this.* "It was the feeling I'd been looking for my whole life," he said. All people with mental illnesses may be drawn to drugs as an escape from the frustration, confusion, and psychic pain caused by their illnesses. But although drugs can make the mentally ill feel better temporarily, they worsen conditions over the long term as they further damage already malfunctioning neurological systems. For example, although depressed people often drink, smoke pot, and use stimulants and other drugs for relief, sustained use can contribute to depression.

Does mental illness cause drug problems, or do drugs cause mental illness? It's almost always a two-way street, though drugs can trigger latent mental illnesses. An analysis published in the medical journal the *Lancet* tied marijuana use to a higher than normal rate of psychotic conditions such as schizophrenia. Matthew Large, the University of New South Wales researcher who led the study, explains that smoking pot not only increases an individual's risk of mental illness but also brings the illness on earlier. He says that the evidence points to marijuana smoking as cause, not symptom. Large offered some reasons in an e-mail: "Cannabis use often starts many years before psychosis; few people with psychosis take up cannabis; half of people who smoke cannabis and then develop psychosis give up smoking; people with psychosis who quit are better; cannabis users with psychosis say they smoke for the same reasons as nonpsychotic people; and the more you smoke, the greater the risk, and the earlier you smoke the greater the risk."

In Large's study, the symptoms of mental illness began an average of three years earlier in pot smokers than they did in those who had not used marijuana. "The link between using pot and developing serious mental illness is strongest in the youngest smokers — twelve- to fifteen-year-olds," he said. It's important to emphasize that the vast majority of people, young and old, who use pot never develop psychosis. However, I've met people whose lives were characterized by devastating mental illnesses that they traced back to smoking pot.

It's no surprise that a person who spends his life in the turmoil and pain of mental illness, and who can't fully comprehend the consequences of his actions because of that illness, will find his way to drugs. It's understandable that he'll use drugs to both self-medicate and escape. A high can be a respite from hell or a net that prevents a person from falling into hell.

Combined Risk Factors

Mental illness, divorce, trauma, poverty, addiction in the family tree. Millions of people have these and other risk factors, and a combination exponentially increases the odds that a person will abuse drugs. Add those to the many other reasons people use: the way drugs can, at least temporarily, treat physical pain and lessen inhibitions; the way they can help people cope with loneliness, insecurity, and stress. For adolescents, there are all of those plus the pull of peer pressure; the innate drives that manifest as curiosity, impulsivity, and a heightened response to pleasure; the cultural acceptance of drugs; and messages in the media. Rather than being surprised that some people use drugs, we should be surprised that some don't.

4

Helping Kids Grow Up

SOME PARENTS ARE NONCHALANT about their children and drug use. They think a little experimentation is inevitable, and occasional recreational use is fine. However, most parents I've encountered are fearful that their kids will use drugs, and they want to stop them. Many are fatalistic, though. The Partnership Attitude Tracking Survey found that four out of ten parents felt they exerted "little influence" over their children's decision to try drugs — and their kids were only in middle school.

Given the daunting statistics about the prevalence of drugs, it's tempting to throw up our hands and conclude that prevention is impossible. But it isn't — once we reject the simplistic and moralistic approaches of the past and replace them with strategies grounded in what we've learned about why people take drugs and why they abuse them. Indeed, it's unsurprising that most past prevention efforts failed so miserably. It's useless to tell a person who's being bullied or is failing in school or is traumatized by family turmoil to just say no. It's pointless to tell people to "make good choices" about drugs if drugs offer them a reprieve from the darkness they feel. Preaching restraint or moderation to someone with a genetic predisposition to addiction is futile. So is warning children that drug use will be detrimental to their future if they feel they have no future. Warnings about the evils of drugs fade into background noise when those who are anxious, overwhelmed, or in physical or psychic pain know they can find immediate respite, even bliss, in drugs.

Protecting Kids

It's no wonder that most prevention efforts have failed, but it's impera-
tive that we keep trying, because if we succeed in preventing use, we can
stop a myriad of other behavioral, health, societal, and personal problems from developing and escalating. It's impossible to overstate the potential benefits of disease prevention when it comes to hypertension,
diabetes, and some cancers and heart problems, and it's especially true
for drug abuse and addiction.

Given what we now know about the trajectory of drug use and the
effects of drugs on the developing brains of adolescents, it's clear that
prevention efforts should focus on children. The onset of the disease of
addiction is so early, it can devastate a person's entire life. As UCLA's Dr.
Steve Shoptaw says, "We have only one brain, and through it we experience the world — every sensation, every image, every feeling — pleasure,
pain, depression, joy. Our brain is of the seat of our consciousness." In
many ways, our brains *are* us. Like the hard drive of a computer, it stores
a lifetime of education and experience. And like a computer's hard drive,
it's vulnerable. All that learning and memory can disappear in a second.
Unlike a computer, however, the brain has no backup. When children
abuse drugs and become addicted, physical suffering, alienation, loneliness, shame, and confusion can characterize their lives and continue
through adulthood — if they make it to adulthood, which many of them
don't.

As I reported, nine out of ten people who become addicted began
using before they were eighteen; a person who gets to age twenty-one
without using is virtually certain never to do so (and only one in twenty
of those who start using after the age of twenty-one become addicted).
The goal of prevention strategies should be preventing all use, but it's
also valuable to delay use as long as possible. An older person who tries
drugs is less likely to have problems with them, and any problems that do
develop are usually less severe. Another compelling reason to postpone
use is that drugs can lead to an earlier onset of psychological problems,
including psychosis, in teenagers. This is rare, but in such cases, "even
if the onset of psychosis were inevitable (for a particular individual), an
extra two or three years of psychosis-free functioning could allow many

patients to achieve the important developmental milestones of adolescence," researcher Matthew Large explained in an interview with CBS News. "That extra time could allow a young person to finish school and gain other skills that might reduce the lifelong disability that often accompanies mental illness."

In spite of parents' frustration, they *can* influence their kids, and so can schools and communities. Effective prevention requires a multifaceted approach. It involves protecting children by untangling and addressing the roots of their problems and offsetting their risks. "Our goal is to change the balance between them," says Dr. Eve Reider, health scientist administrator in the prevention research branch at NIDA, "so protective factors outweigh risk factors."

Offsetting Risk Factors

Rather than fight the teenage brain, we can work with it. We can help kids become immersed in positive (that is, protective) rather than negative (destructive) experiences that can sate their curiosity, engage their passion, and harness their impulsivity. We can try to help lessen the stress on them, and we can teach them ways to deal with the stress they're under. We can guide them so that they'll be in situations in which it's safe to succumb to peer pressure. We can provide them with facts about specific drugs and the way they affect the brain so they can make informed decisions. We can help them find safer and more effective ways to separate and smoothly transition into each new phase of life. Finally, we can diagnose their psychological and cognitive disorders early — and treat them. Only when we do all these things will we begin to turn the tide and decrease the number of people who try drugs, abuse them, and become addicted.

Effective prevention necessitates a full-court press that focuses on strengthening both individuals and families. It requires the participation of parents, schools, and communities. First, parents can learn to be better parents, ones who spend consistent time with their kids, effectively communicate with them, and guide them so they're healthier and better prepared to meet the challenges they'll face. Next, schools can bolster children and families, and communities can support efforts by parents and schools and provide kids with safe and nurturing environments.

"You have to do it all," says Kevin Conway, deputy director of NIDA's Division of Epidemiology, Services, and Prevention Research. "Family-based, school-based, and community-based prevention. The child is in a network of lots of different little communities and they all influence him." He adds that approaches that combine two or more effective programs, such as family-based and school-based programs, have been shown to be more effective than approaches that use a single program alone, and they're even more beneficial if they're practiced throughout the community; for example, in schools, clubs, and faith-based organizations.

What Parents Can Do

Prevention should begin in infancy—even before, because tragically some kids are born into the highest risk groups. Some are born into poor or violent neighborhoods. Some are born into families in which there's mental illness, addiction, and abuse. Some are born into families in which parents simply don't know how to parent. The heartening fact is that all of these risk factors can be offset by protective factors.

Mothers and fathers who aren't prepared to be parents require support and education. A model that's been shown to protect children from infancy onward is the Nurse-Family Partnership (NFP), a program targeting primarily first-time mothers, mostly single and poor, whose kids are in an extremely high-risk group. The program pairs a nurse with a young woman to help her with prenatal care and prepare her for motherhood. The nurse continues to work with the mother after her baby is born, teaching her parenting skills, how to create a safe environment, and how to manage discipline and stress and other problems that arise. The nurse also works with the mother to get her back to school so she can pursue a career that might ultimately make her self-sufficient. According to Dr. David Olds, professor of pediatrics, psychiatry, and preventive medicine at the University of Colorado at Denver, the founder of the program: "During pregnancy a child's exposure to substances, maternal stress and pregnancy complications can damage the developing fetal brain—making the child more susceptible to impulsiveness and under-controlled behavior later in life. These behavioral problems can also be caused by exposure to harsh inconsistent parental care."

Currently, more than thirteen hundred NFP nurses serve twenty-three thousand families. The programs are funded by a combination of Medicaid, Maternal and Child Health Services block grants (Title V), juvenile justice funds, Temporary Assistance for Needy Families (TANF), Child Care Development, Social Services block grants, and the federal Maternal, Infant and Early Childhood Home Visiting Program, in addition to state and local general sources.

I visited a California Nurse-Family Partnership branch that operates out of a nondescript public health office. A coordinator there oversees eight nurses, each of whom has up to twenty-four clients that the nurse visits every one or two weeks, depending on the client's stage of pregnancy or the age of her child.

One NFP nurse, Patricia Reiss, has been an RN for forty years, working in public health for the past seven. She told me that her job with the NFP had been the most fulfilling in her life.

Patricia, about sixty, wore bright colors: a top with blue paisley trimmed in gold, a black jacket with a leopard-skin-patterned collar, and looping necklaces and dangling earrings. She herself is a mother of three children, all of them now adults. Driving to a client's house, Patricia explained that like other nurses who work with the NFP, she went through intensive training. "What we do goes beyond most of the training we get as RNs," she said. Indeed, in addition to monitoring mothers' and babies' physical health, NFP nurses also serve as counselors, advocates, coaches, and confidantes.

Patricia parked in front of a small stucco home at the end of a cul-de-sac and walked to the back of her car. From the trunk she retrieved a nurse's bag that contained a stethoscope, a blood pressure cuff, a thermometer, and other medical tools, as well as a case with a portable scale. In the trunk, there was also a plastic skeleton of a woman's pelvis with a baby doll inside it. She uses this when she's teaching girls the mechanics of childbirth. "It's one of the first things we have to work with them on," Patricia said. "It's one of their biggest fears — childbirth itself."

Inside the home, Patricia met a girl I'll call Martina. Most of the girls NFP serves are teenage mothers referred by their high schools or health clinics, but some are older — Martina was twenty-five.

Martina had deep brown eyes and long spiraling ringlets of black hair.

A silver cross hung from a chain around her neck. At eighteen months old, her daughter, Gabriela, had her mother's dark wide eyes. She wore a SpongeBob shirt, turquoise pants, and bright pink sneakers. Patricia got on the floor and played with Gabriela before beginning an exam. When she grabbed Patricia's stethoscope, the nurse asked if she wanted to hear her heartbeat. Patricia cleaned the earpieces, placed them in Gabriela's ears, and put the diaphragm on her chest. Gabriela listened intently. Martina said to her daughter, "Listen! That's the music your heart makes."

Patricia noted on a chart that Gabriela's heartbeat was strong and her lungs were clear. She measured Gabriela and weighed her. Patricia recorded the numbers on a growth chart she kept in a file. Martina had a copy of the chart too. They compared them and verified that Gabriela was developing normally.

Patricia had been visiting Martina since she was twenty weeks pregnant. The early visits consisted of physical exams, education sessions, and conversations guided by NFP-developed protocols. Before we arrived at Martina's, Patricia told me, "You become part of a girl's life. You want them to completely trust you so they'll tell you if they're struggling. Over two and a half years we become very close." Of course that kind of connection doesn't happen with all of her clients. "There's no warmth with some girls," Patricia said. "They're young, they're scared, they're overwhelmed. They aren't emotionally ready to be mothers. They're just not mature enough. We help them as much as we can."

Nurses are trained to use motivational interviewing (MI), a therapeutic technique that involves asking open-ended questions and never judging the answers. The therapist uses these and other interviewing techniques to help a patient find her intrinsic motivation to change. "We don't tell mothers what to do," Patricia said. "We provide the factual information they need and guide them so they think through the consequences of their actions." Nurses help their clients recognize and monitor the stresses in their lives that might affect their well-being and ability to parent. They also check for unhealthy behaviors. Patricia explained that she asks her clients about drugs but doesn't expect she'll always be told the truth. "But we know what to look for," she said. "One goal is to help girls understand the impact of their choices on their baby. Whether it's nutrition, smoking, or drugs, they have to understand the effect on a fetus and child. Most of these girls just don't know." She and other NFP nurses work to motivate girls who have drug problems to get treatment. They also help their clients evaluate relationships in their lives and cope with stress, whether a girl is distraught after being abandoned by a boyfriend; angry and confused about being pregnant; or worried about supporting herself and losing her freedom. When serious problems arise, the nurses connect their clients with organizations that can help them get the care they need.

NFP nurses also serve as career counselors. "A lot of low-income community moms have assumptions that are self-defeating, and they'll communicate that to their children," Patricia said. "I want to help her realize her own dreams. When she does, she provides a model for her child." Patricia told me about former clients who stuck with plans to go to college and became medical assistants, nurses, and legal assistants, even as they learned to be competent, conscientious, and loving mothers.

After Gabriela was born, Patricia returned for weekly postpartum examinations of Martina and checkups of her baby. The focus of the visits changed over time, evolving from lessons about nutrition, nursing, and child development to teaching communication skills and stress management.

After the physical exam, Patricia asked Martina a series of questions. How's Gabriela's appetite? What's she been eating? Martina explained that her daughter — who at the time was pulling stuffing out of a tiny hole in a couch — was eating "pretty much what the family eats — if we have tacos, I give her the vegetables, cheese, and chicken." Sweets? "No sweets." But then Martina smiled. "Well, when Gabriela got her flu shot, I told my mother she could give her a treat."

Patricia took out a binder. The previous week they'd focused on "loving limits." This week was about discipline. Patricia began by asking Martina what the word *discipline* meant to her. It was a relevant topic, because Gabriela had been hitting and pulling hair. The goal was to teach Martina positive discipline practices and help her monitor her own reactions to her daughter's moods and behavior. "You want to preview times when a mother will be stressed out and overwhelmed, and the last thing they feel like dealing with is a cranky toddler," Patricia explained later. "If they're prepared, they can recognize what they're feeling and react appropriately, rather than angrily."

After Marina defined discipline, Patricia asked her to respond to the prompt "My parents disciplined me by . . ."

Martina said, "I didn't need to be disciplined a lot. I was a quote-unquote good kid. I was easy. If there was a problem, my mother would just talk to me." She mentioned her boyfriend, who'd been spanked. "He thinks you need to spank them."

"Parents who were hit as children may understand that it was destructive, but some learned that it's normal," Patricia explained.

The visit continued for an hour. Patricia and Martina talked about the value of reading to Gabriela at bedtime, of rules — "limited rules but consistent ones" — and of giving her appropriate choices. She could choose which shoes to wear, but not what time to go to bed.

At one point, Patricia spoke to Martina while looking directly at her and then continued speaking while looking away. She asked Martina if she realized what messages are sent by where a person looks when she's speaking to someone. Martina thought for a while and then said, "My father wasn't really there for me in my life. I never felt like he was there. If he ever talked to me, he was watching TV."

Patricia asked, "What did that communicate to you?"

Marina responded, "You aren't worth looking at. That I'm not important."

Patricia said, "What are you telling Gabriela if you're looking into her eyes?"

"That I'm there for her."

"Yes," Patricia agreed. "She feels seen. She feels important. It will stay with her her whole life. She feels as if you're really listening to her."

Martina seemed to be thinking deeply. After a few moments, she told Patricia, "I understand what you're saying."

The remainder of their time together was focused on practical matters. Martina was back in school full-time — she was studying business administration at a community college. Her mother looked after Gabriela, but parenting still presented challenges. "I come home and want to do my homework now and get it done," Martina said, "but I haven't seen

Gabriela all day, so it's my time to be with her. Then I get her to go to bed, and I have to stay up too late to do my homework and then get up early in the morning when Gabriela wakes up."

Patricia asked how she was dealing with it, and Martina said, "It sucks, but that's the way it's gonna be."

Patricia gave her some advice on managing the stress, and when the visit came to an end, the two women embraced again.

Afterward, Patricia reflected on the sad part of her job, when the children in her care reach two years old; that's when the regular visits end, and she has to say goodbye to the mothers and toddlers with whom she's become close. "But our work together stays with her for her whole life," she said. "And her child. At least I hope it does.

"As Martina prepares for the terrible twos, she'll be more prepared to deal with the terrible teens. It's a pattern of learned responses — understanding where a child is coming from, practiced patience and thoughtfulness, learning to listen to your child, value them, look into their eyes. Teenagers are terrible twos all over again. So you want these girls to be competent mothers to make the most resilient teens possible."

The Nurse-Family Partnership is one way that risk factors can be replaced by protective factors that lead to a lower incidence of drug use. Research shows that compared with mothers in similar circumstance, those who've gone through the program have 32 percent fewer subsequent pregnancies, are more likely to hold down jobs (there's an 82 percent increase in the number of months the mothers are employed), and are less likely to commit criminal acts (there are 60 percent fewer arrests). Even more significant, studies showed 80 percent fewer cases of child abuse and neglect among kids whose mothers went through the NFP program. And children whose mothers had been through the program had fewer incidents of running away and being arrested, and an 85 percent reduction of drug use.

Strengthening Individuals by Strengthening Families

Relationships in a family can be the strongest protective factors in a child's life. Protective families can take any form — two parents or one;

biological, adoptive, foster; divorced or remarried parents; with or without siblings and stepsiblings. A NIDA report, "Preventing Drug Abuse among Children and Adolescents," found the following factors to be protective: "a strong bond between children and their families; parental involvement in a child's life; supportive parenting that meets financial, emotional, cognitive, and social needs; and clear limits and consistent enforcement of discipline." By contrast, the report found that kids "likely to experience risk" grew up in situations where there is "lack of mutual attachment and nurturing by parents or caregivers; ineffective parenting; a chaotic home environment; lack of a significant relationship with a caring adult; and a caregiver who abuses substances, suffers from mental illness, or engages in criminal behavior."

Programs like the Nurse-Family Partnership recognize that many parents are themselves in crisis. If they're going to protect their children, they need help for their own problems. A body of research has proven the value of strengthening families by helping parents with substance-abuse issues, problems with anger, and difficulties coping with life events such as divorce, the death of a loved one, the loss of a job, or mental or physical illness. Indeed, parents who abuse drugs or alcohol must get treatment — as I've said, their children are at extremely high risk, and parents lower that risk when they get and stay clean. Parents struggling with psychological problems or traumatic life changes protect their children when they themselves get help. For example, experiencing their parents' divorce is a risk factor for kids, but if individuals, couples, or families who need it go into counseling or therapy, they can assuage at least some of the children's stress. And there's no getting around the tragic fact that poor families have fewer options and must rely on whatever services are available to them. I noted that children growing up in poverty are in an extremely high-risk group — but social services like NFP are protective.

Whether their children are in an obvious high-risk group or not, all parents can protect their kids by improving their relationships with them. Some feel as if their relationships with their teenagers are limited to nagging them, fighting with them, and reprimanding them. Parents become frustrated, the child becomes angry and defensive, and as a result, the relationship simply adds stress to a child's life (and to his parents'). Parents can change these dynamics. One way is to regularly sit down to family dinners. According to a series of studies by CASA, teens who don't eat dinner with their families five to seven times a week are twice as likely to have used alcohol; two and a half times likelier to have used marijuana; twice as likely to have friends who use illegal substances, prescription drugs without a prescription, or over-the-counter meds to get high; and four times more likely to say they expect to try drugs in the future than teens who do.

Presumably dinners are protective because they provide structure, consistency, and a built-in time for children and parents to check in. Another opportunity for that is homework time. A study showed that kids whose parents always or sometimes helped the kids with their homework were half as likely to use than those whose parents never or seldom did. Kids closely connected with their families may receive nurturing that can mitigate or defuse some of their anxiety and stress. According to Dr. Reider, "Family environments teach kids pro-social values, skills, behavior, and promote psychological flexibility."

For many parents or caretakers, regular family dinners and consistent family time are unrealistic — one or both (if there are two parents) are working. But whether it's over dinner or at other times, parents help their children if they spend as much time with them as possible, offer them as much stability as possible, and provide an environment in which children feel heard and protected. The essential point here is that nurturing environments reduce the risk of substance abuse. And by the way, they also lower the risk of other problems, such as antisocial behavior, depression, and academic failure.

There are other benefits to a close parent-child relationship. The more time parents spend with their children, the more they are in a position to recognize dangerous behavior early. In some schools, teachers are simply overwhelmed with more students than they can closely monitor for social or academic problems, so it's left entirely to parents. The professionals advise parents first to pay attention to their instincts. "You know your kids," says Sharon Levy, director of the Adolescent Substance Abuse Program at Boston Children's Hospital. "If you think there's a problem there's probably a problem." Next, the professionals say to rely on physicians, therapists, and other specialists because parents aren't trained — or expected — to diagnose psychological problems, learning disorders, or other conditions that put kids at risk for drug use. Professional intervention, the earlier the better, protects them.

Talking — and Listening

One successful anti-drug campaign directed at parents told them to talk to their children early and often. Talking *to* kids doesn't mean talking *at* them. Kids who are lectured and threatened usually don't listen. Part of the problem with engaging teenagers in meaningful conversation is that they don't necessarily want to talk, at least to adults, and perhaps especially to their parents. When they're cornered or otherwise forced to talk, they may feel defensive and tune out. Adolescents have other agendas — depending on the child, there's schoolwork, sports, dating, friends, Friday night, and any number of minor and serious problems that loom large in the child's life.

The most important component of a conversation with children is listening. It sounds easy, but it isn't. Parents must learn to listen better. It takes practice, patience, and practicing patience. According to Ken Winters of the Center for Adolescent Substance Abuse Research in the psychiatry department at the University of Minnesota, one problem is that "parents in general don't have enough formal education in the challenges of being a parent. They need it." Researchers are developing online parenting classes for future and current parents. In the meantime, there are books and parent-education programs, like Parent Effectiveness Training (PET), that are used to help parents be more successful when they communicate with their kids.

There's a lot of talk about teaching kids to make good choices, but most children aren't making reasoned choices about drugs. They can be helped to. Also, parents can offset risk factors by instilling in their kids a sense that they matter, and that the parents respect and trust them. They can help their children have a deeper understanding of who they are and what they want from life — and how to get it.

It's logical that it's easier for parents to influence younger children than older ones, but underneath teenagers' tough, seemingly impenetrable veneer, most of them crave safety and their parents' approval. In spite of what they say (or think they know), they may be torn between messages from their parents and those from their friends and the media. When parents acknowledge and accept a child's ambivalence and confusion, they're more likely to connect with them.

Michael Pantalon, research scientist in the department of emergency medicine at Yale University School of Medicine and founder of the Center for Progressive Recovery, works with kids and adults who use drugs by utilizing motivational interviewing and communication skills that can be effective for parents too. He begins with statements that acknowledge the child's independence and responsibility, like "While you know that I don't want you using drugs, it's ultimately going to be your decision whether or not you choose to use them." "Why might you decide not to drink or use drugs?" "What kind of things are important to you?" "What kind of person do you want to be?" "How could using drugs keep you from doing those things or being who you want to be?" He explains that these questions are designed to get them thinking, *Hmmm, what kind of a person* do *I want to become?* "We tend to think of children as unable to contemplate questions like this, but they're rarely asked," Pantalon says. He points out that it's easier for a therapist to remain detached from a child's answer than it is for a parent. "If a child admits he's using drugs, parents tend to become afraid, judgmental, angry, or punishing. If they do, the conversation's over." Parents should remember that the answers to the questions themselves often aren't as important as the fact that parents and children are forging trust and a bond, even as parents help kids think more consciously — more maturely — about themselves. When kids do, their choices can be more intentional, their actions less impulsive.

Parents' Values Matter

Studies have shown that children benefit when their parents set limits and consistently enforce them, establishing reasonable expectations for behavior. A CASA study found that "the greater perceived parental disapproval of substance use, the less likely teens are to use." The study found that only around 4 percent of kids who perceived "strong parental disapproval" smoked pot, compared to about 33 percent of those who perceived that their parents "would not strongly disapprove." The research supports our intuition and our hope: parents' values influence their kids.

Many parents believe that teenage drug use, especially of marijuana and alcohol, is inevitable and acceptable. Some parents say, "I smoked and it wasn't a big deal," or "I began drinking when I was sixteen and it's never been a problem. A beer or two is fine." This is a risky assumption because, first of all, it doesn't allow for the fact that their children might use drugs in different ways and for different reasons than they did. It also ignores the fact that today's kids aren't growing up in the same culture, with the same influences and pressures, as their parents did. Nor are modern kids using the same drugs; even the marijuana isn't the same. Now that growing marijuana has become a fine art, laboratory tests have detected three to ten times more THC, the drug's active ingredient, in today's pot than in marijuana from the 1980s.

Some parents allow their kids to drink or smoke as long as they do so "responsibly." Some tell their children that it's okay to drink or smoke pot in moderation but that they're not to use hard drugs. Some tell them it's all right to use as long as they don't get in a car with someone who's high. The parents agree to have parties at their houses because, as a mother who hosted a party where her children and their friends were allowed to drink beer and smoke pot said, "At least I know where the kids are. They're safer at home." But no matter what conditions they impose or rationalizations they make, these parents are sanctioning drug use and drinking. And there's another factor that parents should consider before they allow teenagers to drink or use drugs in their homes: It's illegal, and in many states parents who allow it can face prison sentences and fines. If a child at their house gets high and later has a car accident, the parents can be held responsible.

More faulty logic comes from parents who say things along the lines of "I'd rather have them get used to drinking now, so they learn moderation. Otherwise, when they go off to college they'll go wild." This ignores the research that has demonstrated that postponing use is safer. In addition, there's no evidence that kids who drink and use as teenagers will drink less when they're older. In fact, the opposite is true: Almost every adult who has a drug problem started using as a teenager. Also, it's logical that those acclimated to using drugs face fewer psychological barriers to using more. And if they're using, their developing brains are particularly vulnerable to the effects of drugs on their profoundly changing neurological systems. In addition, drugs compromise kids' social and emotional development — those who haven't used by the time they reach college age are more likely to have learned how to handle stress, failure, and disappointment. They're more likely to have practiced modulating their behavior, and weathering complex relationships. In *Beautiful Boy*, I quoted Robert Schwebel in his book *Saying No Is Not Enough:* "Drugs shield children from dealing with reality and mastering developmental tasks crucial to their future. The skills they lack that leave them vulnerable to drug abuse in the first place are the very ones that are stunted by drugs. They will have difficulty establishing a clear sense of identity, mastering intellectual skills, and learning self-control." Of course, postponing use doesn't guarantee that teens won't use or won't develop drug problems later, but it improves the odds that they won't.

Another question of values comes up when parents decide how to answer their children when they ask if they've ever used drugs. Parents who have used worry that if they're honest they'll lose the moral high ground and be hypocritical for essentially telling their kids to "do as I say, not as I did." They also worry about undermining their own cautionary messages about drugs because their kids can plainly see that, despite taking drugs in their youth, their parents turned out okay. However, parents don't want to lie to their children. They crave honesty from their kids, and isn't honesty a two-way street? It is according to kids; in surveys, kids said it would make them less likely to use drugs if their parents told them honestly about their own use when they were young.

The experts I've polled advise that when (if) the question comes, parents should use it as an opening to a deeper, and ongoing, conversation. Generally speaking, they should answer the question their children ask at a level of detail that seems appropriate to the children's ages and/or experience. But they should keep in mind that a child may be asking this question to assess whether a parent can empathize with his position — curious, confused by mixed messages, concerned about a friend who's using, or surrounded by kids who seem obsessed with using. Candor, even when a parent is uncomfortable and ambivalent, begets candor. If parents admit they aren't perfect, and they're open about their struggles, their children may feel more comfortable discussing their own struggles.

Children Who Are Safe and Healthy

Parents (and this applies to teachers and others working with children) can also help protect kids by teaching healthy ways to cope with stress, channel their impulsivity, navigate challenging social situations, and get high in healthy, rather than destructive, ways.

Meditation, yoga, journaling, creative expression, exercise, and stress-management training have been shown to lessen stress and, as a result, lower drug use and create better overall health. In addition to decreasing drug use, stress-management practices lessen kids' depression and anxiety.

Exercise decreases stress, and it also ignites a blast of neurotransmitters that can ease pain and cause pleasure, much the way drugs do. The increased flow of dopamine, serotonin, and endorphins helps explain why studies have shown that regular exercise decreases drug-seeking behavior in adolescent rats. Another study showed that teenagers — humans this time — who reported exercising daily were 40 percent less likely to try marijuana than teenagers who didn't. Other activities that engage children have also been shown to lower the likelihood that they'll use drugs, whether these are leadership and service programs, kids' involvement in the arts, or "healthy risk activities," as Shoptaw describes them, like motocross riding or rock climbing. Adolescents can be steered toward safe yet intense experiences, places to be impulsive, opportunities to individuate (express who they are, unique from others, and separate from their parents and siblings) — harmless and healthy ways for kids to be kids.

As Steve Shoptaw said, adolescents are wired to taste and experiment. Since they're naturally curious, impulsive, and drawn to intense pleasure, we can "replace the functional value of drugs with something else," says Ken C. Winters, professor in the Department of Psychiatry at the University of Minnesota Medical School. That is, children can be guided toward activities that allow them to safely satisfy their curiosity, express their impulsivity, and experience intense pleasure.

Peer pressure remains a strong force in adolescents — remember all the yellow lights they ran in the study that had them playing a driving game. Giving into the natural impulses to succumb can be harmful, unless the group is a safe one. Exercise and involvement in activities and interests help channel kids' impulses and needs, and they may also lead to safer peer groups. Children can find non-using peers if they are involved in sports, debate, school newspapers, or special-interest clubs; enrolled in outside classes (art, music, science, language); or doing community service.

Exercise and engagement help, but research has shown that computer time can hurt. Facebooking teens are more likely to use, according to a CASA study of a thousand kids between twelve and seventeen. Those who spent time on social-networking sites were five times more likely to report using tobacco (10 percent versus 2 percent), three times more likely to say they used alcohol (26 percent versus 9 percent), and twice as likely to admit using marijuana (13 percent versus 7 percent) than those who didn't. Banning Facebook may seem draconian to some parents, but experts say that it's reasonable — and advisable — to limit time spent online and playing video games. A study showed that kids who were heavy gamers (those who played for thirty hours a week) were more likely to use drugs than moderate players (those who played for nineteen hours a week). They were also more likely to be depressed, anxious, and have social phobias, all of which can contribute to drug use.

Whatever they're doing that keeps them up at night — chatting online, watching YouTube videos, doing homework, listening to music — sleep-deprived kids have a higher risk of using than those who get a full night's sleep. Experts recommend nine hours of sleep for teenagers, which can sound impossible at a time when kids have afterschool sports and several hours of homework, spend hours on the web or texting, and then wake up for school at seven. Plus there's that family dinner to fit in. But a reasonable bedtime (which may mean parents insisting on homework being done immediately after school and confiscating anything with a screen at a given hour) can be a protective factor in a child's life. Children who get enough sleep aren't only less likely to use drugs. They report feeling better and less stressed.

None-of-the-Above Options

Along with working to lessen their kids' stress, parents can borrow directly from strategies taught by the professionals to help children when they face situations where they may be tempted or even pressured to use drugs. If a child enters a room with a bunch of people smoking pot and he's offered a joint, he has two options: succumbing or saying no. In that charged situation, it's unrealistic to expect most kids to decline unless they've learned and practiced strategies to navigate such circumstances. According to researchers who have tested numerous approaches, kids taught none-of-the-above options are better able to resist peer pressure than those who haven't been prepared in advance. "Preview situations in which they may be offered drugs," said NIDA's Dr. Reider. "Kids have successfully negotiated tricky situations by saying they're allergic, that they can't use because addiction runs in their families." One boy told me about the pressure to drink at parties. "Everyone's getting high," he said, adding that he'd felt he had to either go to parties and join the others or stay home and feel isolated and out of it. But then a teacher recommended an alternative. Now he grabs a beer, takes it to the bathroom, pours it out, fills the can with water, and nurses it, refilling it as needed. "No one knows," he said, "and I don't have to feel like the only straight one too uptight to drink."

Dr. Winters teaches strategies to help teens refrain from participating when their friends are getting high. For example, they can tell friends that their parents are drug testing them, even if their parents aren't. "Throw your parents under a bus. They don't mind," he says. Kids who need help extricating themselves from a situation but who worry about standing out or being ostracized for abstaining can call or text their parents with a preplanned "get me out of here" message that contains a code word. Parents see the code word (say, a relative's name or a day of the week) and, as planned, call their child and tell them they have to come home for whatever reason — a family emergency, an early appointment the next day. A child can hang up and complain about his parents, and meanwhile the parents are on their way to pick him up.

What Schools Can Do

The task of protecting kids from drugs falls disproportionately to parents because few schools have programs that help kids deal with stress and social problems or that help identify behavioral disorders and mental illnesses that correlate with drug use. Indeed, one segment of American's education system operates as if its job is to funnel kids into college and careers instead of to make them as healthy as possible. Another segment is doing the best it can with shrinking resources just to stay open and keep kids in school.

School districts and independent schools forced to lay off teachers because of budget cuts often ax PE and art teachers and counselors because they're deemed less important than academic teachers. But exercise, creative expression, and emotional support are more important to kids' well-being than AP courses. Schools can evaluate their priorities and put in place programs that protect kids.

Nearly every school system in America has tried to address the drug problem among its students. Most have a drug-prevention program in place, but many of them are wasting students' time. As of 2008, most U.S. middle schools did not use evidence-based drug-education programs — that is, programs that have been studied and shown to work. DARE — Drug Abuse Resistance Education — is the most widely used program in U.S. schools. It usually involves a local police officer coming to the classroom and lecturing about drugs. Like my own high school, many schools use DARE because they've used it for years, and it's free. But it doesn't work. In fact, numerous studies have shown that DARE not only doesn't lower drug use but may actually raise the rates of use among some of the kids who endure it. In spite of this widely available research, the DARE website claims that 75 percent of America's schools use it.

NIDA's Kevin Conway acknowledges the ineffectiveness of DARE but points out that its popularity "shows that schools and communities want to take this [problem] on. If you can tap into that infrastructure and start delivering a menu of programs that work, we might make progress."

There's ample evidence that schools can put in place programs that protect kids. One such program is geared for kids in elementary, middle, and high schools. Called Life Skills Training (LST), it's an interactive program designed to build social and academic competencies and strengthen kids' self-esteem, all of which lower drug use; as Paulina Kalaj, the LST marketing manager, puts it, the program is meant to "strengthen students' abilities in personal-self-management skills, general social skills, and drug-resistance skills." Teachers trained in LST learn several prevention strategies. Some take the form of classroom activities; one has middle school kids survey their peers about drug use and then tally the results. (Usually they learn that there's less drug use than they thought — plus they hone their math skills.) In another activity, students use role-playing to learn and practice personal-interaction skills so they're better prepared if they, for example, enter a new peer group or arrive at a party where they don't know anyone — both stressful situations that could lead to drug use.

In the South Ozone Park neighborhood of Queens, New York, Our Lady's Catholic Academy, which serves kids from prekindergarten through eighth grade, uses LST. Though the academy is a Catholic school, a majority of its students are of other faiths. The kids are racially mixed, many from families who live in the lower- and lower-middle-class neighborhoods that surrounds the school. On a recent visit to the academy I was impressed by the attention it paid to its students' psychological health as well as their academic success. Each day begins with an activity designed to make children aware of their emotions: they fill out mood charts. Younger kids use strips of colored paper to describe their moods — blue for feeling blue, for instance. Older children describe their emotions in words — *angry, sad, peaceful.* As the children mature, they learn to assess the nuances of their feelings, and their vocabulary expands: "I'm feeling disheartened"; "I'm feeling anxiety."

This seemingly simple exercise makes a profound difference, according to Shannon Pearce, the therapist in charge of the school's drug-prevention program. "The students are learning to check in with themselves," Pearce says. "The exercise teaches self-awareness." It also helps teachers stay better attuned to how the children are doing. Recently a teacher noticed that a young girl indicated that her mood was dark. She spoke to the girl for a while and then escorted her to Pearce, who helped her open up about her struggles; she'd been given up for adoption and separated from her sister. "You can't make their problems go away, but you can help them cope with them."

In addition to conducting the school's drug-prevention program, Pearce sees students individually and in peer groups, counseling them about drug use, bullying, and other common problems. She sometimes includes family members. Once, a young boy came to her office carrying a video-game controller. He handed it to Pearce and said, "I heard you fix things."

Prevention programs in the school are designed to teach kids a broad range of life skills: how to resolve conflicts, communicate better (among themselves and with their families), and deal with anger and other emotions in positive ways. For example, instead of reacting to anger with physical or verbal attacks, a child can talk to friends, write in a journal, punch a pillow, or count to ten. They're taught relaxation techniques as well, like one in which they close their eyes and imagine a peaceful place. "What do you see, how does the air feel, what do you smell?" "Effective drug prevention helps children be stronger," Pearce says. Kids are trained to be more conscious of who they are, how to process what's happening around them, and how to communicate what they're feeling.

The school makes a concerted, multipronged effort to prevent drug use and to address other problems that might lead kids to use, employing a number of evidence-based prevention programs, including Too Good for Drugs and Violence; Protecting Youth; Olweus (designed to prevent bullying); and Project ALERT. The day I visited, Pearce was using Life Skills Training with a class of feisty fifth-graders.

The classroom had a blackboard, walls of books, and signs on the wall: HOMEWORK: DON'T LEAVE HOME WITHOUT IT; FEELING BULLIED, LONELY, ABUSED — TELL A TRUSTED ADULT. The children sat at desks so they faced one another in clusters of three.

Pearce greeted the kids and handed out LST workbooks geared specifically for fifth-graders and asked the children to open them to the first exercise, the subject of which was self-esteem. She asked what they knew about self-esteem, and kids raised their hands. "Sometimes you feel bad about yourself," a boy said. Pearce asked, "When you do, do you have good self-esteem or bad self-esteem?" A few kids answered, "Bad." Another boy said, "You have low self-esteem when people are mean to you." Another said, "Yeah. They call you names." A girl said, "You feel not smart." Pearce acknowledged what each said and elaborated. "Sometimes our self-esteem is hurt because we feel lonely or separate from everyone — that we're different. Well, *everyone* is unique — and that's a good thing. But when we don't remember that, our self-esteem can be low. We can feel alone, left out." She asked, "What do you feel when someone criticizes you?" A child said that your self-esteem goes down. "What about when someone is kind to you or acknowledges that you're special?" "It goes up."

Following the LST protocol, Pearce then asked the children if they knew what good self-esteem felt like. Kids answered, "You feel proud of yourself"; "You feel very happy." Pearce said, "Yes, and if someone is proud of you, your self-esteem goes up. If they criticize you, sometimes it goes down. But you can be in charge of your own self-esteem. How you feel about yourself doesn't have to come from what others say or how they treat you; you can have it inside you so it isn't affected so much by what others say or do."

The first exercise in the workbook showed three triangles that intersected in the center. "Our special qualities make us unique," Pearce said. "You are made in your own special way. No one has the same fingerprints. It's exciting but also a little scary. Sometimes we don't want to feel different. The fact is that we're all alike in some ways and all different in some ways."

She had each child label the three triangles in his workbook: one triangle with his name and the other two triangles with the names of the other two children in the cluster. She then instructed each group to talk among themselves and learn about one another — "who you are, what you're like, what you like, what you care about." If all of the group members had the same answer to a particular question, they were to write it in the intersection of the triangles, which connected them all. If their answers were unique, they were to write them down in the appropriate individual triangles.

The kids got to work. In one group, a child said he liked pizza. The others did too. In the space where the three triangles overlapped, they wrote *pizza*. But they disagreed on what kind they liked best, so they wrote their answers in separate triangle compartments: *pepperonie, saggige,* or *baken.* Children at another table talked food too. They compared their favorite restaurants, agreed that Subway was best, and so they wrote that name in the central shared space. At one cluster, a girl said she was Hindu. Another girl said that she was too. The third girl said she was Catholic. "We're not the same religion," one said. But when they talked about whether they had brothers and sisters they learned, as a girl said, "We're alike!"

When they finished the exercise, the kids shared their answers. Next, Pearce told a story from the LTS workbook. She asked the children to imagine that they were walking in the woods and came upon a unicorn who was crying. She said that the unicorn felt bad because he was different from all the other animals in the forest. "He has low self-esteem,"

Pearce said. "He feels different than everybody else. Maybe you can make him feel better. You can explain that he has some similarities with the other animals. But what about his differences? They make him special. He needs to know."

The workbook page had two columns, one for kids to list ways the unicorn was similar to other animals, and one that identified what made him special.

The kids filled in the worksheets. After a while Pearce asked them to read from their lists. Students said that the unicorn was like other animals because of its four feet, "just like horses," "mules," "donkeys," and, according to two children, "woolly mammoths." A girl in pigtails said, "He lives in the forest and runs like other animals."

Pearce then asked the kids what they'd say to the unicorn so he'd know that it was okay to be different — that his differences made him special. You're special, the children read, because: "You're bright"; "You have many colors"; "You're rarely seen"; "You have a horn"; "You have magical powers."

The class ended, and I asked Pearce if she thought this and similar exercises could actually affect children's decisions about drugs. She answered, "If we do one thing, no. But if we do everything we can to help them learn more about themselves and communicate better, and if we're here when they're struggling . . . Yes, I do. We can help them with their self-esteem, and children with good self-esteem are less likely to use drugs."

"The drug-prevention program is beyond drugs," said Eileen Dwyer, who runs the Program for the Development of Human Potential of the Brooklyn Diocese (Our Lady's is part of the diocese). "It's about strengthening children. The skills they're taught will buffer them so they'll be prepared to handle the risk factors as they get older. Our goal is to mitigate risk factors and enhance protective factors." She explained that protective factors include knowing more about themselves, being in touch with how they're feeling, and having ways to express it through art, writing, or talking with friends, teachers, parents, other family members, or counselors. Studies have shown that Life Skills Training does have a significant impact. One found that those who went through the program had, over the twelve years of the study, rates of drug use 25 percent lower than the control group's (they also did better in school).

• • •

Schools like Our Lady's Catholic Academy, which emphasize kids' emotional health, may sound quixotic, but there are other similar successful models, even some in cash-strapped public school systems. One impressive program is the San Francisco Unified School District's (SFUSD) Wellness Centers, which provide counseling and support groups and offer workshops on reproductive health, family and peer relationships, and drugs and alcohol. In 2011 to 2012, eight thousand students visited Wellness Centers, located in sixteen high schools, for problems with depression, anger, anxiety, grief, trauma, physical and sexual health, and drug issues. Like school districts everywhere, the SFUSD has suffered budget cuts, but the centers have remained a priority for the district and the program's other funders, the San Francisco Department of Public Health and the San Francisco Department of Children, Youth, and Families. In a district survey of students who had participated in wellness programs, 95 percent reported that they used fewer drugs and drank less alcohol.

The program acknowledges that drug use is inextricably tied with other problems kids face, including bullying, gang violence, trauma, stress, poverty, and violence at home. The centers address these issues and others — sexual orientation and gender identity, sexual health, cultural identity — with classroom and schoolwide programs plus individual and group counseling. Students research, design, and present programs to their peers about relevant issues. Full-time onsite licensed counselors offer counseling and therapy. Students can make appointments or drop in anytime. Students can also anonymously refer others. "They tell us they're worried about a friend who's drinking or smoking," says Kevin Gogin, program manager of school health programs for the district. "The student is approached, told that a friend is concerned. They're asked if they're open to talking about it. No one's forced to come to the Wellness Center, but the door is always open."

Abraham Lincoln High School, in San Francisco's Sunset District, has twenty-six hundred students. Inside, up the stairs, and past the bright red lockers lining the hallways, there's an office decorated with posters — WHEN YOU NEED SOMEONE TO TALK TO, THE WELLNESS CENTER IS HERE — and a bright banner painted by students: WELCOME TO THE WELLNESS CENTER.

The Lincoln High Wellness Center is busy; students come and go throughout the day. And the center's offerings spill out to other class-rooms and offices. Down the hall there's a nurse's office and counsel-ing center where two full-time therapists see students for individual and group counseling and therapy, and they lead girls' empowerment, boys' antiviolence, and other groups. In another room a dozen kids are hud-dled over computers, researching and writing presentations they'll give about smoking. A boy named Chris — black hair, dark eyes behind oval glasses — earnestly explains, "People think weed is okay — all-natural, leaves — but they don't know that a lot of it has the same chemicals as cigarettes have. And they use it differently. They inhale pot longer and hold it in their lungs. Some think it's safer than smoking cigarettes, so they should know the facts."

The school district's Wellness Center Initiative is unique its compre-hensiveness and its deep integration into the daily life of the city's high schools. Counselors, social workers, nurses, therapists, and teachers work together to identify kids with problems, including the myriad is-sues that can lead to drug use. There's constant staff training in interven-tion techniques and systems in place for staff members to follow and refer students who need help. According to Gogin, "The culture is built around the assumption that students' health is more important than anything else, and that improving mental health involves an unflagging commitment to deal with whatever students are dealing with. The goal is to create a place where children are closely held and feel safe, where it's obvious and accepted to ask for help when they need it. Kids know they won't be in trouble if they come to the Wellness Center. They aren't in trouble if someone refers them. We're here for small things as well as crisis, whatever you need: someone has passed away in your family, you're feeling like running away, at a party a friend was throwing up and you're worried, you have questions about sex — questions you've always had but never asked anyone."

When kids reveal that they're using drugs or someone else in the community suspects they are, the subsequent process is nonthreatening and nonjudgmental. Gogin explains that therapists are trained in a kind of brief intervention that focuses on quitting or harm reduction, which-ever is appropriate (and feasible). For those who need more intensive intervention, counselors, social workers, nurses, and others associated with the Wellness Centers work with them to find it.

The Wellness Centers, like Life Skills Training, is a school-based program shown to be effective, and there are others. Like NFP, Chicago Early Childhood Centers focuses on low-income kids. Raising Healthy Children, Good Behavior Game, and PATHS (Promoting Alternative Thinking Strategies) target elementary-school kids. Another program for high schools is Toward No Drug Abuse (TNDA). Other programs recommended by NIDA staff, some of which are also for high-risk kids, are Early Risers, Coping Power, ATLAS, and SOAR (Skills, Opportunity, and Recognition). Schools protect children by also offering tutoring, mentoring, counseling, and other academic, social, and emotional support.

What Communities Can Do

Though schools are an obvious place to reach and help kids, others are Boys and Girls Clubs, YMCAs, 4-H Clubs, and community centers where children spend their free time. Kids who attend such organizations already show a lower incidence of drug use. (A study of twelfth-graders who attended 4-H Clubs found that they were half as likely to use drugs as kids who didn't.) Part of the reason is that kids are kept busy, but these organizations also provide healthy communities and peer groups, adult role models, and supervision. Like schools, these organizations are suffering financial cutbacks at a time when they should be expanded. Community-sponsored Big Brothers and Big Sisters programs have also been shown to be successful.

A program that shows how entire communities can organize to protect kids is called Communities That Care, offered by SAMHSA; it involves the building of a coalition of leaders in a city, town, or school district representing schools, health-care agencies, government, business, law enforcement, and others. The Communities That Care program (actually, it's described as a process, not a program) provides a guide for those involved in the coalition to work together to isolate a problem — an epidemic of prescription-drug use, for example, or a rise in pot smoking among middle-schoolers. The program guides these leaders to spearhead communitywide surveys to isolate the dynamics contributing to the problem and to select appropriate responses from a menu of programs (family-based; school-based, like LTS; and others). The next stage is implementing the programs, then assessing their effectiveness and modifying them as needed. A similar program, Prosper Project, is geared toward rural communities. Numerous studies have shown that these kinds of approaches reduce drug use as well as delinquency. In one study of Communities That Care, eighth-graders in towns that had implemented the program were 32 percent less likely than those in the control-group towns to begin using alcohol. (They were also 25 percent less likely to commit their first delinquent act between seventh and eighth grade.)

The Influence of Media

Effective drug-use prevention involves parents, schools, and communities, and it also involves acknowledging and countering a culture in which kids are deluged with positive depictions of drugs. However, most media campaigns to date have been ineffective, and some have actually been harmful.

Many media-based drug-prevention strategies are unsuccessful because they are built on people's best guesses of what might work. Such strategies may be well intentioned, but many are also wrong-headed, simplistic, or both. Some are ludicrous. One public service campaign actually increased drug use. It was an anti-marijuana campaign that ran from late 1998 to 2006 and cost American taxpayers $1.4 billion. The White House Office of National Drug Control Policy and NIDA later contracted with a research firm to study the campaigns' effects, and they learned that the ads had made it *more* likely that kids would smoke pot. The reason, according to a Government Accountability Office report, was that the campaign "may have promoted perceptions . . . that others' drug use was normal," making kids feel more comfortable around drugs and encouraging a common misperception that, as so many teenagers say, "everyone smokes." This and similar ad campaigns helped drugs become accepted, and psychological barriers to use went down; drugs went from verboten to no big deal. The ads merged into a climate that made some kids feel as if smoking was the norm, abstinence the aberration.

• • •

Kids absorb culture — they learn from it and copy it. Countless studies prove this. One showed that four-year-olds have a greater chance of becoming bullies when they're older if they watch a lot of violent TV. Seeing violent behavior on TV or in other forms of media can also make teenagers act more violently. And a study done by the RAND Corporation shows that teens are twice as likely to have sex or engage in specific sexual acts if they see similar sexual behavior in the media.

The media effectively influences kids to have sex, bully, and *use* drugs, but there's scant evidence that it has ever been able to lower drug use. One reason is that kids are too savvy for most of the campaigns that have been tried to date. According to Michael D. Slater, social and behavioral sciences professor at the Ohio State University School of Communication, flawed campaigns "focus on risks that are either already well-known to youth, considered manageable or slight, and . . . appear exaggerated."

Then what might work better?

We can learn from failed ad campaigns. If anything that makes drug use seem normal is harmful, then anything that normalizes abstinence might help. As teenagers, my friends and I used every drug you can name, but not heroin. It wasn't that we thought that LSD, cocaine, and ecstasy were inherently safer. It wasn't that they were cheaper — they weren't. It wasn't that they were easier to get — our dealers would have found us whatever we asked for. No one had to tell us not to try heroin; doing heroin was unthinkable. Other drugs were normal in our sphere of friends and associates, but no one we knew used heroin. I recall consistent subtle and overt messages that glamorized other drugs, but every image of heroin users was bleak and depressing. Heroin was never portrayed as fun, and its users were never cool. At least among our peer group, the *rejection* of heroin became normalized.

Rather than try to scare kids into abstinence, we can use sophisticated anti-drug media to influence kids with subtle — that is, not heavy-handed — images. We can change the association of a drug, connect it not with fun (partying, sex) but with seediness and with values teenagers reject (conformity and submissiveness). A few relatively successful campaigns have shown that it's possible to normalize abstinence.

One successful effort was sponsored by the American Legacy Foundation. Known as the Truth Campaign, it targeted teenage smoking. It didn't vilify tobacco per se; kids know that smoking is bad for them, but the harm is decades in the future, so they shrug it off. Instead, ads showed how tobacco companies manipulate smokers and profit from death. One memorable ad showed demonstrators piling twelve hundred body bags in front of the Philip Morris Company headquarters, representing the number of people killed every day by smoking. A three-year study of this and other Truth Campaign ads showed that kids who had a high recall of the campaign were 25 percent less likely to start or keep smoking than others. Another campaign, Above the Influence, focused on marijuana smoking, subtly challenging kids to do what they wanted to do: be independent, make their own decisions. According to Michael Slater, who conducted a study of the campaign, it had an impact because it tapped into teenagers' "developmentally appropriate goal of achieving autonomy." Slater's research into Above the Influence showed encouraging results: of the kids who saw the ads, 8 percent smoked pot; of the kids who didn't see the ads, the number was 12 percent.

Kids also respond when they're not pandered to but informed. In 2001, a Partnership ad campaign directed at rising ecstasy use was shown to have lowered the use of the drug by as much as 25 percent over four years. There were no don'ts or direct warnings in the campaign; it was straightforward. In one ad, a coroner read the autopsy report of a young girl. Ecstasy was the only drug in the girl's body. She was dead. Viewers were left to draw their own conclusions. "If you put the information out there and it bears up to a little Googling — 'Yeah, that stuff can kill me' — it has an effect on some kids," Steve Pasierb, the Partnership at Drug-free.org president, says.

But if these campaigns work, why is most drug use still rising? Pasierb says it has to do with money. "You've got to keep doing it," he points out. "Every year you have a new wave of thirteen-year-olds you have to hit." At its height, the Office of National Drug Control Policy, which oversees the Above the Influence campaign, had an annual media budget nearing $200 million. In 2010, it subsisted on $35 million for media projects, and more recently its media budget was completely eliminated.

Clearly, money does make a difference, but it's probably possible to spend less to reach today's kids by using digital media instead of expensive television advertising. However, for now, it's hard to imagine that any media campaign can combat the influence of Seth Rogen getting stoned in *Pineapple Express* or Snoop Dogg rapping about gin and juice.

If those in the entertainment business accepted that they're a major influence on teenagers' feelings about what's cool and what isn't, maybe conscientious writers, producers, directors, performers, and others would think twice about the message being communicating. Over the years, actors, filmmakers, musicians, and other artists I've interviewed have maintained, and probably believe, that they're just reflecting drug use, not promoting it. But their works undoubtedly help normalize it. However, since we can't realistically expect that they and the media companies that fund them will choose a more responsible path, parents and teachers must teach children to be critical viewers — to notice when they're being indoctrinated (teaching messages such as the ones used in the Above the Influence media campaigns).

Controlling the onslaught of media that promotes drug use is — at least in the short term — impossible, but that doesn't mean that the effects can't be offset. Still, even the most effective anti-drug-use media campaign would be almost nothing compared to what parents, schools, communities, and the nation could do if we accepted the challenge of fixing systemic problems that contribute to drug use and then established systems to identify kids at risk and help them cope, aided children with emotional problems or mental illness, educated kids and engaged them, redirected teenagers' impulsivity and found safe ways for them to get high, and offered them the emotional support they need.

III

When Drug Use
Escalates

5

Use Becomes Abuse, and
Abuse Becomes Addiction

FOR NOW, WITHOUT MORE effective prevention strategies, more than three-quarters of people under eighteen will try drugs. Some who try them will use once, and some moderately and occasionally. However, others will use more and then more, even as their lives unravel. But the direst consequences of drug use aren't reserved exclusively for those who become addicted. Even first-time users can have heart attacks or seizures. A modest dose (modest compared to an addict's) can lead to overdose in a neophyte. Casual drug use can lead to serious illness, as it did for Ian Sullivan, a twenty-nine-year-old interior designer in Burbank, California, who explains that he used only during a difficult period in his life and never had the hallmarks of addiction. Nonetheless, he contracted HIV, because while he was high, he had unprotected sex. First-time users can wind up in emergency rooms or dead because they take too much of a drug or take a drug that's been tainted or adulterated. One doesn't have to be an addict for drug use to lead to accidents — countless fatalities have resulted from a night of too much drinking or the wrong combination of drugs. The distinction between a user, abuser, and addict is irrelevant when a person is sentenced to prison because he was driving high and killed someone, or when he suffers permanent brain damage or a stroke, or when he OD's. Also, one doesn't have to abuse drugs for them to trigger mental illness, as happens in a small percentage of people who try them. Dr. Vicki Nejtek, clinical researcher at the University of North Texas Health Science Center in Fort Worth, explains that "even marijuana use is like playing Russian roulette . . . you never know whose genetic make-up will make them more vulnerable to negative impacts until they use it, and then it is too late."

Just One More Hit

Dr. Shoptaw says, "Experimenting means you try something two or three times. More than that is using." And after that, there's no clear demarcation between using and abusing. Use is generally characterized by occasional drug taking, but any definition is inexact, and it's dangerous to rely on one. What remains casual use for one person can be harmful to another. Plus, casual users can easily become abusers or addicts.

The distinction between abuse and addiction is even murkier. Until recently there's been an official delineation between the two, at least according to the American Psychiatric Association (APA), the arbiter of psychiatric disorders as it describes them in its *Diagnostic and Statistical Manual of Mental Disorders* (the *DSM*). The *DSM,* considered by some to be the psychiatrist's bible, is used by doctors and other mental-health professionals to diagnosis specific mental illnesses. The inclusion or exclusion of a disease in the *DSM* can determine if insurance companies will cover it and scientists will study it.

In the *DSM-IV,* which was published in 2000, *abuse* is defined broadly as, Steve Shoptaw explains, "a pattern of use over at least a year that causes 'clinical distress.'" Over a twelve-month period, an abuser misses work or school or otherwise fails to meet his obligations, engages in reckless activities (driving while intoxicated, for example), is arrested or has other legal troubles, and/or continues using in spite of social or interpersonal problems caused by drugs. But though abusers get into trouble, sometimes catastrophic trouble, they use sporadically. Typically they go on a binge, get wasted, and as a result get in a fight or get depressed or are arrested for driving under the influence. They sober up and appear to be fine for a while. They may drink casually or not at all. Until the next bender.

Drug dependence and addiction — there's a subtle distinction, but it's not relevant here — are more extreme and persistent; there are rarely breaks in using unless the addict is forced to stop (by an arrest, for instance). The problematic consequences are more consistent and usually they escalate. A key distinction is that a person's motivation changes when he becomes addicted. Abusers want to get high or blow off steam. Those addicted need to use in order to function. If they stop using, they go through withdrawal. And because of the physical impact of drugs on the nervous system, their tolerance increases, so they often use more of a drug, use new drugs, or change the way they take the drugs (pills no longer do the trick so they begin using needles). Their use is compulsive.

The behavioral criteria of addiction includes three or more items from a list that includes exceeding self-imposed limits on drug use, continued use despite knowledge of negative consequences, losing interest in things that were once important, and a "narrowing of their behavioral repertoire," as the Treatment Research Institute's Tom McLellan put it. For example, those who are dependent commonly shed their non-using friends and replace them with ones who'll smoke and drink with them. They're preoccupied with getting high. They spend more time acquiring drugs, talking about drugs, and choosing activities that include drugs. The rituals of drug use (rolling joints, drinking and toasting, cutting lines) become integral parts of their social interactions. They come to believe that drugs make their social activities more "meaningful," whatever they're doing — hanging out, listening to music, and watching movies. They may connect drug use with work, feeling as if they can't perform or create if they aren't high. Addicts routinely lie, many steal, and some become violent. Their actions aren't controlled by their own will. A key factor in addiction is that underlying biology compels a person to use and be consumed with using. An addict's neurology is abnormal; his brain requires drugs — that is, it's dependent on them.

The fifth edition of the *DSM* (the *DSM-V*), to be published in May of 2013, essentially eliminates drug abuse as a stage separate from addiction. The new definition is nuanced but generally states that anyone who continues to use drugs in spite of harmful consequences has a substance-abuse disorder and is an addict, on a scale from mild to moderate to severe. That is, addiction is a continuum that includes all persistent and dangerous drug use.

The revised definition was prompted by a series of studies of treatment and scientific discoveries about the biology of addiction. Tom

McLellan listed some in an e-mail to me: "Some of the more 'severe' symptoms such as withdrawal and tolerance actually came on prior to some of the 'softer signs' — the behavioral signs. If 'abuse' led to 'dependence' this should not have occurred." Another discovery came from research that showed that "regardless of what kind of treatment and regardless of what kind of patient sample was studied, patients with 'abuse' were just as likely to relapse and do poorly as those with very severe 'addiction' after treatment." Other discoveries that influenced the change: Craving, present in both abusers and addicts, existed independent of physical symptoms and could be measured. Basically, the Pavlovian association between environmental and drug effect could by itself produce physical and emotional symptoms in both abusers and addicts. McLellan explains that the new definition of addiction recognizes that many of the former distinctions were arbitrary. Instead, he says, "the new definition of addiction acknowledges that there are mild to serious forms of the disease. It differentiates 'normal use' from use with problems." McLellan explains that in the new *DSM,* the diagnosis of addiction applies if a user has seven to eleven specific symptoms. Two are withdrawal and tolerance. Others are similar to those in the previous *DSM,* including drinking or using more than intended; continuing to use in spite of negative consequences; missing important events or obligations because of using; and family or friends complaining about one's using. "Since you have no basis for ordering or weighting these symptoms, you simply count them, and people with more of them have a more severe diagnosis," McLellan says.

The change in definition is controversial. When it was announced, thousands of psychiatrists and other treatment professionals complained. They and other critics of the revision claim that many people will be classified as addicts who aren't. As Maia Szalavitz wrote on Time.com, this "poses a huge problem, particularly for adolescents and young adults with mild problems who may be pushed to adopt an addict identity and to see themselves as having no way to control their drinking or drug use if they ever 'relapse.'" But Charles O'Brien, a professor of psychiatry at the University of Pennsylvania and one of the psychiatrists who worked on the new manual, believes that by classifying all seriously problematic drug users as addicts, "we can treat them earlier," as he told the *New York*

Times. "And we can stop them from getting to the point where they're going to need really expensive stuff like liver transplants."

There may be other benefits of dispensing with the term *abuse.* Though Szalavitz is correct that it may pathologize some people — she points out that college binge drinkers may now be considered addicts (some of them *are* addicted, but most aren't) — if all problematic use is considered addiction, it may be clearer for users, their families, and society itself that all drug use that causes problems is part of the continuum that can lead to severe addiction. Over time, people may be less likely to dismiss harmful behavior as a temporary aberration, disconnected from addiction, and more likely to see that it must be treated immediately because it could advance to a more serious form of the disease.

Meeting Mr. Hyde

Going forward in *Clean,* I will continue to refer to the traditional classifications of abuse and addiction, because they're still in common usage. The fact is that it *is* a continuum. But then, what causes people to move from one end of the continuum to the other — from use to abuse to addiction? What causes some people to increase their use gradually and some immediately?

Given the current state of science's understanding of addiction, there's no conclusive answer as to why one person's drug use escalates and another's doesn't. Everyone's different, and everyone reacts differently to different drugs, different amounts and combinations of them, and different ways drugs are administered, because of each person's unique biology, psychology, and environment. But some factors that influence the likelihood of addiction are known.

Research has indicated that one of the most important factors is the age of first use. The younger people are when they begin, the more susceptible they are to addiction, because their brains aren't fully developed, and so the impact of drugs on their extremely plastic nervous system is dramatic. It's one reason it's so difficult for doctors to detoxify babies born addicted (each year, more than 13,000 babies are born addicted to heroin, crack, prescription pain medications, or other drugs). Drugs have become an integral part of their nervous systems. Also, early use may cause a permanent deficit of naturally circulating dopamine, making the pleasure caused by drugs particularly potent.

In addition to the age of first use, there are other risk factors. Once again, genetics plays a major role. As I've described, for some, particularly those with psychiatric illnesses like depression, bipolar disorder, or anxiety disorders, continued and increasing use can be an ongoing, desperate, futile attempt to feel "normal" — a sensation that characterized their first use. Indeed, many addicts say they continued using and used more to chase the original feeling drugs had given them. That feeling was no longer attainable because drugs damaged their neurological systems and their tolerance increased, and so they were driven to try — in vain — to attain a satisfying high. It's one reason some users move on from alcohol and marijuana to so-called harder drugs, and why some move from smoking and drinking drugs to snorting and injecting them.

An additional reason some go from use to abuse to addiction relates to the drugs being used. More than 60 percent of those who try heroin will abuse, and almost 30 percent become addicted to it; 45 percent of cocaine users become abusers, and about 15 percent become addicted. Whereas more than 40 percent of those who smoke pot go on to abuse the drug, only about 5 percent become addicted to it. About 40 percent of people who drink will abuse alcohol; about 15 percent become addicted. Contrary to popular belief, it is possible for a person to become addicted the first time he tries a drug. Methamphetamine and crack are particularly addictive to some first-time users.

Warning Signs of Drug Abuse and Addiction

Even while drug use escalates, it can remain hidden. The warning signs, if there are any, may be extremely subtle. Yes, sometimes kids miss curfews and fail tests and skip school, but sometimes they don't. Some adults show up late for work or not at all, and some get DUIs, but for others, even as their use escalates, they remain high functioning, as if nothing's changed. But there are common signs that usually emerge. Kids who are abusing or addicted may become sullen, withdrawn, depressed, unusually tired, silent, uncommunicative, hostile, or deceitful. They're usually less motivated and more lethargic. Or hyperactive. They frequently break curfew, drain money, and avoid eye contact. They're often sneaky; locking doors, hiding conversations, or being vague about where they spend their time. Other signs are periods of sleeplessness or sleeping way too much; unexplained disappearances; the loss of interest in things they used to enjoy and care about; complaints from teachers or coworkers; frequent sickness; sudden or dramatic weight loss or gain; and the disappearance of prescription or over-the-counter pills, alcohol, money, or valuables. If a child displays any of these symptoms, it's time to look closer. If he displays several, he's probably using. Boston Children's Hospital's Dr. Levy advises parents to pay attention to these warning signs; just as they should trust their intuition if they suspect that a child is having social, emotional or psychological problems, they should trust their instincts when it comes to their child and drugs: "If you think your kids are using, they probably are."

Drug Testing

Ultimately, you don't want to guess; you want to know. Some kids will admit they're using if they're confronted, but many — probably fearful they'll be admonished or punished — won't. One way to determine if a person's using is to drug test him. Some parents are loath to do this because they feel it communicates distrust and might anger their child. They refuse even if the child has already proven himself untrustworthy. But testing often entails a welcome irony: it can defuse rather than intensify a climate of distrust. Parents who drug test will know, and they can relax knowing that they'll know. Also, their fear that drug testing children communicates distrust is probably moot. There's a good chance the kids already feel that they aren't trusted. Kids usually sense when their moods, performance at school, or attitudes are being scrutinized. But the primary reason to test is to gather more information, so a parent or caretaker can respond appropriately. And there may be other benefits as well. Some studies have shown that testing can be a deterrent. Kids who go out on a Friday night and know they may be tested when they come home are less likely to use. (Though there are ways to cheat these tests. There are how-to guides on the web.)

Saliva, hair, sweat, and blood can be tested, but urine tests for drugs and breathalyzers for alcohol are the most common methods. Home drug-testing kits are widely available, but Dr. Levy recommends that parents not test on their own and instead rely on testing ordered by a doctor or done in a clinic. "It's hard for parents to get it right," she says. (It's also hard for schools and workplaces to get it right, which is why it's controversial in those settings. Also, the efficacy of testing at schools or jobs is unproven and it can raise civil rights issues.) Whether parents test at home or leave it to the professionals, they should keep in mind that research has shown that testing works best as a deterrent when it's paired with rewards for clean tests — for instance, with restored or expanded privileges. It should also be clear what will happen if a drug test comes back positive. Will restrictions be imposed? A required drug-education course , counseling with a drug-and-alcohol counselor, or assessment by an addiction specialist?

If a test shows (or a parent learns in other ways) that a child has been using (and lying about it), consequences should be carefully considered. Some kids may respond to harsh punishments, but they can also backfire. At the risk of stating the obvious, some parental responses simply don't work. "We know that harsh discipline is a very strong predictor of all kinds of problem behaviors," Dr. Eve Reider says. That's not to say that there shouldn't be repercussions. Grounding is logical for several reasons: kids have blown their parents' trust and for a while they should be restricted and closely monitored. Taking kids out of circulation for a week or two not only deprives them of the opportunity to use but also gives their parents or other caretakers time to regroup and figure out what to do next. In the meantime, children need to know that even though their parents may be concerned, they're sympathetic. They need to know that someone's there if they need help.

Indeed, Michael Pantalon at Yale emphasizes that parents should continue to engage children in conversations similar to the ones that can help prevent use in the first place. "People tend to only listen to one person — themselves," Pantalon says. "So, as frustrating as this may be for a parent who would like to sternly say, 'You can't use!' or 'You have to stop!' and to have that be enough, the real trick to motivating someone is to get them to convince themselves to make a change for their own reasons."

Pantalon employs motivational interviewing to get kids talking about what they'd get if they stopped using. He asks, for example, "Why would you stop if you were going to?" He never judges their answers.

He explains, "People change by hearing themselves argu\
the change. Different wheels start turning, wheels in their \
haven't gotten exercise at all, because they've been defensive. E\
hounding them, but you're not."

Professional Assessment

Drug tests or changes in mood and behavior may indicate a severe problem that requires intensive treatment. The only way to know for sure is
to bring a child to see a qualified pediatrician or psychiatrist for a professional assessment. Doctors may employ any one of a number of screening tools. NIDAMED, at the NIDA website, is one of several designed to
help physicians identify patient drug use early and prevent it from escalating — it includes a web-based interactive screening tool. CAGE is the
most widely used screen for adults, and the Addiction Severity Index
(ASI), though developed for adults, is sometimes administered to kids.
Doctors ask patients a series of questions about their moods, problems
in their lives, and their drinking and drug use. The ASI tells the doctor
where a patient is on a scale of 0 ("no real problem, treatment not indicated") to 9 ("extreme problem, treatment absolutely necessary"). Some
doctors also use a system called CRAFFT to separate low- from high-
risk use in teens. A screener asks a child if in the previous six months
he drank alcohol, smoked pot or hash, or used anything else to get high.
Kids are assured that their answers will be kept confidential. If they say
they've used, they're directed to part B, which explains the acronym.
C: Has the kid ever ridden in a car driven by someone (including himself) who was high? R: Has he ever used drugs to relax, feel better, or fit
in? A: Has he ever used drugs when alone? F: Did he ever forget what he
did when he was high? The other F: Do family or friends ever tell him he
should cut down? And T: Did he ever get into trouble while using? Two
or more yeses suggest a problem and need for additional assessment.

Ideally, the doctors will use a brief intervention strategy if one is required. (If they aren't trained to intervene, they should refer a patient
to someone who is.) One of the most effective approaches is SBIRT
(Screening, Brief Intervention, and Referral to Treatment), developed
for adults but now being tested on children. The assessment stage comes
first. In the offices of doctors trained in SBIRT, patients are asked to

respond to a brief set of questions (verbally, on paper, or electronically) that measure if they're at high, medium, or low risk for drug problems and addiction. A scoring system guides the level of intervention. Those shown to be at no to low risk are encouraged to do what they're doing but monitor themselves. Those with mild symptoms are offered a single, brief intervention, at which a doctor explains their scores and the risks they're taking and attempts to motivate them to reduce use. Those who score at a level of moderate risk are given several counseling sessions that include an assessment of their readiness to change, establishing of goals and strategies for change, and the creation of a follow-up plan. People at high risk with severe symptoms or with complicated psychiatric problems are referred to specialty treatment. Bertha Madras, professor of psychobiology at Harvard and former deputy director for demand reduction at the Office of National Drug Control Policy Research, explains that SBIRT can be "remarkably effective, lowering alcohol and drug use significantly at six months following the intervention." In a study that separated drug and alcohol use, rates of participants' drug use were lowered by 67.7 percent, and alcohol use was 38 percent lower after six months.

It's important to note that these assessments and interventions are still in their early stages of development and implementation. Much more research needs to be done to improve them. For example, there must be longer-term studies of SBIRT to prove that it's effective over time. At present, no assessment tool is foolproof. Certainly no intervention is. Even doctors, the most vigilant loved ones, family members, and users themselves don't always know when use has become abuse or when abuse has progressed to addiction.

"No one knew," says Anna David, author and executive editor of TheFix.com, a website about addiction and recovery. David, sitting in a café in LA, wears all black — a black hooded sweatshirt and black jeans. She has long, dark brown hair parted on the side, with bangs cut just above her eyes. She's confident, funny, attractive, successful. But she wasn't as a teenager, or at least, that's not how she felt. Drinking at parties helped lessen the insecurity she kept hidden. "I felt smart," she says. "Confident." She'd had a crush on a senior boy, and, unthinkable if she'd been sober, she told him so. "I discovered what alcohol could do for me," she says. "I became obsessed with drinking. I loved the lack of self-consciousness drinking gave me. I'd get this euphoric anticipation about the weekend when I'd be able to party. It became the most important thing to me."

At one party she was given a line of cocaine. "It never dawned on me that I shouldn't do it." She used more but told herself it was harmless. By all outward appearances, it was. "I never missed a day of school. I still got good grades."

She drank, smoked pot, took cocaine.

In college she drank even more and used more drugs but was "able to pretend that it wasn't a big deal." After graduating, she got a job as an editorial assistant. When she was working as an editor at a website in her late twenties, she often came into work high. Still, no one knew. Her use progressed. She snorted cocaine all night, took Ambien in the morning, and slept during the day. "Being an addict sort of snuck up on me," she says.

6

Addicts Aren't Weak, Selfish, or Amoral—They're Ill

UNLESS YOU'VE BEEN THERE, you can't imagine what it's like to watch helplessly as someone you love descends into addiction. The transformation defies logic — until you understand that your loved one is gravely ill with a brain disease that's debilitating, chronic, progressive, and, if left untreated, often fatal.

Once and for all, people must understand that addiction is a disease. It's critical if we're going to effectively prevent and treat addiction. Accepting that addiction is an illness will transform our approach to public policy, research, insurance, and criminality; it will change how we feel about addicts, and how they feel about themselves. There's another essential reason why we must understand that addiction is an illness and not just bad behavior: We punish bad behavior. We treat illness.

I understand those who reject the notion that addiction is a disease because I used to be one of them. When my son was addicted, I heard the so-called disease theory in a lecture at a rehab where he was being treated. Later, I heard it at other rehabs and at AA meetings. Still later, I heard it espoused by therapists and counselors.

To me, the adherents of the disease theory were apologists for addicts (often they *were* addicts) who were attempting to rationalize and excuse outrageous, unconscionable behavior, hedonism, and debauchery. To me, when my son was addicted, he wasn't ill, he was an out-of-control, self-absorbed teenager who was looking for a good time and didn't care who he hurt.

During the question-and-answer segment of a lecture I attended about addiction, a father of an alcoholic raised his hand to speak. From his emotional description of sleepless nights and late-night phone calls to the police and emergency rooms, I knew how similarly we'd been suffering. Instead of the anger I'd felt, however, bewilderment was what he described. "This isn't my son," he said. "He wasn't a selfish person. He never lied. He cared about himself and the family and school. Something changed him. He's a different person now. He's ill—very, very ill."

Was he making excuses for his son's behavior? I understood those who took solace in the *rationalization* that addiction was an illness. They were—*we* were—grateful for any plausible explanation of our loved ones' transformation and transgressions. I thought, *Maybe some people dismiss the idea that addiction is a disease until it hits their family. When it does, they embrace the concept because it exonerates their loved ones or themselves. It's easier to believe that a person's behavior is a symptom of an illness rather than a series of reprehensible choices.* But wanting something to be true doesn't make it true. This isn't an issue subject to "belief." We don't *believe* that cancer is a disease. We *know* it is.

The Disease of Addiction

A disease is "an interruption, cessation, or disorder of a body, system, or organ structure or function," according to *Stedman's Medical Dictionary.* It's "a morbid entity ordinarily characterized by two or more of the following criteria: recognized etiologic agent(s), identifiable group of signs and symptoms, or consistent anatomic alterations."

Addiction fits every one of these criteria.

Studies that compare the brains of addicts have consistently identified anatomic alterations. "There are long-lasting changes in the brain, and they're measurable," according to Dr. Susan Weiss, associate director for scientific affairs at the National Institute on Drug Abuse. "The reward system is altered."

The anatomic alterations are mainly in two areas. Both the brain structure and the flow of neurotransmitters through the nervous system are changed. This results in altered brain function, which in turn alters thinking, and altered thinking alters behavior.

Even the most common drugs, marijuana and alcohol, considered by many to be less harmful than others, change the structure of the brain. The gray matter controls muscle movement, sensory perceptions, memory, emotions, and speech. White matter is the network of fibers that link brain regions and allow signals to be sent between them. Anatomic alterations of marijuana users' white matter can clearly be seen in scans and detected in postmortem chemical tests of addicts' brains. The white matter in heavy marijuana smokers' brains has "poorer integrity," says to Susan Tapert, professor of psychiatry at the University of California at San Diego.

What's poorer integrity? Joanna Jacobus, a colleague of Tapert's at UCSD, explains. "A tract of fiber in the brain is judged by how compact and coherent it is. The better its integrity, the better it does its job, signaling between brain areas." The researchers judge integrity by looking at the diffusion of water molecules within the fiber tracts. Dr. Jacobus compares it to a pot of spaghetti cooking in boiling water. The noodles represent the long, thin fiber tracts of the brain. In a pot of boiling water without spaghetti, the water molecules diffuse freely, because there's nothing to restrict them. Put spaghetti in the pot, and the water molecules are hindered. If you start pulling out pieces of spaghetti, the water molecules start to diffuse more freely again. "That's not what you want," she says. "You want to see less diffusion, because it means more spaghetti in there, and more spaghetti means more and better communication within the brain."

Tapert's scans have found *less* compact and coherent fiber tracts in the brains of pot smokers. Their white matter has atrophied. She says, "If there is tissue atrophy in white matter, the brain regions may not be able to communicate as efficiently and as quickly."

These changes appear to be similar to the loss of neurons in the hippocampus region of the brain that occurs as people age. The loss decreases their ability to remember and to learn new information. "Chronic THC exposure may hasten age-related loss of hippocampal neurons," Jacobus says. In one study, rats exposed to THC every day for eight months showed a level of neuron loss equal to that of unexposed animals twice their age.

Tapert has also studied the brains of heavy drinkers, and she found them to be altered too. Once again, her research focused on white matter. She found that heavy alcohol use caused even more pronounced damage than marijuana did. For example, the brains of binge drinkers she examined had "a number of little dings throughout their brains' white matter, indicating poor quality," she told NPR. Alcohol is particularly neurotoxic, according to NIDA's Dr. Baler. "It causes actual degeneration of neurons."

If pot and alcohol cause anatomical changes, it's unsurprising that other drugs do too. For example, by mimicking naturally occurring opiates and binding to opiate receptors, which normally limit, or inhibit, the amount of dopamine released, heroin causes dopamine to flood the synapses. This damages nerve cells in the areas of the brain involved in learning, memory, and emotional well-being. According to Jeanne Bell, professor of neuropathology at the University of Edinburgh, it's similar to damage found in the early stages of Alzheimer's disease. Bell's chemical tests of the brains of young IV heroin users showed "significantly higher levels of two key proteins associated with brain damage." Another study found that drug abuse causes low-grade inflammation in the brain. Bell told the *Scotsman,* "Taken together, the studies suggest that intravenous opiate abuse may be linked to premature ageing of the brain." Similarly, the scans of the brains of methamphetamine addicts and postmortem chemical tests of their brains have shown that meth causes structural changes similar to those seen in people with degenerative brain diseases. Researchers have noted that some neuron ends in meth addicts are essentially singed. Chemical tests of meth addicts' brains showed modestly diminished levels of serotonin and other neurotransmitters and 90 to 95 percent lower levels of dopamine. These findings have led researchers to believe that meth physically changes the brain, more than cocaine, the other drug studied. (There's information about the impact of the various drugs in the appendix of this book.)

While drugs do cause structural changes in the brain, the most pronounced changes are functional. "The brain is hijacked," Baler says.

"Drugs take over the receptors — bind to them. The connections are impaired. The brain becomes dysfunctional."

Indeed, a hallmark of the disease of addiction is the altered flow of neurotransmitters, especially dopamine. I've explained that all drugs change the flow of dopamine — that's how they work. However, with mild drug use and in nonaddicts' brains, the alteration is temporary; the effect of the drug wears off and because of homeostasis, the system returns to normal. However, the brains of those with addiction respond differently. Drugs stimulate dopamine flow, and the floodgates open. For nonaddicts, as homeostasis kicks in, the floodgates close, and the heightened stimulation caused by drugs fades. For addicts, however, the floodgates take longer to close or they cease closing. Rather than recirculating, dopamine repeatedly stimulates receptors. Or maybe the door-opening mechanism becomes ultra-sensitive so that, in the future, even a minuscule amount of any drug causes them to swing wide open again. Either way, the brain is malfunctioning. It never stops "wanting" to heal. More of a drug can send another flood of whatever store of dopamine remains, but the receptors are less and less able to process the chemicals that reach them, if they reach them. Tolerance builds. Damage increases.

Indeed, addiction causes "an interruption, cessation, or disorder of a body, system, or organ structure or function." The American Psychiatric Association's *DSM* describes some functional changes in its definition of addiction. Two of these occur when the addict's brain adapts to the influence of one or more drugs. First, it requires more and then more of a given drug in order to get the same — eventually, any — effect. That functional change, the building tolerance, is a symptom of this disease. Second, the brain becomes dependent on the drug. Dependence explains why addicts can't just stop. It also explains why they experience withdrawal when the system is deprived of the drug. Physical withdrawal is another symptom of this disease.

Other functional impairments caused by addiction include a range of cognitive deficits. For example, the changes in the brain's white matter that Drs. Tapert and Jacobus described correlate with abnormal functioning in the hippocampus — again, a region associated with memory formation. The diminishment of memory in pot smokers has been well established. Dr. Vicki Nejtek, clinical researcher at the University of

North Texas Health Science Center in Fort Worth, adds, "We know the myelin sheath around our brain cells acts like an insulator to an electric cords." The insulator is like the outer layer of pieces of spaghetti. "When that's stripped away, it causes a reduction in brain cell activity. It can cause memory loss; it reduces our ability to concentrate."

Marijuana has been shown to cause other impairments, including, according to Krista Lisdahl Medina, assistant professor of psychology at the University of Cincinnati, "measurable cognitive deficits." Other drugs cause similar impairments—a wider range of them. In many cases, they're more extreme.

A Progressive, Chronic Disease

Addiction is a disease, and one that's progressive and chronic. Progressive diseases are ones that worsen over time if they aren't treated. Like cardiovascular disease and many cancers, unless addiction is being treated, it usually advances. Addiction has also been shown to be a chronic illness, because at least some of the brain changes in addicts appear to be permanent, and even if they're not, the predisposition for addiction probably remains throughout a person's life. Animal studies have shown that sensory input, memories, and stress can cause flies, mice, and monkeys that are "addicts" (researchers have addicted them to a drug) to initiate intense drug-seeking behavior, even after long periods of being deprived of the drug. Human studies have shown that even after years of abstinence, addicts respond to triggers—sights, sounds, smells, and even emotions that they associate with drugs. Their heartbeats and breathing speed up and they can feel intense craving. This craving can lead to relapse. Cancer is another disease that can go into remission but then reappear. The persistent possibility of relapse is another hallmark of addiction, which is why a lifetime of monitoring and treatment may be required.

Along with tolerance and withdrawal and the ongoing potential of recurrence (relapse), the disease of addiction has many other identifiable signs and symptoms. Normally, the nervous system monitors, controls, and balances mood, but addiction impairs that system, so addiction is associated with anxiety, mania, and depression. In addition to memory and cognitive impairments, there can also be impaired motor functions, and addiction can disrupt normal autonomic body functions, including sensory processing, sleep, metabolism, breathing, heartbeat, and blood pressure.

Cognitive impairments caused by addiction explain another hallmark of the disease, a maddening one. We hear about patients' denial of cancer and other physical illnesses. Understandably, seriously ill people are scared, and they might deal with their fear by avoiding or sublimating it. Ultimately, however, it's difficult to argue with x-rays, scans, and biopsies, let alone deteriorating health. Sufferers usually eventually understand that they're ill. When they do, most seek treatment. It's different for addicts, though, because many of the initial symptoms of the disease are behavioral and cognitive. And though many people can't accept that a disease can cause someone to deny that he's ill, one of the symptoms of addiction is anosognosia, a medical condition in which a patient is unaware or does not acknowledge that he's sick.

Like many schizophrenics (an estimated 40 percent of them), many addicts (an unknown number) can't understand that they're ill because the part of the brain that's damaged by the disease is the same part that's responsible for self-awareness and self-analysis. Their impaired insight, another term used by psychologists, explains addicts' denial. The brain differences associated with impaired insight in schizophrenics and addicts seem to be similar — they occur in many of the same brain regions. We don't blame a schizophrenic for refusing treatment; at least we shouldn't, because his or her condition hinders rational thought. Brain cancer or dementia can have this effect too, depending on the disease's location and severity. Like people with a range of mental illnesses, addicts can become confused, irascible, and irrational, because their illness is rooted in the very brain center that normally would tell them that they're in trouble and need help.

The Addiction Gene

It's possible to concede that an addict's brain structure and nervous system are different than a nonaddict's while still rejecting the disease model. Didn't these addicts poison themselves, damaging healthy tissue and circuitry? The answer, which is of paramount importance, is no and yes. It's true that addicts ingested, smoked, or injected illicit drugs into their bodies. However, this action didn't cause the addiction. If it did, all people who took drugs would become addicted, but most don't.

There are two ways people become addicted. Anyone who takes enough of a drug to cause severe structural and functional changes in the brain can become addicted. But most people who become addicted do so because their brains are different *before* they use drugs, not *because* they use them. In fact, there's evidence that addicts' brains are different from birth; they have various neurological and genetic anomalies that, when combined with environmental influences, may cause them to respond differently to drugs than nonaddicts do. A study of cocaine addicts published in *Science* in 2012 showed that neurological abnormalities in addicts appear to predate any drug use. For the study, researchers at the University of Cambridge in England studied fifty cocaine addicts and their siblings who had no history of drug abuse. Karen Ersche, the study's lead author, told NPR that brain scans showed that both siblings — the addict and the one who'd never abused drugs — had brains that were atypical. She said, "The fibers that connect the different parts of the brain were less efficient in both [the addicts and their nonaddicted siblings]." Furthermore, she said that the fibers were ones specifically associated with self-control. "When the fibers aren't working efficiently, it takes longer for the 'stop' message to get through." Both siblings' brains were different from normal brains, and the dysfunction was centered in the braking system. The fact that only one of the siblings became addicted is probably explained by environmental factors, but the addicts' brains appear to have been wired for addiction before drugs were thrown into the mix.

Why would siblings in particular be similarly wired for addiction? It's likely that the main reason is the same as the one that explains why carcinogenic chemicals from household products, cigarettes, or radiation cause cancer in some, but not in everyone. No one would suggest that people who succumb to cancer are weak; they probably developed the disease because of physiological anomalies, environmental influences, and other as-yet-unidentified factors. But there's also a consensus among scientists that genetics determine those who are more likely to get many kinds of cancer, which is why family histories are critical when doctors examine patients. A family history of heart disease indicates a genetic susceptibility to heart disease. Many diseases have genetic components.

And so does addiction. It's been proven that some people have a genetic predisposition to addiction in numerous studies, including studies of twins and siblings of alcoholic parents who were raised separately. A number of twin studies have shown that addiction is about 50 percent genetic (the other 50 percent is environmental). And studies of adopted children showed that those whose biological parents were addicts were twice as likely to become addicts as those whose biological parents weren't addicts.

As I've described, roughly 10 percent of humans have the constellation of genes that predisposes them to addiction. This doesn't mean that those without the addiction gene, or gene set, are immune, just as those without a genetic predisposition to lung cancer can still get that disease if they smoke too much. "Some people have a genetic predisposition to addiction," Nora Volkow said in an interview with *Time,* "but because it involves these basic brain functions, everyone will become an addict if sufficiently exposed to drugs or alcohol." Conversely, having a genetic predisposition doesn't guarantee the onset of the disease. It's not unlike other diseases that are influenced by DNA.

So we might ask why some people take their drug use to greater extremes than others — why do some stop at marijuana or alcohol, some at taking pills, and some at shooting heroin? Again, Dr. Volkow compares it to cancer. "Some cancers are more malignant," she says. "So you do have some vulnerabilities that are much more serious than others. There are people that have grown up in very supportive environments and yet when they get exposed to a drug they rapidly escalate their use, even though their whole social infrastructure is very protective. And then you have individuals who have very little vulnerability perhaps through protective genetic factors, but the environment is so high-risk that it may drive them to take drugs repeatedly and eventually they may become addicted. It's like those individuals that can smoke until they're 100 years of age and they don't die from smoking related consequences, like pulmonary diseases or cancer. It's just they have, for whatever reason, a particularly high resistance to the ravaging effects of tobacco smoking. On the other hand, others may develop cancer from secondary smoke. They don't even get exposed to very high quantities." The variations among people are vast, and so are their responses to drugs.

Variations in individuals' genetic makeup contribute to the severity of addiction, as does environment, and the disease is often compounded by co-occurring psychological disorders. The effect of drugs is exacerbated when those with mental illnesses use them to self-medicate.

A Disease That Mimics Free Will

Fine. The brains of addicted people are different. But in true diseases, there's no volition. People *choose* to take drugs. This is the most common objection made by those who don't accept that addiction is a disease.

"It's true that drug taking begins as a choice," acknowledges UCLA's Richard Rawson, "and one that appears to be a completely selfish and self-destructive one. A disease that causes you to walk into a bar and drink a beer? It's counterintuitive. People choose to walk into a bar or they choose not to. Symptoms of disease are fevers, nausea, hair loss, heart attacks, and seizures. They don't include reprehensible acts like lying and stealing."

But choice has nothing to do with the disease of addiction. Not all those who try drugs and continue to use them have a disease. Eighty percent of adolescents in the United States try drugs. For a variety of reasons, some scientifically proven and explained in this book, and some as yet unknown, only one in ten becomes addicted. Only those who become addicted have the disease.

In the 1920s, a coterie of doctors described alcoholism as a metabolic aberration leading to an inability to process the drug, and some doctors characterized it as an allergy, an idea reflected in "The Doctor's Opinion" section of the Big Book, written by Dr. William D. Silkworth, a colleague of Alcoholics Anonymous founder Bill Wilson. "These allergic types can never safely use alcohol in any form at all," Silkworth wrote, "and once having formed the habit and found they cannot break it, once having lost their self-confidence, their reliance upon things human, their problems pile up on them and become astonishingly difficult to solve."

Addiction isn't an allergy, but there are analogies between addiction and allergy that can help people understand the abnormalities in the brains of addicts. Most people eat peanuts without any negative reaction. Some, however, when exposed to a particular chemical compound in peanuts (generally the protein Ara h1 or Ara h2), go into anaphylactic shock, which can be fatal. Yes, it's a choice to try peanuts; no one would blame a person for trying them — or for the fact that it turns out he's allergic. Even though he chose to eat peanuts, no one would claim that he didn't subsequently become ill. He suffers a disorder of the immune system.

Addicts aren't hypersensitive to drugs the way those with peanut allergies are hypersensitive to Ara h1 or h2, but addicts process drugs in a completely different way than others do. When both addicts and non-addicts get high, they're reacting to a burst of dopamine. After that, the similarities cease; addicts and nonaddicts process the chemicals differently. Neurotransmitters in addicts' brains don't properly circulate and recirculate. The misfiring effectively turns the reward system on full blast and dismantles the braking system.

When an addict takes drugs, it appears to be a choice. One of the many reasons people reject the idea that addiction is a disease is the mistaken belief that people don't cause or contribute to "real" diseases. But they do: Eating fried chicken and pork rinds and doughnuts contributes to the onset and progression of heart disease and diabetes; smoking leads to lung cancer and emphysema. If people don't exercise, they can cause or worsen cardiovascular disease; if they spend too much time in the sun, they can develop skin cancer. In fact, it's possible to argue that choice plays a larger role in some diseases than it does in addiction. The brains of people with heart disease who eat fried chicken haven't been impaired, so they have no excuse. (Actually, there's evidence that neurotransmitter flow may make it harder for some people to follow dietary restrictions.)

Addicts' Behavior Is a Symptom of Their Disease

Addicts' impaired cognition can lead to behavioral changes. Also, with the prefrontal cortex dismantled and the rear brain in control, addicts are literally not in their right minds. The go system is raging, the prefrontal cortex is offline, and, as a result, addicts appear to be pathological narcissists, unable to empathize or sympathize. That's because the reptilian brain can focus on only one thing: the insatiable need for more drugs. In an AA meeting, an addict said, "Everything about my life was about heroin — using heroin, getting it. I was always calculating. Always. At night before I'd pass out, I knew I needed to save two tenths of a gram so I'd have it to wake up. All I was thinking about when I was high was the next high — where I'd score." The unrestrained go system also accounts for what appears to be an addict's unending quest for pleasure — the modulating system is down. It's important to remember that pleasure isn't an end in itself. It's inextricably associated with survival. The brain doesn't merely want more dopamine. It *needs* it. When it gets what it needs, it rewards the addict with pleasure.

The cycle of addiction further explains why addicts do such self-destructive things — turning on the very people they need and love, committing crimes without regard for consequences. Diminished cognitive ability is a hallmark of addiction. When people are addicted, their worldviews are so altered that the irrational appears rational. They justify outlandish behavior. They can feel impervious — immune to consequences. They've been taken over by a single impulse: to use.

All the differences in addicts versus nonaddicts (or "normies," as people in AA meetings sometimes call them) — the genetic predisposition, damaged cellular structure in addicts' brains, misfiring neurotransmitters, the unusual processing of drugs, and more — prove incontrovertibly that addicts have a disease. They also explain why they do things that are outrageous, destructive, self-destructive, and morally reprehensible. Still, although disease isn't a choice, behavior seems to be. However, the same diminishments that cause anosognosia in addicts also cause what appears to be immorality and weakness. In adolescents, it can appear to be willful rebellion.

An unrestrained go system explains behavior that seems to be a reflection of a person's character. We've seen that when the go system blasts, the stop system is repressed. The stop system in the prefrontal cortex that normally regulates impulses and behavior would, if it weren't impaired, moderate the physical compulsion to use. It would also enable clearer, more conscious thinking. The prefrontal cortex is active when a person considering a second or third drink or another hit of coke recalls the likelihood of a hangover or the consequences of driving while high. The stop system isn't working in those who are addicted, which is why they don't consider consequences.

Unlike most other disorders, addiction affects behavior that we think of as free will, which is one reason it's more insidious than other illnesses. Radically disordered brains lead to radically altered behavior and impaired thinking. We think of nausea, tremors, loss of appetite, and fever as legitimate disease symptoms, but we must understand that lying or violence can be symptoms as well.

And the disease has other behavioral and psychological symptoms. One is the reactive component that accompanies addiction. When people are addicted, their consciences are muted but not completely silenced. They feel guilt and shame. Their loved ones can't understand what's happened to them, and neither can the addicts. They're horrified. Retreating from an overwhelming psychological burden, they're even more likely to succumb to craving. Meanwhile, they keep using to prevent withdrawal. And they keep using so they can avoid facing the devastation — the harm to relationships, career, finances, and so on — their drug use has caused.

A common result of this spiral is the addict's tendency to victimize the ones closest to him. The addict lies to his family and steals from them. Family members can't understand why the person they love has turned on them, but there's a certain cruel logic to this behavior: home is familiar — the addict knows where the checks or prescription drugs are stored. And home is safer — he assumes that there's less risk of getting caught. If he is, there's less risk that he'll be arrested and prosecuted — addicts don't think their families will call the police, and they're usually right, at least at first. But when they victimize their families, their shame builds, and it can manifest as hostility toward their loved ones. It would be logical for that shame to cause an addict to keep his bad behavior as far as possible from family members. However, addicts say that their attacks on their family resulted *from* their embarrassment. One man in recovery from his cocaine addiction said, "I would do anything to avoid feeling shame and being judged, so I lashed out at the people who reminded me of what I was doing." This also explains addicts' duplicity—an old (and accurate) adage states, "An addict steals your wallet and then helps you look for it." They want to appear good. They want to be trusted and loved. In the process, they become strangers to others and themselves. But meanwhile, those watching the descent are hurt, confused, angry, and horrified. They think, *What's happened to him? How can she not see what she's doing to herself? How can she not see what she's doing to us? He's become a monster.* Addicts often *feel* like monsters.

They Can't Just Stop

They don't stop in spite of catastrophic consequences. This is another symptom of this disease—continued use in spite of negative consequences. Is it because addicts are selfishly choosing pleasure? They only want to have fun? If addicts were simply set on having fun, why would they continue using when drugs are no longer fun—quite the opposite? But they do. And they continue using even when drugs lead to trauma, physical illness, and a degradation of their lives. There may be a momentary respite the instant the drug effect comes on, but it doesn't last. People aren't choosing to use. Using is a symptom of their disease.

It's true that some people do stop using on their own, suggesting that, in spite of other evidence, willpower is enough, which further suggests that people who don't stop using don't try hard enough. However, longitudinal studies find that only a very small fraction actually quit on their own. In "Exploring Myths About Drug Abuse," former NIDA president Alan Leshner wrote, "To be sure, some people can quit drugs cold turkey, or they can quit after receiving treatment just one time at a rehabilitation facility. But most of those who abuse drugs require longer-term treatment and, in many instances, repeated treatments."

Maybe those who stop on their own aren't as addicted in the first place; they may have mild addiction. As Dr. Volkow says, "There are milder forms of cancer too." Some people with certain personality types, genetics, and socioeconomic situations may be better able to stop on their own, and the ability to stop probably also depends on the specific drugs and amount and duration of use. Family, jobs, and friends likely play a role for these fortunate few, but none of these factors make a difference for most addicts who try to stop, often repeatedly, but are unable to.

"At its core, addiction isn't just a social problem or a moral problem or a criminal problem," said Dr. Michael Miller, past president of ASAM. "It's a brain problem whose behaviors manifest in all these other areas. Many behaviors driven by addiction are real problems and sometimes criminal acts. But the disease is about brains, not drugs. It's about underlying neurology, not outward actions."

For centuries we've viewed addicts as immoral, weak, and pathetic. We told them to just say no, but they didn't. We declared war on them and locked them up, but they kept using. We judged them, vilified them, and banished them, yet they still took drugs. Our best efforts to stop them from using didn't work because we didn't understand the most important fact of the paradigm explained in *Clean:* addiction is a disease with a neurologic basis—a mental illness. When we understand this, we can finally put aside our prejudices and outrage and see that addicts aren't bad people, immoral, weak, or degenerate. Blame, shame, and anger can be replaced by compassion. Most important, when we understand that addicts are ill, we have a model to follow. If someone we love gets sick, we know the course forward.

7

Don't Deny Addiction, Don't Enable It, and Don't Wait for an Addict to Hit Bottom — He Could Die

PEOPLE WITH MOST LIFE-THREATENING illnesses will do whatever they can to figure out what's wrong and treat their disease. Nobody has to convince them to go to the doctor. They *want* to get well. But because of the denial and cognitive impairments that so often accompany addiction, many addicts simply can't do what they obviously need to do: seek help. A twenty-three-year-old Fort Lauderdale, Florida, girl named Kali Spencer, a Roxy addict — Roxicodone is similar to OxyContin — told me that she'd always felt she could stop using whenever she wanted to, "but I didn't want to." Several times, after accidents, stealing from her mother, binges that left her dehydrated and ill — she was five five and weighed 105 pounds; "crackhead skinny," as she describes it — she'd resolve to stop. "I'd make it two or three days," she says, "and then reward myself by getting high. I never understood people who stopped on their own."

It's not only anosognosia that stops addicts from seeking help. For addicts, denial is a self-preservation mechanism that justifies their continued pursuit of drugs even as those drugs are killing them. The twisted logic is a response to the craving they feel — craving so powerful it blocks out other instincts. If not for their denial, addicts would be impelled to do what their bodies tell them *not* to do: find a way to stop.

Addicts can't comprehend that they're ill, and so they do nothing to treat themselves. Some addicts finally end up in treatment only after they've been jolted from denial by one or more tragic events — in the parlance of the traditional recovery movement, they hit bottom. That is, they're brought to their knees when addiction has terrible, possibly life-threatening consequences. For some it's enough to lose a job or a relationship. Some become physically ill and decide to seek help before their health declines further. The cumulative effects of the addiction cycle cause some to find treatment. More often, however, hitting bottom is marked by a traumatic event such as arrest, overdose, accident, or other violence.

Though hitting bottom does describe the beginning of recovery for some addicts, it is a dangerous construct. Many addicts are alive because their families didn't wait for them to hit bottom. And for every person who hit bottom and wound up in treatment, many others kept falling further and further downward. They'd have catastrophes that would have been the bottom for any sane person, but addicts are addicted — many don't stop even after multiple calamities. For many, there's no bottom — it's a bottomless pit. Sometimes people die without seeking help. "I guess that means they didn't ever hit bottom," Richard Rawson, the associate director of the Integrated Substance Abuse Programs at UCLA, observes ruefully.

The danger of irreparable damage or death is only one reason not to postpone getting help for an addict. Another is that when addicts' use continues, their problems worsen. They use more and become more physically ill and mentally debilitated. They may have accidents or develop serious health problems, including heart attacks, strokes, AIDS, or hepatitis C. They may commit crimes and land in prison. The longer they're addicted, the more likely they'll become irrational, refusing help, and the more intractable their addiction will become. As Tom McLellan told me, it's like letting a diabetic lose her foot before addressing her diet.

The belief that an addict must hit bottom before he'll be ready for help grew out of the experience of many people who tried and failed to get addicts into treatment or got them into treatment only to have them leave or relapse. They concluded that addicts can't be helped unless they choose to be. There are many stories that illustrate this; go to an AA meeting, where hitting bottom is likely to be a dominant theme. "My bottom came when . . ." Fill in the blank. "I've been sober since then." The Alcoholics Anonymous Twelve Steps and Twelve Traditions asks, "Why all this insistence that every A.A. [member] must hit bottom first? The answer is that few people will sincerely try to practice the A.A. program unless they have hit bottom. For practicing A.A.'s remaining eleven Steps [following the acceptance of powerlessness] means the adoption of attitudes and actions that almost no alcoholic who is still drinking can dream of taking. Who wishes to be rigorously honest and tolerant? . . . Under the lash of alcoholism, we are driven to A.A. . . . Then, and only then, do we become as open-minded to conviction and as willing to listen as the dying can be."

But science as well as reason contradicts the premise of hitting bottom. As Nora Volkow, director of the National Institute on Drug Abuse, explains, "Research has shown that even addicts who go into treatment only because they've been forced to go — perhaps by a court — have the same chance of getting and staying sober as anyone else." "You want people self-motivated to be in treatment," says Michael Pantalon, "but you can work on that once you get them in."

And no, relapse doesn't mean that a person entered treatment before he was ready (that is, before he hit bottom). Many addicts relapse after treatment, no matter how they got there in the first place. The idea that addicts must "hit bottom" is an archaic and potentially deadly myth.

Impediments to Intervention —
Denial and Codependence

If waiting for an addict to hit bottom is so dangerous, and if their illness prevents addicts from comprehending that they're in trouble, why don't their loved ones do something? They aren't on drugs; they see all too clearly the destruction and danger, because they watch it unfold and are traumatized by it. Sometimes the trauma is severe enough to tear families apart. Divorce is common. So are estrangements between addicts and their siblings and other family members. Addicts' loved ones often don't sleep, some don't eat, and they can become seriously depressed or anxious. As their lives become consumed with another's drug use, they may not be able to fulfill their own obligations — taking care of others in their family, working. They may isolate themselves from their friends and families. They may suffer headaches, nausea, ulcers, and other physical ailments. They can have breakdowns. In spite of all that, they still don't act. Why?

I know why, from personal experience — and I know the ramifications of not acting. It may have been reasonable for me to have dismissed the first time I found pot in my son's backpack — lots of kids try pot. But how could I have excused the missed curfews; an arrest for failing to appear in court after he received a ticket for possession of marijuana; his moodiness, anger, and irascibility? How could I have ignored the implications when I heard from his school that he was skipping classes (he said it was "senioritis")? How could I have believed his excuses and his lies: "It's not my pot. I don't know where it came from." (The pot was in his dresser drawer.) "I didn't take the money." (No one else could have.) "The car ran out of gas and I stayed at a friend's — I didn't call because I didn't want to wake you." (Okay, maybe once, but twice?) "I'm not using!" (He was sleeping all the time, jittery, talking too fast or too slowly.) In a *Simpsons* episode, Homer tells his wife, "Marge, it takes two to lie. One to lie and one to listen." Addicts' family members listen to the lies and often believe them, because they need to. I denied the truth because I was overwhelmed with the reality: my son was out of control, endangering others and himself, and he could die. When we're overwhelmed, another survival mechanism kicks in: part of us shuts down.

I denied what was happening in front of my eyes until I was jolted from denial. Nic had been gone for days and I'd been in an unrelenting hell not knowing if he was alive or not. I had repeatedly called the police to see if there'd been an accident. I called hospital emergency rooms. Again and again. Finally Nic did call. He sounded awful. He told me where he was, and I went to get him. He was emaciated, bruised, sallow, and trembling. When I helped him up, he was so frail it felt as if he could break in two. I couldn't pretend any longer that he was going to be all right. I had to get him into treatment.

I found a program for him, and in spite of the hard evidence of the seriousness of his problem, my denial reappeared. Dropping him off at the rehab was the hardest thing I'd ever done. Though he'd almost died, I thought, *He doesn't need a place like this. He needs to be home with his family.* I ached, desperately wanting to believe him when he said that he'd made a terrible mistake and wouldn't do it again. He said, "I'm not a drug addict! This place is for addicts!" and I thought, *No, he isn't a drug addict. He just let things get out of hand.* He wept and begged me not to leave him there, and I thought, *How could I be doing this to him?* I felt I was abandoning him. I walked out to my car, got inside, and cried.

To avoid having to face that nightmare, we second-guess ourselves. We look for any excuse to backtrack. When our children are hurting, we want to hold them close, not send them away. We're terrified that forcing them into treatment will make them hate us and we'll lose them. We don't act because our hearts break for them. We're overwhelmed by guilt over the mistakes we made or think we made raising them. It's almost impossible to withstand the force inside us that rises up to try to dull our guilt and fear.

But denial is perilous. Every day you wait, addicts' drug use may escalate. By allowing them to keep using, family members conspire with addiction, even encourage it to advance — enabling the addict. As a result of my denial, by the time I got Nic into treatment his addiction had advanced to the point that it had almost killed him. It had advanced to the point that his disease was far more resistant to treatment than it would have been if I'd gotten him help earlier.

In pop-psychology parlance, I was codependent, a word used to describe those who deny a loved one's escalating drug use — those who believe the lies, make the excuses, and meanwhile suffer immeasurably from being addicted to another's addiction.

Though it is a word commonly bandied about, there's controversy about whether codependence exists, at least as a diagnosable disorder (it's not in the *DSM-V*), but from the abundant and packed support groups for codependents, it's clear that it's common for family members of addicts to relate to the term. Every day and evening in most cities there are countless meetings of support groups for codependents, including Al-Anon and Co-Dependents Anonymous. Its sufferers sustain the self-help sections of bookstores stocked with copies of perpetual bestsellers like Melody Beattie's *Codependent No More* (to date, more than five million copies sold).

Doctors who maintain that codependence is a disorder do so because, as one said, "It manifests in common symptoms and can be chronic, progressive, and disabling." But some doctors and researchers criticize the term and believe, as Dr. Rawson says, "There are ways of talking about the unhelpful pathological behaviors and attitudes of family members of addicts without invoking this un-definable term." Also, some addiction specialists see the obsessive preoccupation with another's well-being as a symptom, not a cause. They say that many of those who describe themselves as codependent have underlying depression, anxiety, or other disorders, including dependent personality disorder. The last, though, is a chronic condition in which people depend too much on others to meet their emotional and physical needs, whereas codependents — or whatever they should be called — need to be depended *on*.

I've spoken to psychologists who reject the concept of codependence because it pathologizes genuine caring and rational worry, but there's a difference between, on one hand, concern and obsession with trying to help a loved one who's dying, and, on the other, enabling him. Indeed, it's impossible to worry in moderation when a child, spouse, sibling, parent, or close friend becomes addicted. It's understandable and rational that people try to control loved ones who are killing themselves — even if they sacrifice their own well-being in their efforts, and even if they're continually disappointed, hurt, and angry. Lennard Davis, author of *Obsession: A History,* says that codependency "describes a certain kind of behavior if you're looking through a really stupid lens." His criticism comes from a view that, he says, "we pathologize behaviors and feelings that for many people are normal." Wendy Kaminer, in the *New York Times Book Review,* noted that Melody Beattie defined *codependence* as being affected by someone else's behavior and obsessed with controlling it. Kaminer then asked, "Who isn't?" Yes, who isn't or wouldn't be affected by someone's behavior and obsessed with controlling it (or trying to) if the behavior could easily lead to death? And this person is a parent or husband or wife or brother or sister. Or child.

Indeed, there's research that suggests that codependence is neither a discrete disorder nor a manifestation of an underlying psychiatric disorder. The most instructive are several studies by Rudolph Moos, emeritus professor in the department of psychiatry at Stanford School of Medicine, that have shown that people with symptoms that we describe as codependent are responding rationally to the irrational behavior of addicts in their lives. He came to this conclusion after his studies showed that, for example, the wives of alcoholics who exhibited signs of dysfunction were fine once their husbands got sober, suggesting that their dysfunction was a reaction to the insanity of living with a using addict. Moos wrote to me in an e-mail, "Spouses and families of individuals who continue to misuse alcohol experience some deficits in functioning, whereas spouses and families of 'recovered/remitted' individuals appear to function 'normally.'" That is, when they're not living with using addicts, they're fine. It makes sense, because living with an addict is inherently traumatic; those who do often feel as if they're living in a war zone, because they're dealing with someone out of control, irrational, and threatening, who is self-destructing before their eyes — and this is someone they love. Dr. Rawson observes, "When an individual becomes addicted, family members do their best to adapt. They try to protect the addict, they try to discipline the addict, they try to reason with the addict, they try to compromise with the addict. All of these are reasonable and rational coping responses under normal circumstances. When these techniques don't work, they try them again and they try them more intensely . . ." However, he continues, though their reaction may be a rational response to an irrational situation, "after years of being alternatively disappointed and terrorized and feeling encouraged, the behaviors become more extreme and in some cases really distorted and maladaptive — and also damaging to the addict." And, he acknowledges, "There are people among the family members who do have serious psychopathology (as in any group of people) and surely there are cases where the pathology of the family member can really make the situation even more crazy."

For the purposes of this book I'm using the word *codependence* as shorthand, not for the rational preoccupation with trying to help a loved one who's ill, but for the enabling behavior of family members who wait for a crisis before they try to get the addict in their family into treatment. It's codependent, and harmful, when they deny the addict's problems; excuse the behavior, no matter how appalling; cover his tracks (pay the bills, bail him out); and ignore or believe the addict's lies. People described as codependents sometimes even excuse outrageous violence, even when it's directed at them. In fact, an addict's cruelty may only intensify a codependent's devotion. And codependents suffer greatly. They can become debilitated with their obsessive preoccupation with the addict they're trying to save.

These codependents and addicts feed off one another. When they do, the addiction cycle worsens. If addicts are treated as if they can't take care of themselves, they may well become less likely to take care of themselves. Also, an addict trying to separate from a person when the ties that bind feel oppressive may use *more* drugs because of the stress that's inherent in codependency. It's ironic, because when codependents protect an addict from the consequences of his actions, it seems that they'd be relieving an addict's stress. But the addict pays the price in guilt, which is a trigger for drug use.

Treating Codependency

Since there's no consensus among doctors about what codependence is, it's not surprising that they don't agree on treatments. The most popular "treatment" for codependence is Al-Anon (and Alateen for teenagers) and similar support groups, including Co-Dependents Anonymous (CODA) and Adult Children of Alcoholics. Indeed, people in despair can find solace, support, and advice in Al-Anon meetings (they're related to Alcoholics Anonymous meetings) that help them manage. Al-Anon works so well for some that they don't seek other treatments. For others, it has a role in treatment, and still others reject it.

Some doctors prescribe behavioral approaches similar to ones that are used to treat addiction. These include family or couples therapy, assertiveness training, and a combination of therapy and medication.

Therapy will often include education about the fact that rather than helping the loved one, codependents' overinvolvement undermines an addict's recovery when they enable him. Codependents can be taught to erect boundaries so they can get an addict the treatment he needs while not enabling him. It's not easy to know what to do, and even when you know, or think you know, it's not easy to act. At one point, when Nic was on the streets, I realized, after attending Al-Anon meetings and speaking with a therapist, I was enabling him by continuing to go and get him when he called and allowing him to come home after promising he'd go into treatment. He'd sleep off his recent binge and then forget about his commitment. He'd leave again. Another relapse.

After numerous such episodes, Nic was again on the streets. Again I was desperate to know where he was, whether he was alive or dead. After another two weeks of the hell of not knowing, he called again. "Dad, I'm in trouble. I need help."

How many times had I gone to get him? How many times had I believed him when he said he wanted to stop and would do it on his own? I'd let him come home to sleep it off. I'd trust his promises and believe his remorse. Mostly I'd be so worried that I'd do anything to return him to safety, even if it was a short-lived respite.

But it hadn't worked. And so when Nic begged me to help him, pled with me and sobbed, against every parental instinct I said, "I'll help you get back into treatment. I'll drive you there."

Then he became annoyed and angry. "I'm not going back," he said. "I've been there, done that. Those places don't work for me. I messed up, but I'm going to stop on my own."

I took a breath. "Nic, I love you so much. Take care of yourself. Please. Call me if you'd like help getting into treatment." And I hung up.

That's not what I wanted to do. I wanted to go out and find him and hold on to him. Instead, I hung up and cried. I didn't know what would happen next. I didn't know if he would make it another day, another hour. I didn't know if I would ever see him again.

The next time I heard from Nic he was ready to enter treatment. I went to get him, drove him to a program, and checked him in. Because that sort of tough love seemed to work, it might seem as if I'd look back and know that I'd made the right choice. But I look back and still don't know. My doubts come because of stories I hear from others. Some of them had had experiences similar to mine — they drew a line and their loved one went into treatment. But others will never forgive themselves for trying that sort of tough love and having it fail: when their loved one — most were children — died.

My conclusion is that there isn't a definitive answer. I never found a doctor with one. It depends on the child. It depends on his circumstances. It's a decision that shouldn't be made without consulting a specialist. Addiction counselor Diana Clark teaches family members to set limits on what they will and won't do for an addicted loved one. Some of her patients have such a difficult time setting boundaries that she makes a pact with them to call her before they agree to a loved one's request, so she can help them assess whether granting it would help or hurt. For example, "a lot of dads have enormous trouble stopping the flow of money," Clark notes, "because that may have been their primary way to show love." Refusing to give money makes sense — it's often said that giving money to a using addict is like giving a loaded gun to a suicidal person. But we'd never kick a child out of the house if he had cancer.

Effective codependence treatment may involve confronting deep fears and working to change lifelong patterns. There's relief as people untangle their enabling and denial from their rational and healthy concern. When they're treated, they continue to love and care about the addict in their lives, and they can participate and help in a person's recovery. And treating codependency doesn't help only the codependent. When a loved one stops enabling an addict, the addict is more likely to agree to be treated.

When codependents are doing better, they may suffer setbacks if the objects of their obsession react negatively to the changing relationships. An addict's problem may worsen, and there can be crisis, unconsciously motivated by a need to draw the loved one back into the unhealthy cycle. Paradoxically and perilously, codependents may also regress when their loved ones improve. They can be threatened when an addict makes progress. They're probably aware of only their worry and desire to save the people they love, but there may be another motivation, albeit an unconscious one: They may be deeply afraid of losing the addict, to either his addiction or his recovery. If they're no longer needed, codependents think, where will they be then — *who* will they be then?

Whether you call codependence a disease or not, it can be a torturous state. As I said, people can be overwhelmed by anxiety, deeply depressed, and physically ill. Treatment doesn't stop those affected by their addicted loved ones from worrying, but their suffering can lessen and — critically — they can stop enabling the addicts and work to get them into treatment.

8

Intervention

In the living room of a stone house in a quiet neighborhood in the Chicago suburb of Oak Park, a fire crackled. The only other sound was sobbing.

Joan and Richard Laurel huddled together on a couch. Earlier, when Joan arrived home from work (she's a commodities broker), she'd gone upstairs and changed into a light blue cardigan and beige slacks. Richard, an attorney, didn't have time to change out of his gray suit and white shirt, but he'd loosened his necktie.

Joan had set a silver tray on the glass coffee table. There was green tea in a cast-iron Japanese teapot, rice crackers, and almond cookies. She had been composed but wasn't for long. She sobbed, and Richard put an arm around her. He was near tears himself.

Joan whispered, "Our poor baby."

Richard looked at her with incredulity. "*Poor baby?* She's out of *control.* For God's sake, Joan, your poor little girl is *shooting heroin!*"

Joan said, "I can't send her away. She needs her mother."

"She *hit* you," Richard countered. He looked at his wife. "What's it going to take? It's for her own good. We've gone over it a thousand times."

A chime. Richard rose, went to the front door, and let in a gray-haired man in a business suit and a seventeen-year-old girl hidden inside a pea coat — his brother and niece. She had short, chopped, bleached hair and dark eyes. Her father looked at Richard with sympathy and sadness. The brothers hugged. Marc said, "It's going to be okay." Joan didn't get up, but Marc and her niece Tami came over to her. She hugged them, managing to say, "Thanks for coming." Looking up at Tami, Joan said, "It'll mean a lot to her that you're here."

The room was rearranged, the couch pulled back along one wall. Oak dining chairs and metal folding chairs had been placed in an imperfect circle around a scarlet area rug.

Another girl arrived, Bridget; she was Richard and Joan's youngest daughter. There had been a discussion about whether or not to include Teddy, their twelve-year-old son. They'd decided that it would be too confusing for him, so he was spending the night at a friend's.

The door opened again and a sylphlike girl with wispy blond hair entered and hugged her father. May, the Laurels' eldest, was pre-med at the University of Chicago. She kept clutching her dad. When finally she pulled away, she had tears in her eyes too.

The next to arrive, a man in his late thirties, took off a parka to reveal a mud-colored corduroy jacket and starched black jeans. He circulated through the room shaking hands, hugged Richard and, when she approached, Joan. "I know this is hard," he said.

Addressing everyone, Miles Grissom, the therapist hired to guide this intervention, said, "Let's all sit down."

Everyone did. Grissom leaned forward, his elbows on his knees. "So Elizabeth will be here soon," he said. "We've rehearsed, but that doesn't mean it will be easy. Do your best to sit quietly. From experience, I can tell you what helps." He looked around the room. "Breathe."

Joan was crying again. Richard edged closer and took her hand. May was holding back tears.

The door opened. The first one in was Richard and Joan's other son, Mac. He was broad shouldered and thick necked. He looked around the room, focused on his parents, his sisters. He was followed in by Elizabeth; tiny; gaunt; coffee-brown hair with short and uneven bangs. A thigh-length gray wool jacket. Her black eyes flashed around the room. "What the fuck!" Her eyes bulged. "You gotta be fucking kidding."

Grissom stood and approached her. Elizabeth looked at Mac. "Did you . . . ?" He backed away. "Motherfucker."

She eyed her parents. Ice. "You mother*fuckers*." Louder, fiercer. "*Fuck you!*" Then, as she turned: "Fuck all of you." With his massive body, her brother blocked her exit. "Please," he said. "*Liz.*" Tears streamed down his cheeks, but he didn't move from his place in front of the door.

Staged interventions like Elizabeth's — or those on a number of television shows — are actually rare. Most addicts enter treatment after less formal pressure from loved ones, or on their own, when they're tired of the physical effects of using or they're worried about the consequences. Addicts enter treatment in many different ways. For Luke, the boy from Sonoma, California, the journey toward recovery started in his high-school gym.

Luke had continued using, huffing and taking other drugs, anything he could find — cocaine, meth, pills, but mostly ecstasy. He smoked pot every day and drank whatever liquor he could get his hands on. He was dealing, outrunning police; his grades were falling. His skin was ghost white, his skeletal face was hidden under long greasy hair, and his expression was fixed in a glare. At fourteen, Luke looked aimless, but he had a plan. He wanted to run away to San Francisco with his friends and live on the street. He knew he could get high easily because San Francisco had way more drugs than Sonoma.

Luke's high school has an impressive gym: shiny floors freshly lacquered, and long rows of blue bleachers. Luke went to the gym with his parents for an evening event about drugs. He didn't usually read much, but over the previous few days he'd read the book *Tweak,* my son's story about his meth addiction. Luke related to the feelings of isolation and depression Nic described, and to the way that drugs helped the pain he felt. Like Luke, Nic discovered that his relationship to drugs differed from other kids'. Nic's first experience drinking with a friend was identical to Luke's. He was twelve too, and he and a friend stole liquor and filled up a glass. His friend hated it, but Nic — like Luke — drained the glass. Nic's drug of choice was meth; Luke's was ecstasy. When he read the book, Luke says, "I was almost vibrating because I thought I was the only one [who felt this way]."

Nic and I had been asked to speak to a gathering of teachers, students, and parents at Sonoma Academy. We read from our books and answered questions. Then we listened as students and parents told about their own struggles with drugs and alcohol. The event ended and we talked with the people who came up to us. One boy in the audience waited to talk to Nic until everyone else had gone. I noticed that he and Nic spoke for a while. After they talked, Nic signed the boy's book, and we left.

Luke didn't look at his book until he got home. He opened it and read what Nic had written: *Dear Luke, everything is going to be all right.*

"I hadn't cried for two years, and I started crying," Luke told me later. "Every time I felt like I was going to cry, for my whole life until then, I'd just go numb. That was the first emotion I had felt in so long, so I just started crying and I couldn't stop."

That night, he told his parents that he was addicted to drugs. In the morning, he went to school and waited in front of the office of the dean of students — the one who had almost kicked him out. When she arrived, he told her he needed to go into rehab. She said, "Thank God."

Legally, parents have the authority to place their kids in treatment, but adults must enter voluntarily unless they're deemed a threat to themselves or others. If they are, many states have statutes that allow doctors, law enforcement officers, judges, or other professionals to force them into treatment, but the "hold" is usually too short to do much other than address an immediate crisis. It's ludicrous to think that anyone can help an addict in a couple of days. "Releasing them is heartbreaking," a nurse at a psychiatric hospital told me. "Some are admitted over and over again, and, as we know from police and social workers, some leave and overdose or kill themselves." But in a hospital, under the care of doctors, social workers, and therapists, an addict may agree he needs help and decide to continue treatment. For children under eighteen, these holds can be used as an interim step toward forced treatment.

Informal Interventions

Begging, cajoling, or threatening sometimes will get an adult addict to go into treatment, but one who becomes angry or feels bullied may flee. Less confrontational approaches are more effective. A series of conversations, or even a single conversation, can make the difference. Family, friends, bosses, coworkers, or other relatives can sometimes convince an addict to enter treatment. It's worth reiterating that you shouldn't wait for your loved one to hit bottom.

It's almost never productive to talk to addicts while they're high, when they're likely to react with denial, lies, or aggression. Many addicts don't spend much time completely sober, though. One doctor told me that when addicts are coming down and feeling ill, emotional, and remorseful, they may be vulnerable and more open to responding to their loved ones' entreaties. In spite of the general advice to stay as neutral and as unemotional as possible in these conversations, I've heard addicts say that they went into treatment because a husband, wife, or other loved one drew a line and issued an ultimatum. "After everything we'd been through, I knew she wasn't bluffing," a man in rehab said of his wife. "She was ready to walk." A woman in her twenties had told her father that she'd no longer visit him unless he got help. Parents threatened to withdraw a child's financial support. A man threatened to sue for full custody of the child he shared with his addicted wife. I've met people in treatment who were there because their bosses had given them a choice between getting help and getting fired.

Some addicts are forced into treatment. After an arrest, an addict may be given a fait accompli by a judge: court-ordered treatment, or a choice between treatment and jail. I've met parents who called the police on their addicted children in hopes that a court would force their kids into treatment. It's a scary, risky move, but as one mother told me, "Jail was safer than where she was. She was on the streets, shooting drugs, hooking. I couldn't believe I was calling the police on my own daughter, but I did." On my Facebook page, a woman described her anguish after convincing her addicted son to turn himself in to the police (she didn't specify the crime he'd committed). A man posted a comment and consoled her by telling her to keep in mind two words that had helped him when his own addicted son was in prison. "The two words are 'Protective custody,'" he wrote. "Sometimes it's good when people are protected from themselves."

To appease their families, when they're confronted, addicts may admit they've been using and promise to cut down or stop. They need to know that it usually takes more than their willpower or the best intentions to do so. If addicts can be made to understand they're ill, they may be more amenable to entering treatment. Family members can offer to aid and support an addict, to help her find a doctor trained in addiction medicine. If the addict is in imminent danger and there's no time for a consultation with a doctor, loved ones should offer to drive her then and there to be admitted into a program to detox, if detox is necessary, or to residential treatment.

There may be other opportunities to guide addicts into treatment, such as when they become ill, overdose, or have accidents and wind up in an emergency room. They may be motivated to get help on their own, or family, doctors, nurses, or social workers can encourage them. An ER nurse says, "I do everything I can to get addicts from the ER into treatment programs. A lot of times their resistance is down, because they're ill and scared."

Unfortunately, most doctors, nurses, cops, probation officers, and others who frequently come into contact with drug users don't know how to intervene. "Normally when someone's in an ER or they enter the criminal justice system, they're harangued — pushed to change, confronted, but the opposite is what works," says Yale's Michael Pantalon. "In fact, what works is more about what you don't do than what you do." Pantalon uses motivational interviewing with addicted probationers in the criminal justice system and patients in emergency rooms (no matter what brought them to the hospital) to induce them to willingly enter treatment. "When a person's arrested or lands in the ER, we have a few minutes," he explains. "We're not going to reverse an addiction. We want them to go somewhere where they can work on reversing addiction." In clinical trials, even brief sessions — as short as seven minutes — convinced many people to go into treatment. Pantalon says that most addicts have already been told to stop, and have told themselves to stop, "but we're not telling them to do anything. We ask, 'Why might you get help for your drinking?' 'What are you losing because you're using?' 'What would you get if you stopped?' We're opening a window. They look through it and, possibly for the first time, think, *Hmmm, why would I decide to get help?* Their mind is headed in a new direction. *What* would *I get if I stopped?*" If the addict says he doesn't want to get help, Pantalon responds, "I didn't ask if you're going to get help, but why you might decide to get help if you ever do." He explains, "Because the question is hypothetical and surprising, the person's defensiveness is lowered." The patient may say, "I guess I'd get help if I couldn't stop," or "Maybe if I lost my job." The point isn't the specific answer, but the fact that something new has been introduced: the notion that there's another way forward. Envisioning that, the addict can begin to contemplate stopping.

Whether the tactic is MI or other intervention strategies, ER visits and post-arrest periods are opportunities to interrupt use and get a person into treatment. It's also possible to reach addicts who go to needle-exchange programs, doctor's offices and health clinics because they're ill, or food banks or shelters.

The process of getting kids under eighteen into treatment is different, at least in most states; parents can usually forcibly admit them into a program. The legal right to commit a child to treatment is one thing. Sometimes kids agree when they're told they have to go, but it's often not that easy.

It's legal to force kids into treatment in some states, and in some it's also legal for parents to have their children forcibly extracted — essentially kidnapped — and brought to rehab. Some rehabs have employees on staff or can recommend people who will grab a child, sometimes handcuffing him, and then "escort" him into the program. Such aggressive tactics can backfire, but in some situations they may be justified — if a child left on his own on the streets is in imminent danger, it's usually safer to get him into a hospital or treatment setting. These extractions may in general be legal, but only if legal tactics are used. Violence is illegal, and moreover it's counterproductive.

People who've forced their unwilling loved ones into rehab describe the experience as harrowing, but when they were successful, they were relieved, because they'd gotten their loved ones into treatment. Even if the addict didn't stay, at least he was removed from a dangerous environment and deprived of drugs for a while, and interrupting drug use for even a short time can be lifesaving. In many cases, the intervention reversed an addict's self-destructive trajectory. Recovery began.

Formal Interventions

It's preferable for an addict, no matter his age, to go into treatment willingly. A formal intervention is an alternative that works in some cases.

It can be expensive, it can fail, and it can backfire. Before trying one, it's important to meet with a therapist or counselor, who can help family members weigh their options and make a plan.

Not all orchestrated interventions are the same. Sometimes families, friends, coworkers, and others plan interventions themselves, but that route can be risky. As I said, users confronted by anger, blame, or chastisement may become angry and defensive. A trained interventionist can be a referee, guiding the process. Even in the hands of a professional, an intervention may cause the addict to bolt or be even less open to entering treatment in the future. Formal interventions can be traumatic and can fail, but when things are already dire, they're less risky than doing nothing at all. But someone trained in the process should lead them.

Guided by a therapist, a family prepares for a formal intervention in advance, and then an addict is lured to a location where the family has gathered. When he arrives, he's confronted, as Elizabeth was. Family members talk about their fears and how the addict's behavior has affected them. Interventionists may require family and friends to read impact letters they've written. The intervention shouldn't be characterized by anger, blame, and threats, which can alienate an addict who already feels defensive and attacked, but by expressions of love, concern, empathy, and support. The goal is for an addict to accept that he needs help, to know that help is available, and to understand that he'll be supported by his family and friends. Writing in the *New York Times,* Maia Szalavitz cited a 1999 study that compared the traditional confrontational intervention approach to a less truculent one known as community reinforcement and family training, which, she explained, is "aimed at helping the family nurture the addict's own motivation." She reported that in the study, "more than twice as many families succeeded in getting their loved ones into treatment (64 percent) with the gentler approach than with standard intervention (30 percent). But," she said, "no reality shows push the less dramatic method, and it is difficult to find clinicians who use it."

"These formal interventions often work," according to Marvin Seppala, chief medical officer of Hazelden. "In a properly planned and executed intervention, an addict feels vulnerable in the presence of his family and friends. He may agree to go [into treatment] because of guilt or shame or because his loved ones break through his denial and defenses, at least enough so that he can glimpse the truth of his circumstance. There's resistance, but somewhere inside he knows that the people who love him would not lie. They are motivated by one thing. To save him."

The Intervention

There's no specific interventionist credential, and not every therapist with a degree and a license actually knows how to handle the process. Some rehabs and treatment centers provide referrals, but these must be checked with independent sources; some organizations get kickbacks from interventionists they refer. Indeed, I've heard people in the addiction-treatment field express the concern that some treatment facilities support interventionists because, as Dr. Rawson says, "they bring in business and [the facilities] don't have to deal with the consequences of the failed and counterproductive interventions."

Regardless of the style of intervention, the object of it isn't to instill guilt or reinforce isolation; addicts already feel guilty and isolated. Instead, the goal is to help the addict understand that he is loved; that those who love him are desperately worried; and that the problem is serious enough that he must enter treatment right away. After all participants have said their piece, it's usually explained that, in light of the seriousness of the problem, there's no time to waste — he must leave for treatment immediately. A bed in a hospital or other treatment program is waiting. Sometimes, that's it, but sometimes the message comes with an "or else." That is, the addict must go into treatment or else. The "or else" shouldn't be presented as a punishment, but as a simple fact: "I can't live this way anymore, not knowing if you're going to come home stoned or not at all. If you don't go into treatment, I'm moving out. If you do go, I'll be here and support you in whatever ways I can." "I'm so worried about you that if you don't agree to check into rehab I won't pay your rent or college tuition any longer. If you do, I'll help you through this and help you get back into school when you're healthy again. But it's your decision." A father told his son, "It breaks our hearts to make you go, but we don't want to lose you. We'll be there for you." He said, "You have to try it. Let's see how it goes for a few days. We're here with you — we're going to help you figure this out." Of course a few days in treatment isn't enough, but if it's necessary, detox can begin. And treatment can begin. A few days can become a week, a week a month, a month many months — whatever's deemed necessary.

Elizabeth was blindsided. After her angry stream of curses, she looked up and saw her mom. Joan was in tears, and Elizabeth looked horrified. Her knees gave out, and she would have fallen to the floor, but Mac caught her. Joan came over and put her arms around her daughter. She and Mac led her to a chair in the circle with the others. She was trembling. She took out a cigarette and lit it.

One by one, her family members read letters they'd written. The letters told about their worries, their nights without sleep — their anguish. And they expressed their love.

The interventionist interrupted Richard when he veered from his composed letter into a tirade: "How could you do this to your mother?"

"That's not helpful," Grissom said. He spoke evenly but firmly. "This isn't about blame and guilt. I imagine Elizabeth already feels guilty enough." He looked at Elizabeth, but she was staring at the floor.

Richard said, "I'm sorry, but I'm furious." Turning on Elizabeth, he said, "We've given you everything. You have the opportunity to do whatever you want in life but you're throwing it away."

Elizabeth wept. When finally she looked up at her parents, she appeared docile, like a wild horse that had been broken. Her mother begged her to go to rehab. Joan sobbed uncontrollably.

Finally Elizabeth said she'd go — "If it'll make you all feel better." Her parents, sisters, and brother walked her outside, half holding her up. They put her in Grissom's car, and he drove her away.

Remember that however an addict gets into treatment, he's almost always safer there than anywhere else, as long as the program is run by professionals qualified to care for him. And remember that whether a person goes willingly, is coerced, is bribed, or is forced into treatment, there's now an opportunity to change his path from a vicious cycle of use, debilitation, and damage to himself and others to a road that can lead to healing and health.

IV

Getting Clean

9

Finding Treatment

TEN DAYS EARLIER, IMMEDIATELY after the intervention, Elizabeth had been brought to a treatment program that was recommended by the interventionist, who in turn had been recommended by a family friend. Elizabeth wasn't allowed visitors for her first week in treatment. She spent it detoxing. Richard and Joan called to see how she was doing. The on-duty nurses reassured them that their daughter was doing fine. After another week, they were finally allowed to visit her, but Elizabeth barely spoke. She was dispirited—not angry, not remorseful. Nothing. Her parents were discouraged, but a counselor reassured them. "She's been through a lot. She has a lot to process."

Four days after they saw her, they were called by the director of the program and told that Elizabeth had run away. They were aghast. They went to the center to learn what had happened. The director said, "She was doing better. Sometimes they run when they're doing good. Facing life sober can scare the hell out of them." A tech who'd worked with Elizabeth was in the meeting too. "She wasn't ready," he said. "Wasn't ready?" Richard asked. "To be sober," the tech said.

The Laurels went home—angry, confused, distraught, overwhelmed. Scared. Joan said that sometimes she and Richard consoled each other, and sometimes yelled at each other. "We wanted someone to blame."

They cried a lot—both of them.

Whenever the phone rang their hearts pounded.

Five days later, Elizabeth finally called.

She sounded weak. She told her mom she was okay, she was sorry, she just couldn't take the rehab anymore. "It was bullshit. They're all creeps. I couldn't stay." She said she was going to stay clean on her own, needed time to figure things out. She was slurring slightly, and Joan knew that her daughter was high.

"Oh, Liz . . ." Joan cried.

"I don't need any trips laid on me."

"Where are you?"

"I'm fine. Met some good people. I gotta go. I'm fine."

And then she hung up.

Another interminable week passed. Her parents waited for the phone to ring. Were terrified that the phone would ring. When Elizabeth finally did call, she said she needed help. "Will you get me, Mama?"

Joan picked Richard up at his office and they went to get their daughter, who was waiting in front of a Target store. They drove up and saw her sitting on a concrete wall. Her face was streaked black; she was skinny and pale. She got in the backseat of the car and didn't speak. She stared blankly out the side window.

At home, in the bedroom she'd had since she was a little girl, Elizabeth slept. Richard and Joan sat at the kitchen table. He called the interventionist and then called two therapists recommended by friends. He wrote down the names of treatment centers and began dialing one after the other. He took notes. The admissions director of one program listened as Richard told her about Elizabeth. When he finished, she said, "I think we can help her. She's a good candidate for our program." The program didn't take insurance; the Laurels would have to pay $10,000 for the first month and $8,000 a month after that. One of the therapists Richard had consulted told him, "She should stay for a while. See how things go, but plan on a minimum of six months. These problems don't develop overnight and they aren't solved overnight."

Few doctors and other professionals know where to refer people in need, partly because there aren't many appropriate options. This is one of the treatment system's greatest failures. Effective treatments exist — I'll get to them — but they're difficult to find and access. Joan and Richard Laurel found Elizabeth's initial program through the therapist they'd hired to stage the intervention. He'd been recommended by a friend who'd gotten the name from a colleague who had a child with drug problems.

Later, Elizabeth charged that she'd run away from the first program because she and other patients were treated "as if we were a bunch of fuck-ups." She said that counselors yelled at her and the others. She claimed that patients earned points when they did chores — scrubbing pots and pans, cleaning the floor — and demerits when they were late for or missed AA meetings or when the pots weren't clean enough. Accumulated demerits resulted in punishments: extra chores, isolation, or the "hot seat," where they were berated by counselors. She claimed that one girl beat up another resident, and as punishment the girl herself was beaten. She said there were groups each day in which "we all talked about how fucked up our lives were and ragged on each other for, like, using someone else's towel in the bathroom." She claimed that she never once saw a physician and had no individual therapy. She was, she said, grabbed, thrown to the floor, and then tied to her bed after being caught walking through the halls late one night.

Richard called the interventionist who'd recommended the program and asked about Elizabeth's charges, and he responded, "It's a good program. I don't think you can really trust what she tells you. She wanted an excuse to leave and get high."

Richard didn't know what to think but, he said, "This guy was the expert, we were paying him to help us, he sounded as if he knew what he was doing."

The next program Richard chose was, he said, "better, thank God." There was no yelling, no violence, and, according to Elizabeth, had good therapists who helped her. "But how are you supposed to know?" Richard asked. "We just know Liz seems to be doing better." She completed the program and moved from there into a sober-living house, where she now lives. She's attending college, studying to become a teacher.

Richard's grueling, hit-or-miss experience finding treatment for his daughter is all too common. Countless others have had similar experiences. A father named Gary Mendell is one of them.

I wish all parents who think their children are immune to addiction could see Brian Mendell when he was young. I wish they could stare into his eyes, as I have seen them in photographs that chronicle his life. In the photos, his eyes are joyful, and sometimes there's a mischievous and irresistible glint. The pictures show Brian in dinosaur pajamas brushing his teeth. Standing jubilant atop a pile of fallen leaves. In jeans, shirtless, with his brother, Greg, both of them soaking wet: a water fight. Fishing. Dressed as a pirate for Halloween. Stuffing s'mores in his mouth around a campfire. Tailgating at a Giants' game, whitewater rafting, and on a golf course with Greg and his father. Lovingly with his arm around his grandmother, and beaming in a portrait of his family. These are photographs of light and promise.

Brian was born in Bridgeport, Connecticut, on December 26, 1985. His family lived in a bucolic woodsy suburb. His father, Gary, had built a business that owned and operated hotels throughout the United States.

When Brian was five, his brother, Greg, was born. In spite of their age difference, they shared a deep love for the outdoors: they picked berries; went fishing and camping; and often just chased frogs, squirrels, and geese in the woods. Brian's parents divorced when he was seven. The boys lived part-time at each parent's home, which were less than a mile apart. Eventually both his parents remarried.

From the beginning of grade school, Brian struggled. He had a hard time holding his pencil and had poor balance and coordination. He was taken out of class two days a week to work with a specialist on his coordination. By middle school, he began to struggle academically and socially. In eighth grade, for language-arts class, Brian wrote an essay titled "Crazy." "It's just the way I am and the way I was meant to be," he wrote. "It can be bad because it gets me into trouble because no one understands me."

He was the last one picked for kickball. He felt as if he didn't fit in. In class he had trouble paying attention and was eventually diagnosed with ADD and put on medication. He was also diagnosed with learning disabilities and given accommodations in school — help with his homework and extra time for tests. During middle school when all the other children got on the bus to go home after school, Brian stayed each day to work with a tutor.

Brian found comfort in the outdoors. He and his friends would hike through the woods to a nearby farm, where they'd sneak in, pick raspberries, and eat them until their stomachs ached. They'd slip through a fence and fish in a neighbor's pond. They looked for hidden treasures in the woods. And like so many teenagers, Brian and some of his friends tried pot.

In the beginning of his freshman year of high school, an educational consultant recommended that Brian transfer to a private school. Psychological tests indicated that he had a high verbal IQ, but with his ADD, he'd be able to learn much better in smaller classes and with a more structured program. Brian liked the idea, and his parents explored the options. They decided that the best choice was a nearby boarding school, and they began to make plans to send him there.

Two months later, Brian's parents got the first indication that he was using drugs. They got a call from his school: he'd been caught selling a Tylenol with codeine tablet to another student. They were dumbfounded. The school suspended Brian for one month, the police arrested him, and a judge put him on probation. Brian's parents took him to a psychiatrist, and she recommended that Brian continue with the plan to switch to the boarding school. She didn't express any concerns about all of Brian's risk factors for drug use — his ADD, learning disabilities, and the fact that he'd been caught selling a pill. Sending a child with these particular issues away to boarding school, where he'd be isolated from his family, was a misguided recommendation. Connection to one's family is a protective factor that has been shown to lessen drug use.

Brian was accepted at Suffield Academy, a boarding school a little more than an hour's drive from his home. He adapted well to the new school, but his parents didn't know until later that their son was regularly smoking pot and had started selling it. They found out near the end of Brian's junior year, when they were called by the dean of students and told that Brian had to withdraw or be expelled.

Brian's parents researched what to do next and chose Second Nature, a wilderness-therapy program in Utah, which was recommended by a psychologist. Parents of patients in the program were asked to write their children impact letters. In his letter to Brian, Gary described the steps that led him to send his son to treatment: the "bad decisions . . . putting you on a path to a very unhappy life." Gary wrote that he hoped that in the wilderness program Brian would come to understand why he had made such bad decisions. "I am hopeful that you can understand yourself better and feel better about yourself." He concluded, "Brian, you know I love you and you love me. It is with this love that I have sent you to Second Nature."

There were no phones in the wilderness, so Brian and his family wrote each other weekly. In one letter, Brian wrote home that he was in "No Man's land." "I am in a group of 7. My pack weighs 60 lbs." With sarcasm, he described the "important life lessons" he was learning: how to make a campfire without matches, how to distill water from urine, and how to make jewelry out of bark and yucca fiber. Brian wrote that there were new arrivals to the program, and as a result, "there is less food and more really screwed up kids who get the whole group consequences. For example, our whole group is now in a 'push-up intervention.'" His resistance melted over time, though. Later he wrote, "I am learning how to handle anger, frustration, depression, sadness, loneliness and fear. And the way to do this is to accept these feelings." He ended this letter: "Tell bro I say yo, tell Janet and the kids [his stepmother and her children] yo. . . . Mom and Dad — I don't think I've ever missed you more or realized how much you do for me and I want you to know I know all your decisions are out of love. Love, Brian." In another letter he explained: "Out of all the emotions which I feel, powerlessness and hopelessness bother me the most. For some people, managing these emotions is simple." And later, "I really miss both of you and I don't like being away. When I was little, you used to be more sad than me when I was away, but I think the tables have turned. I also learned a lot about relationships between brothers and how much I affect Greg. Tell him I miss him. Dad — Happy Father's Day. I'm sorry I'm not there."

Greg, much younger than Brian, didn't understand why his brother wasn't home. He did know that his parents were stressed and that their worry centered on Brian. "I always just tried to grow up and do everything I could to keep my parents happy, to do the right thing," Greg says. "I knew they had a lot on their hands worrying about my brother and I didn't want to have to have them worry about me."

As the weeks went by at Second Nature, Brian started to write to his parents about the future — going to college. In one letter Brian asked for an assortment of books that suggested that he was searching for meaning in his life: the Tao Te Ching, *The Four Agreements*, *The Road Less Traveled*. He described being moved by Viktor Frankl's *Man's Search for*

Meaning. He responded to what he read of Taoist philosophy in a note to his parents: "'Emotion which is suffering ceases to be suffering as soon as we form a clear and precise picture of it.' It's similar to what I'm working on." Brian concluded the long, thoughtful letter with stark honesty: "I am really confused."

Gary encouraged Brian. "I can feel the progress you are making by the growing perspective you have in your letters," he wrote. "I cannot pretend to know all the emotions you have felt over the past weeks and how hard it has been. What I do know is how much I love you. And what I also know is all the wonderful qualities you have to offer yourself, your loved ones, and your friends . . . With love, Your Dad."

The program ended and, following the recommendation of the program director, Brian's parents sent him to a therapeutic boarding school called Hidden Lake Academy. "At the time I questioned the capability of the therapists and did not get a good feeling," Gary says now. "But I had nothing to compare to and followed the advice of the so-called experts. I later learned that there was fighting and bullying in the dorms, and there were many other issues I was unaware of."

Brian kept the abuse from his parents until he escaped and ran away. He called Gary, who brought him home. Two years later, a federal class-action lawsuit was filed on behalf of parents of students who'd attended the academy, accusing it of "tragic mistreatment of troubled teenage students and families." The lawsuit settled out of court, and the school was subsequently closed.

Brian moved home and appeared to be doing better. Although there were bumps along the way, Brian did well in school and excelled in English. He began college, where he had a successful first semester. However, unknown to his parents, he was using alcohol and drugs, and his use intensified in the second semester. That summer he lived in the dorm and worked at one of his father's hotels nearby. In the beginning of August, Gary received a call that Brian had been arrested for dealing out of his dorm room. After Brian was put on probation, his parents were again at a pivotal decision point. They researched programs that promised to help kids with their drug problems and chose NorthStar Center in Bend, Oregon, another boarding school for troubled teens that focused on addiction treatment and relapse prevention. Gary was told that before Brian could come to NorthStar, he'd have to attend a wilderness program "to stabilize." Brian returned to Second Nature, where he wrote his parents, "Thanks for sending me here. I know it must suck for you to go through everything you have . . . If I work hard, NorthStar will 'fix' me and we can all finally relax and be happy. . . . I want you to know that I am trying my hardest."

I have examined binders filled with letters, medical records, e-mails, and other documents that chronicle both these and the next few years of Brian's life. His life was trying—for him and for his family. He'd do better, then he'd relapse, and then he'd return to treatment in a series of residential and outpatient programs. During this time his father wrote him, "You should feel proud of yourself. Like all of us, you have things that are difficult for you and things that you are great at. Don't let yourself forget that. . . . You are one great son. . . . I am very proud of you."

By then, Greg was a teenager and understood that his brother was in successive rehabs for his drug use. Of course, it confused him. "Then when he would come home he'd be clean and sober for a little time," Greg recalls. "Each time my parents would convince me, 'He's sober; try and fix your relationship.' We'd go on fishing vacations and golfing, and for a while it was like nothing is wrong. We'd be brothers. But then he'd relapse again, and I'd get mad and not talk to him for six months. It happened again and again."

Greg felt what siblings often feel—mystified, worried, resentful. "I was always kind of mad at him because I didn't understand what was going on," Greg says. "From my point of view, he had a simple choice. Take a drug, or don't take a drug. Why was he doing this? I spent a lot of time mad at him." When Greg's friends asked how Brian was doing, he'd respond, "He's been sober for six months but he's probably going to relapse again." He says, "I didn't trust it." But he also vividly recalls times when Brian was home, and they were together. "Sometimes Brian would say, 'I'm sorry for everything, bro. I know I screw up a lot and I'm trying hard.'" The more Greg has thought about it, the more he's come to understand that it wasn't that Brian *chose* not to stop; he couldn't. "A lot of kids try drugs and don't get addicted. That's something he had that he couldn't help."

After yet another relapse, Brian was sent to the adolescent program at Hazelden, one of the most renowned and respected drug-rehabilitation programs in the country. Gary says that Brian was allowed to make a few trips to the gym each week, but other than that, he was confined to one building for four months. Afterward, the counselors recommended that Brian move to a halfway house, Fellowship Club, also owned by Hazelden. After four weeks there, Brian was caught taking a Vicodin. Gary was called and told that Brian was being kicked out and had to leave the next day.

The main problems with America's addiction-treatment system stem from its roots in the archaic notion that addiction is a choice, not a disease. One common symptom of the disease of addiction is relapse. Kicking an addict out of treatment for relapsing is like kicking a cancer patient out of treatment when a tumor metastasizes.

How are diseases treated? Many addicts describe programs like Elizabeth's in which "therapies" included group sessions during which patients were encouraged to denounce and rebuke one another — the goal was to break them. The philosophy behind such "treatments" is that addicts are undisciplined and morally bankrupt, so they have to be punished. In many treatment facilities, patients are lambasted, criticized, and berated. They're told they aren't going "with the program" and scolded for their bad attitude or arrogance. In the *Congressional Quarterly*, former congressman Patrick Kennedy, who's been open about his addictions, summed up the problem with sad, hard-won eloquence: "I've made a very close personal analysis of treatment centers. I've gone to the best in the country myself . . . It's all based upon . . . treating your weakness instead of your strengths." I've never heard of any disease that responds to censure, blame, or denial of treatment.

Over the course of centuries, medicine has evolved from a disorganized and dangerous realm dominated by guesswork, received wisdom, faith, and fear into a comparatively reliable and effective means of dealing with a wide array of illnesses. It's now grounded in evidence-based approaches — also known as evidence-based treatment (EBT) or evidence-based programs (EBP) — ones developed by doctors and researchers and proven effective in clinical trials. EBT is the paradigm that defines treatment in *Clean*. People choose proven treatments, not shots in the dark.

The current addiction-treatment system *is* based on shots in the dark, at least most of the time. There's a standard model used for other illnesses. A patient sees a doctor and explains his complaint. A history is taken, and that's followed by a physical examination. There are ancillary tests if needed, diagnosis, treatment, and then follow-up care. But patients with drug problems are rarely examined at all by a medical professional. If they are, the physical comes after they've been diagnosed, often by people without any credentials whatsoever, based solely on the addicts' behavior and their own descriptions of their drug use. Or they aren't really diagnosed at all; everyone who walks in the door is presumed to be a drug addict, as if there's only one form of the disease, and the addict is sent to generic rehab, as if there's one form of treatment.

If you're looking for treatments supported by evidence, the system is fraught with challenges, because, compared to other illnesses, there's still not enough empirical evidence to offer a clear course forward. Many questions about addiction and treatment simply haven't been answered categorically yet, and there's active debate over the most basic assumptions about treatment — whether inpatient or outpatient programs are more effective, for example; what's appropriate for adolescents and adults; whether (and when) medication should be part of treatment; how long treatment should last; which therapy models work and which don't. It's further complicated by the fact that most addiction treatments (indeed, most treatments for psychiatric problems in general) involve therapy, but there are limitless varieties of therapy. The evidence that supports or discredits each method is often inconsistent. Also, proven treatments may be poorly administered. Addiction medicine isn't an exact science, and it's still a relatively new one.

Go to the Doctor

The medical model for treating illness should be applied to addiction. Patients should be evaluated on a case-by-case basis. The initial step should be assessment, but it can be hard to find a doctor who can help. A Center for Addiction and Substance Abuse (CASA) survey found that only 6 percent of primary care physicians recognized alcoholism in patients, while the majority missed or misdiagnosed the signs, and 41 percent of pediatricians failed to recognize drug problems in teenagers. "Many doctors never learned to screen for drug problems," Dr. Ken Winters of the Center for Adolescent Substance Abuse Research explains. "They miss the warning signs."

One reason they miss them is that so few medical schools offer, never mind require, courses in substance abuse. "It's woefully under-emphasized," according to Jim Flack, assistant medical director of the Menninger Clinic in Houston. "The only time most physicians run into addiction is at two in the morning when Uncle Joe comes into the emergency room for the twenty-third time — angry, smelling, cussing. They're not interested in treating something they consider self-induced."

This is slowly changing, as a growing number of hospitals are introducing residency programs in addiction medicine. The American Board of Independent Medical Examiners now recognizes addiction psychiatry as a specialty. Organizations such as the American Society of Addiction Medicine (ASAM) and the American Academy of Addiction Psychiatry (AAAP) are growing too. Increasingly, people are training to be psychologists, psychiatrists, and counselors specializing in addiction. And in some medical schools, students are required to take courses in addiction medicine. In the meantime, some practicing doctors are taking it upon themselves to learn to diagnose, if not treat, addiction. Fred Holmes, a pediatrician in St. Albans, Vermont, did so after facing a stream of teenagers coming into his office addicted to pills. "I was literally clueless," he said. "Well, doctors have our egos. We think, *I can do it.* But this wasn't like diagnosing pneumonia or an ear infection." He decided to learn more about addiction, and now his practice is devoted to helping kids with drug problems. "We see physicians as being important triage people for screening individuals to see whether or not they might have a problem with using drugs or alcohol," says Dr. Kevin Conway of the National Institute on Drug Abuse. "One, they don't know what to ask about or how to ask it, and, two, they don't know what to do once they get the answers. We're trying to bridge that gap."

Patients and their families must be their own advocates when it comes to finding qualified doctors. As I warned, beware of the web. Some hospitals have referral services, and some have their own addiction specialists on staff. Teaching and research hospitals with programs in addiction medicine, usually in their departments of psychiatry or psychology, can be good sources for referrals.

According to ASAM, evidence indicating that a physician has adequate training to diagnose addiction and recommend a treatment course includes completion of a residency and fellowship in addiction medicine or addiction psychiatry; board certification in addiction medicine by the American Board of Addiction Medicine; subspecialty certification in addiction psychiatry by the American Board of Psychiatry and Neurology; certification in addiction medicine by the American Society of Addiction Medicine; or a certificate of added qualification in addiction medicine conferred by the American Osteopathic Association. ASAM maintains a list of resources that include licensed physicians who have completed an accredited residency or fellowship program in addiction medicine, who practice addiction medicine full-time, or who have been credentialed in addiction medicine. The ABAM website also has a physician directory, and ABAM doctors have been credentialed in addiction medicine. Both the ABAM and the American Academy of Addiction Psychiatrists (AAAP) websites also have a physician directory, and ABAM doctors have passed exams in addiction medicine.

People without financial resources or good insurance have fewer choices for general medical care, and the same is true for addiction care. Still, as flawed as the system is, even those without money or insurance can usually find at least some medical care. But it's harder for addicts. Few hospitals would be unconcerned about a patient having a stroke, but most ERs pay minimal attention to addicts. No police officer would take a person suffering hypoglycemic shock or a heart attack to jail, but many addicts in crisis are arrested rather taken to a hospital for medical treatment.

Even those who do have insurance often have no or limited coverage for addiction treatment. The lack of adequate insurance coverage for addiction has led to horror stories. In 2007, I interviewed a mother named Roberta Lojak for a book that was a companion to the HBO documentary *Addiction*. I wrote about her daughter Ashley:

Roberta Lojak says that her daughter Ashley was "a blessing from the day she was born. She never got into trouble. She was helpful around the house. She came home when she was supposed to come home."

Ashley began experimenting with drugs when she was a high-school senior. "She changed her friends," her mother says, "and became different." Roberta found drug paraphernalia in Ashley's car, and her daughter admitted that she was using ecstasy and heroin. Eventually Ashley told Roberta she needed help. In a letter, she wrote, "I don't want to turn out like some of my friends — I don't want to be some dopehead. I haven't seen anything in this world so far and I want to."

Roberta found an inpatient program and provided the family's insurance information and Roberta was told that Ashley was approved for admission. "I was hopeful that Ashley would finally get the help she needed," Roberta said.

A week later, someone from the program called and told Roberta that Ashley was being released because the family's insurance wouldn't cover any more time there. Roberta was stunned. "I was told, 'When the insurance is declined, there's nothing we can do.'" The program cost six hundred dollars a day.

Roberta picked Ashley up. Back home, she frantically searched for another place to send her daughter. The following morning, Roberta went to wake Ashley up, but she was unconscious. Her fingers and lips were blue. "I tried to do CPR on my daughter," Roberta said. "But she was already dead."

Two weeks after her daughter died, Roberta received a letter from the insurance company. It said she had the right to appeal the company's decision. The Lojaks' insurance policy did cover addiction treatment, but it was inadequate. It's a common deficiency. Some companies cover only the initial stage of treatment, detox. Some plans cover a limited number of therapy sessions or brief outpatient programs, and others cover twenty-eight-day residential programs — though those are usually inadequate. At present, the beginning of the proccess for those in PPOs is to attempt to find in-network doctors on the ASAM and AAAP websites. A number of insurance companies allow subscribers to go outside the network if the companies don't have a contract with a specialist they need. Medicaid and Medicare cover addiction care; their coverage is limited, sometimes to detox only, but it can include assessment, outpatient programs, and residential treatment for pregnant women and adolescents. Medicaid and Medicare coverage varies from state to state, for inpatient and outpatient programs, depending on the treatment setting (whether in a hospital or not). In a statement, ASAM called for less disparity in Medicaid and Medicare coverage of substance abuse and other medical conditions, saying, "Coverage for 'substance abuse services' is not at a par with coverage for other medical/sugical services. The result is that patients with diseases affecting one region of their brain, e.g. Huntington's chorea, receive different coverage under Medicare and Medicaid for diagnostic and therapeutic health care services than patients with diseases affecting another region of their brain, e.g. cocaine dependence." Some HMOs have procedures in place for subscribers searching for addiction care. When Luke Gsell was desperate to go into treatment, his school counselor worked with his parents to find a rehab. There weren't many choices, especially for a teenager. The family's insurance, the HMO Kaiser Permanente, denied authorization for Luke to go into a residential program, approving only an outpatient program that involved three or so meetings a week. Luke's father called other doctors. Finally, one doctor met Luke and grasped the severity of his problem; he understood that Luke had to be confined and separated from the community where he was dealing and using. The doctor got the required approval for inpatient treatment. "If I'd had to go to outpatient treatment I never would have made it," Luke says. "I'm a hundred percent certain." As Luke's case shows, it can take a patient advocate to get the kind of treatment that's called for, but it's possible.

As I said, with any other ailment, a doctor will listen to a patient's complaints, take a history, and conduct a physical exam. The last part is critical for addicts, because they're almost always in bad physical shape owing to the drug use itself and to the array of physical problems, ranging from malnutrition to hepatitis to HIV, that drug use frequently leads to. The doctor will then recommend the next step. Options range from Twelve Step meetings and drug-and-alcohol counseling to therapy to outpatient treatment; from sober-living houses and therapeutic boarding schools to residential programs. No matter which of these treatments are recommended, there's an essential first step for those who are physically dependent on alcohol and drugs. They must get drugs out of their systems and become physically stable. They must go through detox, the initial stage of evidence-based treatment.

10

Detox

Toughing It Out

The addict's nervous system adapts to the presence of drugs. Inside an addict's brain and body, a transformation has occurred. When drugs are withheld, the addicted brain goes into a kind of shock. The system is starved for dopamine and other neurotransmitters. It's not quite as serious as oxygen deprivation, but it can feel like that — as if death is imminent. In distress, the entire body system now has one purpose: to return to equilibrium by finding more drugs to stimulate dopamine flow. Addicts can feel as if they're fighting for their lives, and they may be.

Most addicts enter treatment after weeks, months, or years of using, and often immediately after long binges. Many are still high or just coming down. There's no easy way to detoxify the system; cells are dying and neurons misfiring, which can cause tremors, nausea, anxiety, hallucinations, fever, and disorientation. But that's not all. The heart rate can rise dangerously, and the addict has a high risk of seizures, which are sometimes fatal. Detoxing from alcohol — the DTs (delirium tremens, also known as the shaking frenzy or the horrors) — and benzodiazepines is particularly dangerous. Withdrawal from heroin, prescription opiates, and stimulants like cocaine and methamphetamine can cause a variety of symptoms, including restlessness, insomnia, irritability, loss of appetite, diarrhea, headaches, abdominal cramps, nausea, sweating, and chills. Intense anxiety and depression accompany most detoxes, but these are particularly acute in withdrawal from methamphetamine and

other stimulants. Some people maintain that there's no physical withdrawal from marijuana, but there's a body of evidence that supports
cannabis withdrawal syndrome, which can include depression, sleeplessness, and anxiety.

Most of those addicted to so-called hard drugs will supplement them
with booze and weed; this means detox is required for multiple drugs.
Unsurprisingly, the more drugs the addict was using, the more traumatic the detox can be.

Reject Cold-Turkey Detox

Before the mechanism of detox was understood, addicts were told that
they had to just stop. Dr. Benjamin Rush, who in 1809 first described
"inebriates" as addicts, instructed them to "abstain . . . suddenly and
entirely." However, he didn't offer any way for them to do so other than
what we now call cold-turkey withdrawal, "white-knuckling it."

The classic depiction of the addict withdrawing has him locked in a
room, tied to a bed, sweating, hallucinating, kicking walls, pleading for
drugs. Think Ray Charles and Johnny Cash in biopics. Or Sinatra in
The Man with the Golden Arm. Despite their histrionic torments, these
movie-version addicts always heroically tough it out and sober up on
their own. But outside the movies, a lot of them don't make it.

Though it's dangerous and only a minority of addicts do make it to drug-
free status using a cold-turkey approach, it's still advocated by some so-
called addiction experts, and it's the only option offered in some programs. It still exists because of the regressive belief that a person will get
and stay sober only by enduring the agony of withdrawal; that way, he
won't ever want to go through it again. As I heard an addiction counselor say at an outpatient rehab meeting, "You must be humbled. You
must be brought to your fucking knees." An even more insidious ethic
underlies the reasoning of why addicts must suffer through cold turkey:
They must be punished for their debauchery.

The science-based approach rejects cold-turkey detox. Toughing it
out is archaic, ineffective, and dangerous. A new approach to detox has
been developed, tested, and shown to work. It's practiced in hospitals

and some rehabs by doctors trained in the process. Called medical detox, it's an evidence-based treatment that's not only more humane but safer, and far more people make it through the process.

Medical Detox

Medical detox is based on the fact that getting sober isn't about character but about chemistry — the removal of a toxic chemical from a compromised system that has become dependent on it. An initial assessment will determine if detox is required. If it is, it should be done in a hospital or some other facility where patients are under doctors' supervision. Throughout the process, they must be closely monitored.

A patient who enters detox should be freshly assessed and given another physical exam. Many addicts arrive malnourished, anemic, dehydrated, or suffering from other illnesses. In addition, an admitting nurse or doctor should take another history. Patients are drug tested to confirm their self-reported histories and to determine the variety and volume of drugs in their systems.

Medication is integral to medical detox. Many rehabs reject the use of medication in any stage of treatment, including detox. Theirs is an outdated, doctrinaire, and counterproductive policy. There's a risk when using any medication, and there's a fear of transferring one addiction to another. However, most medications used in detox aren't addictive (those that are, such as benzodiazepines, are used in moderation), and, in any case, trained doctors should always control dosage and monitor patients, adjust medications as required, and taper use.

The medications used depend on the drug or drugs abused. Doctors prescribe anticonvulsants, sedatives, and, for opiate addiction, agonists or partial agonists that block craving and make detoxification faster and more tolerable by interacting with opiate receptors, replacing heroin or other drugs. For some addictions, medications are used to moderate craving and control or prevent many withdrawal symptoms, including ones that can be life-threatening. Some medications have antidepressant effects. Other drugs may be used to block withdrawal symptoms, and still others to treat anxiety. Withdrawal from alcohol is aided by controlled doses of sedatives and antipsychotic medications. There cur-

rently aren't replacement drugs for stimulants, but sedatives, mood stabilizers, and antianxiety medications can increase the odds that people
addicted to those drugs will make it through.

Rapid Detox?

Proponents of rapid or ultra-rapid detox claim that the process can be
completed faster, even in a matter of hours. Patients are usually given a
general anesthetic and high doses of a cocktail of medications including
the opiate blocker naltrexone and drugs to treat withdrawal symptoms.
Rapid and ultra-rapid detox are expensive, and there's scant evidence
that they're effective. In fact, in a number of studies, rapid and ultra-
rapid detox weren't shown to lessen the severity of withdrawal, and
some people experienced severe complications from the general anesthesia. "They claim you'll sleep for a while, wake up, and be drug free,
but you can wake up in florid withdrawal," says the Menninger Clinic's
Jim Flack. According to a study reported on in *USA Today* in August of
2005, "The [rapid detox] technique can be life-threatening, is not pain-
free and has no advantage over other methods. . . . The method also
did worse when it came to keeping addicts clean. Eighty percent of the
anesthesia patients in this study dropped out of follow-up treatment, a
dropout rate slightly higher than for another method in the study."

No experts I polled advocated rapid detox. They did all agree on
the three most important pieces of advice regarding detox in general:
Toughing it out and cold turkey should be rejected in favor of medical
detox. Decisions about detox should be made with the advice of professionals. Medical detox must be administered and supervised by doctors
who have been trained in the procedure.

Detox Is Only the Beginning of Treatment

Detox is essential, and completing it is a triumph, but without next-stage
— sometimes called primary — treatment, most addicts will relapse. Every specialist I interviewed agreed that detox isn't enough, and yet some
rehabs — and some insurance companies — perpetuate the myth that
people who make it through detox are fully treated and are ready to
rebuild their lives.

It may seem that completing the hellish process of detox would keep people from backsliding; who would want to go through it again? But the pain of being and staying sober, coupled with persistent craving, can be a powerful force. Indeed, after making it through detox, most people feel depleted and depressed, and many are still ill with complications of the process or with sickness that predated detox. They feel compelled to use; paradoxically, an intensified craving is often a result of detox. If an addict was depressed before he began using, his depression may return, possibly worse than before. In fact, depression is common even for those without a prior history of the disorder. "The opposite of the euphoria caused by the drug is the dysphoria that is inevitably experienced afterwards," says Christopher J. Evans, director of the UCLA Brain Research Institute. "After a drug binge you're left with a dysphoric state that can last hours or even weeks. . . . The dysphoric state may be reversed by taking the drug again, but by doing so the brain adaptions become more pronounced and the recovery of the brain to respond normally more difficult to reestablish."

If an addict's drug use was a response to being overwhelmed by his life, he's probably more overwhelmed now. If he had problems with relationships, he may feel further alienated and alone. After detoxing, one addict said, "Welcome back to the fucked-up life that made me use in the first place." In addition, sober for the first time in months or even years, he's probably horrified about how he behaved while he was using, frightened of relapsing, and terrified of the future. It's a sad fact of addiction: getting clean is traumatic, and the reward can be the very hell the addict was running away from in the first place.

However, though waking up from months or years of addiction can be devastating, it's also an opportunity, possibly the first opportunity ever, for a person to address lifelong problems and move forward to the critical next stage of treating his illness. In many cases, especially for those who began using as adolescents, it may be the first time underlying problems can be recognized, because, for years or decades, drugs hid them. These problems can include serious psychiatric illnesses. The positive news is that when an addict is drug-free (or mostly drug-free; often residual drugs remain in a person's system after detox), real treatment can begin.

V

Staying Clean

11

Beginning Treatment

THERE'S WIDESPREAD IGNORANCE and confusion about post-detox treatment, often called primary treatment. There are countless options, a dizzying range of proven and unproven alternatives practiced (or malpracticed) by an equally bewildering variety of doctors, counselors, therapists, and others.

Some people in the recovery community maintain that after detox, addicts can stay clean by attending AA and working the Twelve Steps. That's enough for a small percentage of people, and so it's reasonable for addicts to try AA if they're willing. It's ubiquitous and free. Dr. Keith Humphreys, professor of psychiatry and behavioral sciences at the Stanford School of Medicine, has researched the effectiveness of AA, and he says that he advises that addicts go at least a few times and try different meetings. "Think of it like a date," he says. "Just go to dinner and see if it works. If you go to a bad movie, you're out ten bucks and an evening. If you go to an AA meeting and don't like it you're only out an evening. Give it a go. See if any of it sticks."

Some addicts aren't open to trying AA; some have tried it and weren't helped by it and aren't willing to go back; and some aren't in good enough physical and mental shape to go — they need a more intensive intervention. Similarly, some newly detoxed addicts do well in counseling or therapy (sometimes in addition to AA), but many require more aggressive treatment. They should be guided by professional assessments and recommendations, and they should get second opinions. Ideally, there'll be a seamless handoff between the detox site and a treatment program.

Some institutions provide both; patients can be transferred from de-tox to the primary treatment ward. This doesn't mean they should be, though. Not all primary programs are right for all addicts. Some aren't equipped to deal with patients with, for example, co-occurring disor-ders, poly-drug abuse, or a history of multiple relapses.

Inpatient or Outpatient?

A patient's physical and emotional state after detox, plus her history of drug use and other factors, will inform a doctor's recommendation about the next step. One of the first decisions people must make re-garding primary treatment is whether to choose an outpatient or a resi-dential program. In the former, addicts live at home (or perhaps in a sober-living halfway house) and go to a therapist's office or treatment center for a prescribed number of sessions a week. Addicts in inpatient or residential treatment live in a rehab or hospital. Many inpatient and outpatient programs offer at least some of the same therapies, though the frequency and duration differ. Inpatient programs are usually far more intensive. Generally there are multiple individual and group ther-apies throughout the day; outpatient programs usually include only one session a day several times a week. Residential programs often add ther-apies that aren't practical in outpatient settings. Some of these therapies — art therapy, anger management, assertiveness training, and various treatments for trauma, for example — plus activities such as yoga and exercise have been shown to be effective treatment components .

In some cases, inpatient rehab is the only viable option. After detox, some addicts shouldn't return to their old environment, where stresses like family conflicts or the prevalence of drugs would make staying clean virtually impossible. Some can't participate in outpatient programs due to physical, emotional, or psychiatric problems, or they need continual monitoring for medical conditions. Also in need of inpatient treatment are many of those people with both addiction and severe psychiatric disorders, a combination of issues that would make it unlikely for them to follow through in an outpatient program. And some patients have nowhere to go. Jeanne Obert, cofounder of the Matrix Institute on Ad-dictions, an EBT-based outpatient program in Los Angeles, says, "We work to get people with severe dependencies into inpatient programs when their circumstances warrant it." An example: "Women who don't have a safe place to live — when it isn't safe for them to go home because of an abusive or addicted partner, or they are homeless." Of course those in imminent danger of harming themselves or others should immediately be admitted to psychiatric hospitals or other institutions equipped to care for them. Family members should use any means, including legal means, to institutionalize a suicidal or violent patient. As I explained, the legal process that allows forced institutionalization differs from state to state.

Other than in these extreme cases, there's no foolproof formula to determine whether an inpatient or outpatient program is called for; the answer depends on the individual's needs and circumstances plus the available options. Even experts disagree on whether residential or outpatient care is appropriate for a particular individual.

Professionally run inpatient programs, if they're staffed by qualified people and employ EBT, can provide a safe and controlled environment where a patient can be closely monitored. Addicts (usually) can't score drugs in inpatient programs; they're supported twenty-four hours a day through crisis and craving; they're contained, monitored, and occupied; and treatment can be consistent and intensive. It's asking a lot for many addicts, especially adolescents, to adhere to an outpatient program when they're surrounded by the same friends, living in the same neighborhood, and dealing with the same pressures that led them to become addicted. Inpatient programs are usually safer in that regard. Adolescents are especially susceptible to environmental and social cues. There are many more opportunities for an addict in an outpatient program to slip and relapse even as he remains in treatment.

There are concerns about inpatient treatment, though. First, it's expensive. Second, some addicts simply refuse to go (those under eighteen may not have a choice, but in most cases, adults cannot be signed in by others); they're more open to treatment if they can return to their homes and families, school or jobs. Ian Sullivan, the Burbank-based designer in treatment for meth addiction, said, "I knew that I needed to maintain as normal of a life as possible. Still going to work. I mean, we needed the income. I had no disability insurance. I knew that if I threw myself into this depressing inpatient treatment center I wasn't going to make it. I'd be completely freaked out."

Some doctors discourage most patients from seeking inpatient treatment because it's a radical and, they maintain, usually unnecessary intervention. They argue that if an addict needs intensive inpatient treatment down the road, he may be resistant to it because he's already found it irrelevant or useless. "It doesn't work for me." Or "I hated it. No way I'm going back in." Some experts believe it's an unduly aggressive approach, akin to putting a cancer patient in the hospital for months on end when his disease could be treated with medication and weekly or monthly doctor visits. That said, some advanced-stage cancer patients need treatments they can't get at home. They need to be hospitalized and monitored twenty-four hours a day. It's the same with some drug addicts.

For patients who don't meet the specific criteria for inpatient programs that I list above, many doctors suggest trying an outpatient program first to see if it works. If a patient doesn't respond, she should then enter residential treatment.

A number of studies have compared the effectiveness of inpatient and outpatient treatment, but the results have been mixed. Overall, they support inpatient treatment for those with psychiatric disorders or severe problems in their lives. One study showed similar abstinence rates for inpatient and outpatient programs except for certain subsets of patients, for whom residential treatment "significantly predicted a higher post-treatment abstinence rate than outpatient treatment." The subsets included patients who had histories of suicidal thoughts or attempts and, as the study's lead researcher, Patricia A. Harrison, adds, "Having what the study classified as severe problems in at least four of five areas." She lists alcohol use, drug use, psychological distress, social isolation, and employment problems.

Another study compared patients who went from a residential program to an outpatient program with ones who began treatment in an outpatient program. Those who were in residential programs first had "somewhat" better outcomes. The study, conducted by Stanford's Dr. Moos, was done with VA patients, so, as he clarifies, "It is not clear how well these findings would generalize to community treatment programs." He concludes, "In general, existing research suggests that individuals who are experiencing more severe alcohol or drug use, who have been diagnosed with a serious psychiatric disorder, who are more socially unstable, and who have more severe family, legal, and/or employment problems tend to benefit more from an initial episode of inpatient/residential treatment than from an initial episode of outpatient treatment."

Other than in clear-cut cases, however, Moos says, "If there is initial doubt about treatment . . . the more prudent course would be to engage first in the less restrictive treatment option; that is, outpatient treatment rather than inpatient/residential treatment."

Helen M. Pettinati, professor in the department of psychiatry at the Perelman School of Medicine at the University of Pennsylvania, has a different view. Pettinati conducted an inpatient/outpatient study years ago (in the 1990s) that dramatically supported inpatient as opposed to outpatient treatment. In it, "outpatients, regardless of level of psychiatric severity, were four times more likely to be early treatment failures."

Pettinati explains that the study was conducted at a time when managed-care companies were entering the insurance market and looking for ways to save money. Inpatient care was more expensive (though, Pettinati maintains, it's more cost-effective than outpatient programs because of its greater efficacy). The insurance companies pushed the industry from what was then standard — residential treatment — to the newer model of outpatient care. This push wasn't inspired by money alone, she says, but by a reasonable concern that patients in residential programs were in "an unrealistic world," and so they often relapsed when they were discharged from treatment.

The problem, Pettinati maintains, wasn't the fact that these patients were treated in an institution; it was the lack of transitional programs — aftercare, such as outpatient programs, follow-up monitoring, or sober-living environments. "But inpatient care offers structure to patients who desperately need it," she says. "A lot of people with addiction problems live in an unstructured world. They do drugs when they get them, they don't sleep or eat regularly. In an inpatient facility, people sometimes begin to clean up just because they have structure for the first time. Also, though you can't guarantee that drugs aren't ever snuck in, people in inpatient programs have a chance to feel what it's like to be abstinent. People get terrified — I mean really terrified — when they think they're going to lose their best friend: their drug. The thought of going without it for one day terrifies them. But in a structured situation, where they have no drugs, one of the first things they learn is that they can be abstinent and their world isn't going to crash in around them. And in addition to being protected, of course they can get far more treatment in a residential program than a few hours a week in an outpatient program." Yes, she concedes, sustaining the lessons of inpatient treatment is the next challenge, but that's what the relapse-prevention stage of treatment is for. "I saw the benefit of inpatient treatment then, and I see it now," she says. "We lose people every day because they can't get inpatient treatment — they have no access to programs like those at Hazelden and Betty Ford. Residential care should be available for everyone who needs it."

Yet Yale's Michael Pantalon is far more reluctant to recommend residential programs. "Of course, inpatient rehab is absolutely necessary for some," he says. But he cites research that contradicts Pettinati's and indicates that residential treatment doesn't work any better than outpatient care. He says, "Additionally, it can be rather ineffective and potentially harmful for [some patients], such as those with less severe problems (i.e., not at the level of abuse or dependence), adolescents, and those who need more intensive individual counseling. I say this because I've heard some very troubling rehab stories from each of these groups. For example, less severe people say that rehab made them feel their drug use was not that bad when compared to others in rehab and that this comparison led them back to use." This is especially true of adolescents, he says. "Adolescents frequently tell me that they learned new strategies for procuring and using drugs in rehab, most notably how to use drugs intravenously." Another problem, he says, is that "those who need more professional individual counseling, such as those who are anxious in groups or those with co-occurring psychiatric (e.g., anxiety, depression, PTSD) and substance abuse problems, may only get an hour a week of such treatment. And according to a number of my patients, that hour frequently only focuses on acceptance of the Twelve Steps discussed in groups, rather than on evidence-based psychotherapies for both addiction and other psychiatric issues." This can be true in outpatient programs too, but he says, "In many intensive outpatient programs, there is a greater focus on individual treatment that is based on scientifically supported treatments, including medications (which are also much less available in rehab) and better tailored to the severity and needs of the client."

Pantalon concludes, "We have to balance being off the street for a while (provided they stay in the program, which many do not) vs. inadvertently learning other bad behaviors, getting very little individual contact with professional, licensed counselors, and being turned off by the emphasis on Twelve Steps that predominates the rehab system, which turns many off to treatment in general. In my experience, and provided there isn't a medical need for inpatient rehab, the more science-based, motivational and individual outpatient treatment with a licensed professional, the more likely clients are to achieve and maintain abstinence."

Dr. Pantalon's arguments notwithstanding, I've heard from a substantial number of people who regretted choosing outpatient programs because they or their addicted family members dropped out of treatment (or weren't helped enough by it) and then suffered relapses, including overdoses, some of them fatal. Of course there are no guarantees that they would have done better if they'd chosen inpatient programs — people flee residential treatment too — but in a good inpatient program, these addicts would have been in more intensive therapy; they would have been more closely monitored and better protected from the environments in which they were likely to relapse.

Overall, the consensus of experts advises neither overreacting or underreacting when it comes to choosing treatment. As always, my first recommendation is that people work with addiction specialists to decide about inpatient versus outpatient programs. After weighing the opinions and evidence, if there's doubt about which approach is required, I'd advocate speaking with the consulting doctors to see if they recommend an outpatient approach as a first step for patients who aren't at high risk of relapsing, whose drug use is relatively mild, who don't have serious psychological disorders, and who live in relatively stable environments. For others, however, though all approaches have risks, given that relapse rates are highest in the earliest stage of treatment and the fact that any relapse can be deadly, I'm biased toward erring on the side of caution and strongly considering an inpatient program for most severely addicted patients — of course, it must be a good one staffed by professionals who practice EBT.

How Long Should Programs Last?

Outpatient programs last anywhere from several weeks to three, nine, or twelve months, or more. Many inpatient programs last only twenty-eight days, even though research has shown that a month is rarely enough. A problem with longer inpatient stays is that they're prohibitively expensive for many people, especially since insurance plans often don't cover them or don't cover them at a level that makes them affordable (despite the fact that even the most expensive residential treatment programs are less expensive than inpatient hospital care for other diseases). But while an addict may become well enough in four weeks to understand the need for ongoing care, he may not be well enough to follow through on it. More time is usually required. There's no scientific evidence that supports the twenty-eight-day limit, according to UCLA's Dr. Rawson, Treatment Research Institute's Dr. McLellan, and other experts. The research does support primary inpatient or outpatient programs of at least ninety days. A NIDA-funded project called Drug Abuse Treatment Outcome Studies found that addicts who dropped out of treatment before ninety days had relapse rates similar to those who'd stayed in treatment only a day or two. After ninety days, however, patients' relapse rates dropped steadily the longer they stayed in treatment. One possible reason: Yale University researchers concluded that it takes at least three months of abstinence for the brain's prefrontal cortex to be able to process the kinds of information related to decision making and analytical functions. After that amount of time, some addicts who begin in residential programs can be safely transferred to outpatient or extended-care programs.

Selecting a Program

Determining whether an addict should go into outpatient or inpatient treatment is only the beginning of the trying process of choosing a primary care program. The next challenge is finding one that fits a particular patient's needs. It's the same process used for finding a good detox facility but much less straightforward because there are so many more variables to consider.

Once again, the decision should be made with the counsel of professionals. Once again, second opinions are advised. In addition to doctors and therapists, consultants can help families weigh options and make decisions. Like other experts, they must be licensed professionals. Anyone can call himself an educational consultant and charge sometimes hefty fees to help place addicts — or generic "troubled youths" — in appropriate programs. Unconscionably, just like some interventionists, some consultants get kickbacks from programs to which they refer business. However, a professional and credentialed consultant can provide an invaluable service for those who are overwhelmed by the myriad options. Rather than relying on self-reported statistics and staff credentials listed online, the best of these consultants frequently visit programs to be sure they're doing what they claim to be doing, and doing it effectively. Whether he's an educational consultant or a trained counselor or a therapist, a professional can, following an assessment, help decide on the appropriate course and guide people away from ineffective or potentially harmful programs and outright scams.

There are online directories of treatment programs, but most are unreliable, and some are insidious. The latter appear to be nonbiased guides, but they're owned by programs or they list rehabs that pay to be included on the website.

There are independent sources too. A SAMHSA website has three types of directories — an Opioid Treatment Program Directory, a Substance Abuse Treatment Facility Locator, and a Buprenorphine Physician and Treatment Program Locator — but the government agency doesn't endorse these programs. At this time there's no reliable source to guide people to programs that have been vetted and are monitored. EBTs haven't made it into many rehabs, and in many cases, practitioners haven't been trained in them; it can be hard to trust their claims. Some programs are in the exploitation business, which is no surprise in a multibillion-dollar industry (it's projected to have revenues of $34 billion by 2014) that's largely unregulated. They prey on people's fear and desperation.

In any field of health care, patients should seek professional help but also advocate for themselves, be wise consumers. In an e-mail, Dr. Rawson suggested some considerations for choosing a residential treatment program. First, it should be accredited or licensed. He says that "the most trustworthy" accreditation comes from the Commission for the

Accreditation of Rehabilitation Facilities (CARF) and the Joint Commission on Accreditation of Healthcare Organizations (JCAHO). The "next best" accreditation is a state license. A general certification means less. "If they don't mention anything [regarding their accreditation or license], stay away," Rawson advises. Next, the program's staff should include doctors trained in addiction medicine (as evidenced by membership in AAAP or ASAM, or certified by ABAM). Prospective patients should be sure these doctors are onsite frequently: "daily is best, two to three times a week isn't great, and 'as needed'" — Rawson says it again — "stay away." Therapists should be licensed psychologists, licensed clinical social workers (LCSWs), or licensed marriage and family therapists (LMFTs). Again, check to be sure these professionals are full-time and don't just stop by weekly. Counselors should also be licensed or certified. "I would use a rule of thumb that [a program] should have more of these professional licensed staff than they have acupuncturists, massage therapists, Reichian experts, horse therapists, etc.," Rawson says. "I would caution that too much of that stuff is a sign that they're more of a resort than a serious treatment program. If you look at the website for McLean Hospital at Harvard — probably the best psychiatric hospital in the U.S. — you don't see anything about metaphysical astrology."

Patients should receive psychological evaluations and medication, if necessary. Of course, programs should offer EBT. However, trying to find an evidence-based program is problematic because, as Rawson says, "Anybody can say they do CBT, MI, and the like, but without a research team going in to measure fidelity of the intervention it's impossible to know if they are really using it." He advises people to look at a program's daily and weekly schedule and ask who runs the various activities. "If they have a CBT group that's run by a licensed psychologist, MD, LCSW, or LMFT, it's good, but 'by counselors', it isn't as good." It's also critical to be sure programs include continuing-care plans for patients when they leave the program. Rawson suggests finding out if residential programs send patients who need them to outpatient treatment and halfway houses and those on opiate medications to outpatient programs that will continue their treatment. He adds that an inferior approach is when programs recommend that their patients who leave attend alumni group meetings and Twelve Step meetings without other ongoing treatment. He also holds that a valuable component of a good treatment center is a structured program of post-discharge checkups, ongoing telephone support, or web-based support resources. Finally, he suggests that people ask if a program has treatment evaluation reports they can see. "No (not good); yes, done by themselves in house (better, but they need to have a written report, not just a few numbers off the top of their heads); or an outcome or performance program by an outside university or independent group with a written report (best)."

Pediatrician Fred Holmes adds that programs should have a team approach to treatment. (This applies to both inpatient and outpatient options.) Dr. Holmes says, "It isn't one doctor, not one set of ideas or beliefs or one kind of professional training." Holmes says that this model exists throughout the world of pediatrics (and other medical specialties), but rarely with addiction. "With other diseases, there's a well-established protocol," he says. "There's evaluation. As a result of the evaluation, the level of service that's needed is determined. The team members consult and adjust treatment over time." A team can involve a medical doctor, behavioral therapist, family therapist, psychiatrist, and other specialists. "No one physician is capable of doing all that," says Dr. Holmes.

In sum, those discussing treatment options with their doctor should consider:

- It should be evidence based. SAMHSA has online a National Registry of Evidence-Based Programs and Practices. (This is different from the SAMHSA listing of rehabs I mention above.)

- A physical exam by a physician should be routine. Patients should be monitored frequently by an MD and RNs while they're in the program. It's still possible for them to have seizures or other life-threatening events during rehab.

- Patients should be screened or rescreened for co-occurring psychiatric disorders by psychiatrists or psychologists trained to identify patients with dual diagnoses. Patients with co-occurring problems — eating disorders, attention disorders, mood disorders — must be in programs that treat them as well as their addictions.

- Programs should continually evaluate patients and adjust treatment as needed, and if a program identifies a patient who requires treatments beyond or outside the program's expertise, it should work with the patient (and her family) to identify appropriate care and should coordinate a seamless and safe transition into the new program. Patients should never be discharged without a solid plan in place.

• Therapists and counselors should have degrees in counseling, clinical psychology, social work, or similar relevant specialties. A therapist's or counselor's former addiction is *not* a qualification by itself. As Walter Ling, professor of psychiatry and director of the Integrated Substance Abuse Programs at UCLA, said ruefully of some programs, "The more of a drug addict you were, the more of an expert you become. Having cancer doesn't enable you to treat cancer." Also, programs should have adequate numbers of these professionals so patients can meet with them regularly. Bonding with a therapist can be a critical part of treatment, so patients should meet frequently with one primary therapist.

• There should be a team approach to treatment. This applies to inpatient as well as outpatient treatment. As needed, MDs, therapists, registered nurses, and counselors should consult with one another about an individual patient. As needed, they should also consult with other specialists.

• All support staff working with patients should be well trained and closely supervised.

• Teenagers should be treated in programs designed specifically for them. Many programs throw adult and adolescent addicts together, and some counselors believe that teenagers should learn from older addicts who have suffered addictions that began when they themselves were teenagers. The experts I polled disagree. If they're in treatment with adults, some kids will be intimidated and less able to participate in and benefit from therapies. In addition, some treatments developed for adults backfire when they're used with kids. And kids can dismiss the idea that they're addicted when they compare themselves to older addicts; further, they might want to emulate older hard-core addicts who've used more drugs and more varieties of drugs.

- Ideally, patients should enter programs adapted for them, depending on their race, religion, sexual orientation, or culture. Some addicts should be treated in single-sex programs.

- Programs shouldn't offer one-size-fits-all treatment. They should be able to tailor the treatments they offer to meet individual needs.

- One qualified person — a case manager or primary therapist, for example — should work with each patient to coordinate and oversee his treatment, monitor progress, and be sure she gets the specific help she needs.

- Programs should evaluate whether it would be beneficial for family members to be involved in treatment.

- Program staff should be capable of identifying patients who require care that the program can't provide. In such cases, they should help patients find appropriate care and help with the transition to the new program.

Reject Programs That Use Tough Love and Other Confrontational Approaches

I've described detox programs that rely on a rigid, paternalistic model that features a confrontational approach and force patients to detox cold turkey — and I have rejected them because they've been shown to do more harm than good. Many primary programs, especially residential programs, are also modeled on a tough-love approach. Some are dangerous. Numerous studies have shown that they rarely help and can hurt addicts. "People dig in their heels more, become more angry, or more into denial," said Dr. Lisa Onken, chief of NIDA's behavioral and integrative treatment branch. People who are ill should be treated with compassion, not judgment and vilification.

Compared to traditional confrontational and aggressive approaches to treatment, evidence-based behavioral treatments begin more gently, recognizing a patient's fragility and history. Another on the list of ASAM guidelines for qualified doctors: They must "demonstrate an empathetic, positive, and hopeful attitude toward the person with a substance related disorder, as well as toward family members and significant others." When taking the Hippocratic oath, doctors promise to treat all patients with compassion. Addicts deserve and require no less.

I've learned about inpatient programs like the one Elizabeth described, where patients were yelled at, restrained, and forced to scrub toilets when they broke rules, and the now-shuttered academy where Brian experienced bullying and abuse. There are practical reasons for both inpatient and residential programs to set rules and define expectations. Patients who relapse can threaten the sobriety of others. Patients in all programs must be protected from those who are in any way threatening or toxic to them or the group. However, there are alternatives to punishment and rejection. Relapse and rule breaking are indications that current treatments aren't working. Treatment should be reevaluated and intensified or modified. As I said, if a program isn't equipped to help a particular patient, its medical staff must find another program that is, and help with a safe transfer.

Wilderness Programs and Therapeutic Boarding Schools

Some inpatient programs are hospital-based; some are standalone rehabs. Some therapeutic boarding schools and wilderness programs offer intensive addiction treatment. Both of these usually focus on treating teens.

Research into the effectiveness of these programs is limited. Like at any rehab program, highly trained therapists and counselors are critical. It's also necessary that programs have physicians and psychiatrists either on staff or on call — in California there's actually a statute (widely ignored) that prohibits a residential program from employing doctors (a remnant of a time when most rehabs focused exclusively on Twelve Step treatment). Effective therapeutic schools and wilderness programs must use evidence-based approaches, including ones I describe later in *Clean*. And doctors I've spoken to say that neither therapeutic boarding schools nor wilderness programs are appropriate primary treatments for many of those with concurrent psychological disorders.

Wilderness programs in particular are gaining popularity among parents who seek treatment for their children, partly because there are many of them and they appear to have big advertising budgets; search *addiction treatment* online and many pop up. And they make extravagant promises that many parents find hard to resist.

It's also true that some parents prefer to send their children to camp-like environments rather than to institutions, and they're convinced that it's good for their kids to be out in the woods or up in the mountains. There's anecdotal evidence about the effectiveness of these programs — testimonials galore — but little empirical evidence that the great outdoors is therapeutic. Also, while camping in the woods may be fun and even inspiring for some patients, for others it could be nightmarish and hence counterproductive. People need to be engaged in treatment, not traumatized in an environment they abhor. And be aware that some outdoor programs are based on the philosophy that kids who are using drugs just need some tough love. Some have military-like rules and mete out harsh punishments, tactics that are ineffective and, in some cases, harmful. Children should be treated with gentleness and compassion. Some of these, advertised as boot camps, claim they treat kids' drug problems, but they can be dangerous. The National Mental Health Association reports that "employing tactics of intimidation and humiliation is counterproductive for most youth" and points to research that "boot camp graduates are more likely to be re-arrested or are re-arrested more quickly than other offenders." It states that "the use of this kind of model has led to disturbing incidents of abuse." In 1998 a U.S. Justice Department investigation concluded, "The paramilitary boot camp model is not only ineffective, but harmful."

Use caution when selecting therapeutic boarding schools or wilderness programs. I've gathered enough anecdotal evidence to conclude that some of these programs are effective — I interviewed kids who attended therapeutic boarding schools where they worked consistently with therapists for a year or more and at the same time earned their high-school degrees — but some are dangerous. Programs should be accredited or licensed and run by people who know what they're doing; they should hire and monitor trained and licensed therapists, have available physicians and psychiatrists for patients who need them, and — even for kids backpacking in the Sierra — have a program of EBT. Never choose a program that isn't recommended by experts experienced in addiction medicine. Always get professional opinions before sending a child away, even for a short time.

Reject the My-Way-or-the-Highway Approach

While he was in the inpatient program, between therapy sessions, Ian Sullivan went out for a beer with his friends. Someone took a picture and posted it on Facebook, tagging Sullivan. A counselor was alerted to the photograph and confronted Sullivan, who explained that yes, he'd gone out with his friends and had a beer, but he rarely drank and never got drunk, and it was no big deal. "He was mean and nasty and accusatory," Sullivan said of the counselor. He had broken the program's strict no-drugs policy and was summarily thrown out.

Relapse isn't the only grounds for expulsion from some programs. When visiting one rehab, I sat talking with a group of patients outdoors on a picnic bench. Raised voices came from inside a residence for participants in the twenty-eight-day program. We heard the voice of a counselor, whom I'd met earlier. He was a hefty 220-pound recovering heroin addict who had recently celebrated his twenty-fifth year sober. His tone was firm, irritated, sighing, indicating a sad resignation. "Pack your things. Ten minutes."

We then heard a patient (a man I later learned was a high-school teacher addicted to alcohol and pills) tearfully pleading with the counselor to let him stay.

In a while the teacher walked through the door with the counselor. He lugged a black garbage bag that held his possessions; not much, just some clothes, basically. He was a fortyish man with long hair brushed straight back. Standing on the grass, he displayed some bravado — lots of *fuck you*s and *asshole*s — but it was undercut when he began silently crying and wiping tears on his shirtsleeve. "What the fuck am I supposed to do?"

The counselor turned his back and walked inside.

Afterward, when I challenged the counselor, he told me, "You have to be humble if you're going to succeed here. He's not ready to be sober. His ego is in control. I've seen a million like him. He's cocky, thinks he's above the steps, think he knows better than all of us. He isn't ready to do what it takes. He'll be back when he is."

The patient was kicked out because of his bad attitude — his failure to get with the program. The *Los Angeles Times* reported the story of a man who was kicked out of Promises, a rehab in Malibu, "for belligerent behavior." The program refused to refund the $42,000 he paid up front. My son Nic was kicked out of a program called Life Healing Center in Santa Fe, New Mexico, in which he was making great strides forward, for breaking a rule that prohibited male and female patients from fraternizing. Kicking Nic out (especially without facilitating a transition into a new program) was unconscionable, and it could have been lethal. And this happened at a reputable program that was staffed by highly qualified (and effective) therapists. Here again addicts — already judged and shamed — are punished like bad children for their bad attitudes or breaking rules. Addiction is the only disease whose patients are refused treatment for showing their symptoms.

"No one gets kicked out of here," says social worker Joe Schrank, the owner of Loft 107, a sober-living house in Brooklyn. "We understand people fail. You're not booted out on the curb. You're not banished from the kingdom." His policy doesn't mean that relapsing addicts are allowed to stay even if their presence is detrimental to other residents. However, Schrank says that in such cases, he and his staff work with the patient to return him or her to more intensive treatment, possibly at a residential program. Sometimes they try other options, such as assigning a relapsing addict a sober coach or sober companion (the latter is almost like a bodyguard, except instead of protecting a person from outside threats, he protects him from his own disease).

The Cost of Treatment

Finding treatment is one thing. Paying for it is another. There are free and low-cost inpatient programs available for people who have limited resources, who are on public assistance, or who have minimal insurance. If recommended programs are out of a patient or family's financial reach, they can ask if the programs offer sliding scales. Some will negotiate prices and payment plans. Some free programs — publicly funded or run by charities — also have highly qualified staff and offer EBTs, but many don't; it's a severe failing of the system that quality addiction treatment is inaccessible to so many people for purely financial reasons.

A model example of a free, licensed, sixty-bed residential program for indigent and homeless people is San Francisco's Father Alfred Center, which is associated with the St. Anthony Foundation. The all-male program lasts a year or more and includes assessment, individual and group counseling (counselors are certified drug and alcohol counselors), and Twelve Step work. Patients who need it also see licensed therapists through St. Anthony's mental health services. Social workers help patients with nonmedical needs too, such as legal aid and vocational training. Patients are offered computer classes, job-search counseling, and life-skills tutoring.

The St. Anthony's program is comprehensive, but many free or subsidized programs are bare bones. They may include a meal, a place to sleep, and AA meetings. Even then, some have months-long waiting lists. It's tragic; an addict should enter treatment when he or she needs it. So many things can go wrong if an addict has to wait.

At the other end of the spectrum, some inpatient programs cost tens of thousands of dollars a month; a few run as high as $100,000 a month. Outpatient programs are usually cheaper, but even these can cost thousands of dollars a month, though there are many less expensive options, and some of these programs are free. Some high-end programs — inpatient rehabs, hospital-based programs, therapeutic boarding schools — offer comprehensive, evidence-based treatments practiced by trained therapists and have physicians and psychiatrists on staff. However, a high price tag doesn't guarantee high quality; along with offering massages and gourmet meals, the program may employ untested treatments. Top-tier residential treatment programs that treat addiction and co-occurring psychiatric disorders cost about $1,300 a day. This can sound outrageous until you compare it with the cost of a hospital stay for patients with other diseases. In 2005, the average cost of a day in a hospital was anywhere from $1,629 (for for-profit hospitals) to $2,025 (for nonprofit hospitals). For cancer patients, the average cost was $3,000 a day. The disease of addiction should be covered at rates similar to those for other illnesses.

In the past, most insurance companies haven't covered addiction treatment, or they've covered it inadequately. As I said, some cover only detox and some cover only a twenty-eight-day program. Former congressmen Patrick Kennedy and Jim Ramstad championed the Mental Health Parity and Addiction Equity Act (known as the Parity Act), which became law in 2008. It states that group health insurance plans that cover mental illness and drug addiction must cover them to the same extent that they cover other medical issues. However, it doesn't mandate that insurance companies have to cover mental illness or drug addiction at all.

A number of therapists suggest looking for appropriate clinical trials in research institutions, because they may employ the latest EBTs, and they're sometimes free. (There are online directories of ongoing clinical trials.) Other options: community health-care organizations, treatment programs run by charities, and clinics for programs that are free or offer sliding scales.

I've met patients who, because of tireless advocacy and even filing lawsuits, got insurance companies that had denied coverage to reverse their decisions. In some cases, however, it was too late. It was for Ashley Lojak.

People who are sick need treatment, the best care possible. There should be more options, but addicts can't wait for them to arrive; they need help now. People who need it should aggressively challenge county, state, hospital-based, and nonprofit agencies to help find affordable programs that offer science-based treatments.

Safe, Not Sorry

Regardless of a patient's finances, there's no surefire course of treatment for addiction, because this disease has unusually complex physiological, psychological, social, environmental, and behavioral components, and there are as many permutations of the disease as there are addicts. The science-based approach tells us to rely on professionals, and we should. But it's true that this isn't an exact science, and treating addiction isn't like treating other illnesses. The fact is, given the current state of addiction science — not only what's known, but what *isn't* known — sometimes there's no clear course forward even for those being advised by highly skilled doctors.

In spite of this, people in need of treatment must make choices. Where there isn't definitive research, they must rely on whatever research exists and they must rely on experts' advice. And though science doesn't trust anecdotal evidence, sometimes it's all there is to tip the balance when hard evidence doesn't lead to a clear conclusion. The anecdotes I've gathered inform at least some of the conclusions I've drawn. They certainly inform my conclusion about the treatments I would choose for my son if I had the chance to decide again.

I'm often asked what I'd do differently if I could relive the years of my son's addiction. I wouldn't deny the signs in front of my eyes. I would intervene immediately. I'd also intervene differently.

First, I would learn about risk factors and work with doctors to identify and minimize the ones that applied to Nic. Next, I would bolster Nic in whatever ways I could to help him be as resilient as possible. I would also keep in mind the fact that parents are allowed to force their children into treatment as long as they're minors; this window of opportunity closes the day the child turns eighteen.

In his last year of high school, Nic was exhibiting signs of extreme, dangerous drug use. If I could do it over again, I would immediately bring him to see a psychiatrist specializing in addiction medicine. I'm still astounded that during that time, Nic saw therapists who didn't even recognize that he was stoned in their offices or, if they did, didn't alert me and insist that we find him treatment for his drug abuse.

I would have Nic assessed by the psychiatrist and proactively request psychological testing to determine if his drug use was connected to a psychiatric illness like depression or bipolar disorder. (Later, Nic was diagnosed with both.) If after assessing Nic, a doctor confirmed that he was using and needed treatment, I would follow his recommendation — up to a point.

If Nic was in the early stages of his drug use, I would agree if a doctor recommended that he enter therapy or an outpatient program that included drug testing. Doctors would probably have advised trying those approaches to see if they could slow or stop his use. But if it didn't stop immediately — if drug tests were positive and his drug-related behavior continued — I wouldn't go slowly, no matter what the experts advised. I'd waste no time in choosing a program. Contradicting the advice of some experts, I would choose a long-term residential program, one that lasted for at least six months, with the option of extending treatment to a year or more. Of course, I would use great care in choosing a treatment program — it would be accredited or licensed and staffed by licensed psychologists, psychiatrists, and therapists trained in addiction medicine who worked regularly and closely with patients. (I would follow Rawson's guidelines.)

Sending a child away for six months or more goes against every instinct a parent has. But I would still do it, even against the recommendation of experts, because if you underreact and wait, you may lose the chance to stop drug use from escalating. I'm not alone in questioning the experts on this. I've talked to many people whose loved ones' addictions led to overdosing, running away, getting arrested, stealing, and terrorizing their families. Or to death. And all of these people agree with me: It's better to be safe than sorry.

12

Primary Treatment

ONCE THEY'VE FOUND A program, patients are admitted. Experts recommend that patients be given a physical exam (another one, even though they probably had one where they detoxed) performed by a physician. After detox, depending on the drugs involved and other factors, there's still a risk of seizure, strokes, and other life-threatening events. Patients must be monitored. It's easier to track patients in residential treatment, but outpatient counselors and therapists must also follow patients' progress in regularly scheduled sessions. Patients should understand the risks of relapse and be instructed about what to do if they feel vulnerable (or if a relapse occurs). They should be encouraged to check in with program counselors or therapists whenever they need to.

By the time addicts make it to treatment, they're usually beginning to become more conscious of the consequences of using. They may be facing deteriorating or defunct relationships, physical impairment (caused by illness and/or injury), harm to their careers, financial worries, or legal complications. Also, they're confronted with all the time they lost while they were high. For teenagers especially, that lost time can be crucial, as they could otherwise have been maturing, learning to handle disappointment, and building relationships. Meanwhile, they're still feeling withdrawal symptoms that can last for weeks, probably some levels of depression, exhaustion, anxiety, cravings, severe cognitive impairment, and protracted brain dysfunction. It's no wonder that addicts who arrive in treatment feel miserable, physically depleted, sick, and scared. Many are seriously depressed; some are suicidal.

The first days in primary treatment should be designed to help patients become mentally and physically stronger, so treatment should be focused on easing anxiety and providing encouragement. Sleep, nutrition, and, if they're able to do it, exercise can help. Also, experts say that palliatives such as massage, acupuncture, and yoga may increase the chances that an addict will stay in treatment. Carefully monitored sedatives may help patients stabilize and reach the point that they can focus and concentrate and participate in therapies.

How People Change

Since there are physiological and psychological components to addiction, it isn't enough to treat the physical dependence or to work with therapists to change patterns; it isn't enough to put a person in a new environment; it isn't enough to administer medication to block craving; and it isn't enough to teach addicts how to survive sober. It often requires all these things.

With detox, physical dependence on drugs can begin to lessen, though there's a long way to go before the nervous system normalizes, so craving continues. There are other reasons that it's so difficult for addicts to stay sober. One is the complex internal process that has become linked to, and drives, drug use. Behavioral therapies work to unlink them.

Whether in inpatient programs, outpatient programs, or therapists' offices, behavioral treatments are practiced in individual and group situations. They differ from one another in their methods but most have the same goal: to help addicts change by interrupting the physiological and psychological pathways connecting triggers to drug use. As I've explained, for addicts, taking drugs isn't actually a choice but a subliminal reaction that has become automatic. Numerous behavioral therapies teach and train addicts to make conscious what had been unconscious and to interrupt automatic behaviors that lead them to use.

Therapy should be introduced gradually and reflect a person's ability to engage. Scans have tracked the slowly repairing functioning of addicts' brains, and treatments that require concentration and rational thought should be phased in as patients can manage these cognitive skills. For example, one researcher told me that for meth addicts with cognitive impairments caused by that drug, frequent fifteen-minute therapy sessions are better than the longer but less frequent sessions that are common for treating other addicts. Having people begin slowly keeps them in treatment. In fact, one reason some leave or quickly relapse is that they're expected to do things they can't do, and when they can't, counselors angrily confront them. It's common, but as I've said, research has shown that the more patients are provoked or antagonized, the more likely they are to drop out and relapse.

The wiring gradually repairs itself once a person is off drugs, and therapies aim to reroute thinking patterns once tied to the addiction. The goal is to replace the addiction cycle with a cycle of healing. Along with psychological and behavioral change comes physiological change; the longer an addict is clean, the more the brain heals. The more the brain heals, the easier it is for the addict to stay clean. Patterns of use cause physical damage, and patterns of abstinence reverse the damage.

Education

Ian Sullivan entered the outpatient program for treatment of his meth abuse after two life-threatening experiences, but before that, he was, he says, a user who had "never missed work, kept hidden the fact that I was shooting meth." But he had a minor heart attack when grains of meth clogged a vein, and, later, he had a psychotic episode after a weekend of shooting up. "I was paranoid — hearing things, thinking everyone was looking at me and could see through me," he says. "I was in the shower and had a knife and was going to kill myself." Sullivan told his physician, who referred him to Steve Shoptaw, whom he saw for weekly therapy sessions. Sullivan also began outpatient treatment. One of the first components of the care he received was education. It seems counterintuitive that learning about a disease can help treat it, but it can. From experience, addicts know how drugs affect them, but they can be helped to understand the chemical reaction of various drugs with their nervous systems. Sullivan learned how drugs caused brain changes that led him to his physical and emotional crises. If addicts see how drugs change their thought processes and realize that their behavior is altered by physiological and psychological forces, not conscious choice, they can begin to commit to treatment in a new way — no longer feeling weak, shamed, or inadequate. They can understand the seriousness of the illness and its chronic and progressive nature, but also that, and how, it can be treated.

Sullivan asserts that the education he received was critical for him. "I needed something tangible," he explains. "I needed to understand the effect meth was having on my brain. I needed to know what happens to the brain of people who continue to use. When I understood the damage meth causes, it became very real. I didn't want to risk being unable to complete a sentence or do a math problem. I learned that I could be clean for six months and everything would seem to be fine, but then if I used again the damage would worsen. I understood what had caused the paranoia, and I didn't want it to happen again. Putting it into practical scientific terms made me able to see the truth, which I hadn't been able to do. It helped change my motivation."

As they learn about the symptoms of their disease and the effects of drug use, addicts can begin to understand denial, why it's been so difficult for them to accept that they need help. They learn how their mental illness, or brain disease, causes cravings that lead to repeated use and relapse. They learn about the mechanics of addiction — what precedes use and how triggers can lead to a biological change that will, if it isn't interrupted, cause a relapse. This knowledge lets addicts participate more willingly and effectively in their treatment. It's also useful for them to know where they are in the process — why, for example, they're feeling depressed, or why cravings intensify after having abated. A key fact they must understand is that the biological system is dynamic, which means it can be altered — repaired. Addicts can gain hope from learning that treatment gets easier over time, partly because treatment literally heals the brain.

Behavioral Therapy

Education is vital, but understanding how addiction works isn't enough. Behavioral therapy trains addicts to recognize condition cues that cause relapse and shows them how to interrupt the automatic process by which cues lead to craving. It can help desensitize them to these cues, and it encourages them with rewards that build their motivation to change. Addicts learn to interrupt their normal reactions to anger, disappointment, and other emotions. Therapies continue to teach new behavior patterns. New behaviors eventually acquire the force of habit.

Motivational Interviewing

Before a person will change his behavior, he has to want to change it. Earlier I described motivational interviewing; it can be used to prevent drug use and to stop it from escalating. MI is central to many addiction-treatment programs. It's designed to help addicts clarify their thinking and heighten their motivation to change. It helps empower them with an understanding that change is possible. A person who's motivated to change will fully engage in therapies that bring about change.

As I've described, in MI, patients aren't judged or confronted. Instead, they're guided to work through their denial, to envision a future without drugs, and to set a course toward that future. Some therapists pose questions in therapy sessions. Some have patients write down their answers during therapy or between sessions. "Writing makes their thinking more concrete," Dr. Lisa Onken says. "As it becomes concrete, awareness leads to changes in your thinking that can then lead to changes in your behavior."

The goal of MI at this stage is to help addicts understand the conflict between their life goals and their drug use. They're guided through a process that helps them clearly see the positive and negative consequences of their choices. One doctor told me that, using MI, he asks patients to think about how much they want to keep getting what they get from using. At first, they usually want it all — the relief that comes from drugs, the escape into temporary euphoria, the circle of friends. They're next guided to explore the price they're paying. Maybe they feel guilty, scared, anxious, or depressed. They may be spending too much money on drugs. They may often feel sick and, when they can't get drugs, suffer withdrawal until they score again. They may be damaging their relationships. They may come to see more clearly that getting high isn't as great as it used to be or as they imagine it is, and that their problems are terrible and escalating. Then they're helped to envision life sober. A person who imagines himself in a different future can feel that it's possible to attain it and be further motivated to make it real.

Patients are reminded that change is hard. It will take work and time, but it's possible. This can give addicts hope and encouragement when they're at their bleakest and don't believe that things can get better.

Cognitive-Behavioral Therapy

Cognitive-behavioral therapy (CBT) is an umbrella term for a number of related therapies that train addicts to be aware of the thoughts and feelings that have led them to drug use and teach them how to interrupt them before they use drugs again. Addicts are given tools to change these thoughts and feelings and break the link between them, craving, and drug use. By identifying feelings that in the past led to using drugs, addicts can reduce their power; they recognize that they don't have to lead to use. Sometimes recognition isn't enough, though. Addicts must learn to consciously change their thought patterns or actively choose a constructive behavior.

One cognitive therapy focuses on recognizing and changing maladaptive thoughts. Research has shown that people with depression, for example, think of themselves as incapable, unlikable, unlovable — "I'm a worthless person," "I'm hopeless," "They think I'm disgusting and they're right," "I can't cope" — thoughts that perpetuate their depression. Addicts usually engage in similar defeatist self-talk. In cognitive therapy, people learn to identify these harmful thoughts, to become aware of when they're reinforcing their self-loathing and anxiety. They're trained to stop these negative thoughts or substitute them with positive ones. As a result, anxious and depressed moods, which are common triggers of drug use, can subside.

Cueing

Cueing occurs when an addict encounters a stimulus that triggers — *cues* — a cycle of intense craving that often ends in using. For example, addicts can feel intense craving when they're at a street corner they associate with drugs. Dopamine can begin pumping even when they see a photo of that corner. The heart rate and respiratory rate quicken, and they go into drug-seeking mode. Using PET scans and MRIs, researchers have recorded the brain activity addicts experience when they are

Diffuse anger   CBT

anticipating drugs. The scans showed that the parts of the brain that moderate behavior become subordinate to the pleasure-seeking center. "The craving caused by condition cues doesn't only come from a psychological association," researcher Ulrike Heberlein explains. "It has a biological basis."

Cues don't have to be as obvious as the sight of a street corner or the smell of pot. Emotions are potent cues. Drug-seeking behavior can be triggered by anger, disappointment, frustration, panic, stress, hunger, fatigue, or embarrassment — any emotion that the patient associates with the relief that can come from drugs. Some addicts associate drugs with sex, so anything from pornography to an intimate sexual situation can be a powerful trigger.

Addicts are taught to avoid these cues when possible. When the cues can't be avoided, the addicts learn to interrupt the cueing process before it leads to drug use. Sometimes recognizing the feelings is enough. Often, an addict, aware that the cue has been triggered, reaches a "choice point," as Dr. Rawson calls it, when he can select an alternative behavior to defuse the trigger. For example, he may go for a run to cool down. Or he may call a friend, therapist, counselor, or, if he's in AA, his sponsor. Or he may attend a Twelve Step meeting.

In a sense, CBT reprograms addicts so that they become inured (or at least less susceptible) to triggers, whether physical, sensory, or emotional. For the last, addicts can be taught to recognize, for example, escalating or sudden anger, to notice what causes it and how it feels, so they can defuse it. Once again, the idea is that the impulses that lead to behavior, including those that seem automatic or compulsive, can become conscious and can then be interrupted. Eventually, cues can be neutralized as the brain rewires itself, weakening their power.

Thought-Stopping

Triggers lead to drug use. Burn your finger on the stove, and you jerk your hand away. Encounter a trigger, and the craving hits. "From there you're on the bobsled ride," says Michael McCann, codirector of the Matrix Institute.

There's a visceral reaction to a thought, an emotion, a person, rubber band on wrist

place, or thing associated with drug use. Various versions of cognitive-behavior therapy begin similarly with training to help patients recognize a trigger at "the first inkling," McCann says. There are variations that mostly differ in the way that patients are trained to interrupt cues. As I've said, some focus on emotions rather than external triggers. Some train patients to tolerate the feelings — to accept them. When they do, the feelings dissipate. Some train patients to take active steps — call an AA sponsor, go for a run, or focus on some other preplanned activity. One therapy used by Matrix trains addicts to stop a craving by preempting it. The approach is called thought-stopping.

"The goal is to stop a craving before it has a chance to take over," McCann says. "When the thought hits, you don't start negotiating with it. You don't engage in an argument: 'I shouldn't.' 'I can't do it because of my family.' 'Maybe it's okay if I use just once.' 'Just a drink, nothing else.' The argument itself churns up the physical craving, because it itself is associated with using; it's a familiar pattern that hasn't worked before." Thought-stopping is designed, McCann said, "so it never gets that far." That is, patients learn how to stop the bobsled before it starts.

Thought-stopping is exactly what it sounds like: stopping the thought process that could lead to a full-blown craving. What works is different for different patients. At the first inkling, some Matrix patients literally say "Stop" out loud. "It can get to the point that that's enough," McCann says. One way to stop the process is by having the addict literally snap out of the unhealthy thoughts. An addict wears a rubber band on his wrist, and when he catches his mind wandering from the present, he snaps the band. Presumably the sudden physical sting takes a person out of his head and into his body, interrupting the cycle. It may be hard to believe that something so simple works, but clinical trials support the intervention. Other thought-stopping techniques: picturing a stop sign; imagining a switch going from on to off; pulling out a photograph of one's family. The instant the thought is stopped, it is replaced with an image: a meadow, ocean waves, the face of a loved one. Creating a new connection further interrupts the negative thought and redirects it. This form of CBT teaches those who are addicted that they're in control — they can nip a craving in the bud.

coping strategies

Dialectical-Behavior Therapy and Mindfulness

I've explained that anger, anxiety, sadness, feelings of being overwhelmed, and grief can be tied to using. With dialectical-behavioral therapy (DBT) and mindfulness therapy, addicts are trained to accept and tolerate the feelings rather than medicate them. Research has shown that mindfulness meditation, as one version of therapy is called, effectively interrupts cues. Addicts are taught to recognize and sit with their feelings — to experience them with curiosity and acceptance rather than react impulsively to them. This makes them better able to defuse their triggers.

To learn about their triggers, addicts may be given homework. They're told to chart their moods, responses to situations, and reactions. In individual and group therapy, they're also taught coping strategies — various ways to interrupt and divert the feelings that could lead to relapse. In addition, addicts learn to mentally prepare for situations that could trigger emotions. For example, an addict can prepare in advance for a meeting with her boss that's likely to make her angry, or a family gathering that will arouse feelings of guilt and anxiety. She imagines those feelings so that she can recognize and process them when they occur, accepting them but not reacting automatically to them as she would have when using. *I'm feeling angry. I knew I would. It's okay. I can tolerate it. From the past I know that the feeling will lessen and eventually disappear.* Similarly, an addict can recognize craving and learn to tolerate it too. *Here I go again. I'm dying for a drink. This feeling won't last either.*

In DBT, addicts may record their feelings between sessions to keep track of thoughts or behaviors counterproductive to staying sober. They write negative feelings down and analyze what sparked them. In therapy sessions, they examine their experiences and learn to respond to their anxiety, depression, or similar feelings and thoughts associated with drugs — the onset of craving. They can use mindfulness and similar practices — emotional regulation and distress tolerance are two — to dispel them. Over time, DBT and mindfulness help addicts refine their sensitivity and change their responses to emotional triggers so they can disable them.

Priming Therapy

In CBT, patients are trained to understand and interrupt another component of addiction, priming (as in priming a pump, when a small amount of water is used to start a steady flow). I've described the switch in an addict's brain that, once turned on by a drink or a hit of pot, can be almost impossible — without treatment — to switch off. The pump would be primed and that would be that: a full-on relapse would probably ensue. Priming therapy allows addicts to recognize what's happened — "I've relapsed!" — and interrupt the cycle. Instead of proceeding in their old patterns, they can reset the switch.

Scheduling and Skill Building

One benefit of inpatient programs is that they contain addicts in a safe environment where they're unlikely to relapse. In outpatient programs, there are no walls between patients and drugs, so there are limitless opportunities to score. If someone is in outpatient therapy for ten hours a week (it's often much less), he has 158 hours left in the week when he might relapse. Scheduling helps addicts manage those dangerous hours and keep relapse at bay.

In individual or group therapy, an addict writes down a detailed plan for the days until the next session. Patients are kept busy, focused, and safe, with a pattern of regular events that become, as Steve Shoptaw describes it, "scaffolding for a sober life." Scheduling is one success-oriented practical skill; others are time management and breaking tasks into manageable pieces.

The purpose of scheduling is straightforward. Idle hands are dangerous for addicts. An hour with nothing planned is an hour that could lead to relapse. Matrix's Jeanne Obert says that scheduling can include exercise, spending time with family or friends, and other healthy activities. She explains, "Follow the schedule and you won't relapse. It's a skill clients learn and can use later if/when they are feeling vulnerable. You use the rational part of your brain to do the schedule, so following it helps prevent the addicted brain taking over. Just don't allow your brain to operate on automatic or you risk relapse."

Adapting Therapy as Needed

Remarkably, behavioral change can lead to physiological change. Dr. David Shurtleff, acting deputy director at NIDA, explains, "The system is dynamic. There's synaptic plasticity. And neurons come and go. Stem cells continue to turn over in the brain. It's not a static system. The brain is constantly changing, forming new connections. Just as drug abuse leads to changes in the brain so that a person becomes wired for addiction, behavioral treatments change the brain so a person is less vulnerable to triggers." As addicts gain strategies and learn to respond differently to cues and priming, the brain is changing; new connections are strengthening. "You're putting in thicker brake pads," says Joseph Frascella, director of NIDA's Division of Clinical Neuroscience and Behavioral Research.

The various forms of CBT are closely related, and many therapists combine them. I saw this when I visited the West Los Angeles location of the Matrix Institute for an evening group therapy session. At 7:00, a dozen patients — Matrix calls them clients — filed into a nondescript building; it could have been an insurance company or a law office. They walked purposefully down a hallway and entered a rectangular office that had a desk cluttered with papers and books, a computer, a bookshelf, and a semicircle of cushioned chairs. They retrieved blue binders from the shelf and then sat. There was small talk. A woman said, "God, do I need to be here today." Another responded, "I hear you."

The walls were white, and slatted blinds were drawn so the only light came from a pair of floor lamps. A young man with a clipboard came in and nodded meaningfully at a few of the patients, who dutifully followed him out of the room to a bathroom, where, as required, they peed in cups — the program includes random drug testing.

The participants settled in when a woman in her late thirties entered. She had dark hair, bangs, squarish glasses, and looked a little like Lois Lane, or at least the actress who played her in the 1980s Superman movies. She turned out to be the group's therapist. I'll call her Ruth. She greeted her clients and took a seat.

At the previous session, Ruth had asked the group members how they'd feel about a journalist sitting in and observing a session, assuring them that their identities wouldn't be revealed. The patients assented, and at the first meeting I attended, she asked them to introduce themselves to me. There was a man who described himself as "an artist, alcoholic, addict — here by the skin of my teeth." There were coke addicts, alcoholics, two meth addicts, and three people who had been strung out on OxyContin, Vicodin, and other prescription medications. An attractive middle-aged woman introduced herself as a "banker and crack addict." She wore an Ann Taylor suit and matching heels. A male patient, muscular and athletic in bike pants and shoes, said he was a college professor addicted to heroin, but, he said, "I'll take what I can get." There was a dentist who said, "I'm a cliché. I started on nitrous oxide, a perk of my profession. But I took everything — pills, coke, ecstasy, weed, and lots of champagne."

The session began with Ruth checking in with the patients to see how they were doing and to learn if anyone had been struggling or if anything had come up since the previous session. Diane, a woman sitting on my right, spoke up. She was fortyish with sandy-blond hair parted in the middle. She wore a black T-shirt and jeans. She was a stay-at-home mother of three, a boy and two girls, from six to twelve years old.

She said she'd been having a particularly difficult time. She was, she said, "stressed — my mother, the kids, John [her husband] . . . It's been really hard." She looked up, surveyed the faces in the circle. "I love the kids, but sometimes it can be too much," she said. "You've all heard a lot about the problems I have with John. I'm sure you're sick of me complaining. It's been worse. He's been coming home angry — really angry." She was holding back tears. "He doesn't talk, has a couple drinks, watches TV, goes to sleep. He's been coming home really pissed off, always about something — someone else's fault, someone at the office. I ignore it as best I can, take care of the kids, get them to bed, but then it all comes out in the middle of the night, those thoughts — those thoughts are the strongest trigger for me. I freak out, and in the old days [I] would go downstairs and open a bottle of wine and you know how that goes. More wine. Dope. Then I'm wasted and freaking out because I had to get up with the kids, but it would be too late by then to stop. I'd be so fucked up I just kept getting high."

The central focus in the early-recovery Matrix groups is teaching the addicts the basic skill of thought-stopping, but therapists employ other treatment styles as needed. That is, though the Matrix program is run by the manual, its therapists respond to their clients' needs of the moment.

Ruth asked Diane to say more about what she was feeling in the middle of the night.

She thought a moment before answering. "My shrink just says it's depression, but I'm on Paxil and I tried Prozac and Celexa and Xanax. I'm just . . . It doesn't help. I get in these spirals." Her eyes drifted to the ceiling, then around the room, then to her folded hands on her lap. "My mind doesn't stop. I think about everything. It's like falling into a tunnel. I worry about the kids. John."

No, she hadn't been successful stopping the thoughts.

"When was the last time you saw your psychiatrist about your depression?" Ruth asked.

Diane said it had been a few months.

"Maybe it's time for you to check in, to talk about your depression, how it's managed, if everything's like it should be. It sounds as if it's been worse recently."

Then Ruth asked, "What happens when you experience those triggers in the middle of the night? Walk me through it."

Diane took off her glasses, rubbed her eyes, and sat quietly for moment.

"So say I'm up at night, and I start getting that feeling like I'm going down. I just want it to stop. I know that getting high will make it stop. Actually I'm not thinking, *Getting high will make it stop*. It's more of a hunger."

"Before that," Ruth said. "Before the hunger. Tell me more about the feeling of — you said you're 'going down.'"

"Yeah. If I succumb, I'll fall in." Diane stopped, put her glasses back on. She stared at her hands. Her fingernails were trimmed, painted pale pink. "I guess it starts in my head and goes right to my throat because it constricts, and I think I can't breathe."

"Your throat — it constricts?"

"Yeah, tight. And there's like this feeling of intense — I don't know. Panic, I guess. I'm breathing hard."

"What else do you notice?"

She said, "Mmmmm . . . my heart."

"You're breathing hard, and it feels like you can't breathe, and your heart is beating fast?"

"Yeah."

"What else happens?"

"What do you mean?"

"You're worried about whatever it is, and you're breathing fast or you worry that you can't breathe. Your heart is racing. What else?"

"My mind. One thing, the next. Work, the kids, John, my mom, the bills, the car. Money's tight now." She sat up straighter. I could see that Diane had become more anxious. Ruth noticed it too.

"Are you feeling that nervousness now?"

Diane nodded.

"Can you sit for a minute and feel what you're feeling? Pay attention. What's the feeling in your stomach? Your head? Your heart? What are you thinking? How does your chest feel? Your breathing? Get to know this feeling. Get comfortable with it. Recognize it."

Diane sat still, closed her eyes.

"Now slow down your breathing," Ruth said. "Just a little. Start with a slow deep breath. Feel what happens. Can you slow your heart down so it's not racing?"

A moment passed, then Diane opened her eyes. "I slowed it down." She looked calmer, even a little excited. She had glimpsed something.

"The next time you wake up in the middle of the night, Diane, try not to run away from what's happening. Stop it if you can. If you can't stop it, you can stay with it, pay attention to it. Think, *Okay, here it goes. Here it comes. Let's watch it come, watch it take over. What am I feeling?* Feel it. Take a breath. Tell yourself, *Okay. The kids are asleep. They're okay.* One thing at a time. *Ah, I know this feeling in my chest. And there's my heart going.* Take a deep breath. What else is going on in your head? *Money's tight.* Feel the breathing quicken, the heart beating. Sit with it. Take a deep breath. Feel things calm down. Take another deep breath. See if you can let the anxiety go. Think, *This isn't about money. It's not about the kids. It's about me — the way I freak myself out. It's what makes me use, but I'm okay. It's okay to feel scared like this. I can deal with it. It'll go away.* Pay attention. Feel what's going on in your body and listen to what's going on in your head. There's an entire book-length monologue going on in there between the trigger — that worry, that anxiety — and using. The self-talk winds you up and you get tense and scared and your heart races. Get inside that book, examine each page, read them, sit with them, examine the feeling in your head and your heart and your chest and your legs and get inside the book page by page — and it's not as overwhelming if you're looking at a page at a time — and breathe, and keep breathing, and pay attention, and you'll see that the self-talk changes, and you relax. What do you think?"

Diane said she'd try; it made sense. But she didn't know if she could do it.

"That's okay," Ruth assured her. "It takes time to change, but change comes."

To the group Ruth said, "It's not only addicts who are controlled by visceral responses to fear or a smell or a scene in a movie. Everyone is. It's just more dangerous for addicts. But you don't have to be controlled by craving. You can change your reaction to the craving and then it's not in control of you, you are in control of yourself. Breathe through it. Sometimes that's enough. Think, *I can help it go away,* and you can. You can't control the universe, but you can control your breath." This reflects something McCann said: "Addicts feel they can't control their addiction. That feeling of being out of control terrifies them, but they can learn to be in control."

Ruth continued, "Take that slow, deep breath. Sometimes that's enough. Sometimes it isn't. If it isn't, what can you do?"

Near Diane, a man named Bob — a bond trader — said, "That's when you call your sponsor. . . . Or when I feel it, I throw myself into doing something. It almost doesn't matter what. Not sitting there banging my head against the wall."

A girl said, "Go to a meeting, go to a movie, go see friends. I just go as far from dope as I possibly can."

Ruth asked, "What else can you do?"

A young girl — she'd said she was a student — suggested, "Just get out of bed and go watch TV. Because it takes a while but then I'm into whatever's on — it doesn't matter, some stupid show. But it gets you out of your head."

"That can work too," Ruth said. "You interrupt the train. Stop it. Change it at one of those . . ."

"Switch stations," another girl said.

"Yes. Diane? You're a runner. What happens when you run? How do you feel? Do you feel like using?"

"If it's during the day, maybe I'd go for a run, but in the middle of the night I can't."

"In the middle of the night, what can you do to interrupt the train, change its course?"

A man said, "Just take a shower. Call someone. Make a sandwich."

A woman who hadn't spoken before said, "I freak out at night sometimes too. I get up and clean the house. I get tired and go back to sleep, and in the morning I have the cleanest damn house."

Diane said, "I think just getting up, moving around, might be enough. Or sit in the living room and do the breathing."

"Try it. See what works. Let us know."

Referring to their binders, patients talked about their triggers and their success preempting them — stopping them — or their inability to stop them. The triggers they listed included beer commercials, the smell of chemicals (on a client's construction job), "worry about my kids," "anywhere near where I'd meet my dealer," stress, sadness, anger.

Diane said, "It's a minefield."

"What is?" a man named Jack asked.

"Life."

When Rosalyn, the crack-addicted banker, spoke, the session again veered in a new direction. She was concerned about the coming weekend, when she was obligated to go to an office party. "I'm heading into a room full of triggers on Friday night," she said. "They'll all be gathered there waiting, like an ambush. Pretty freaked out about it."

Someone asked if her colleagues at work knew she was an addict.

"Tell them I go home at night and turn on the TV and smoke crack?"

"Can you make an excuse?"

"I have clients I had to invite. I can't not show up. They're big clients."

The bond trader said, "Sometimes, you may have to make choices between two things that are important. You weigh them. 'I have to go to the office party.' 'If I go to the office party, I'm going to relapse.' It becomes pretty clear. The office party? Dying?"

"Maybe there are other choices too," Ruth said. "Can you think of any?"

Rosalyn said, "I think about just calling in sick, but it would be pretty bad. And what about next time? These parties, work dinners . . . They happen all the time."

Ruth spoke directly to Rosalyn. "Let's assume you decide you need to go this time. What can you do to go to the party and make sure that when you come here on Monday you'll test clean? Tell me what you see when you walk into the room and the party's going on. What do you see? And pay attention to what it feels like."

Rosalyn described the party — walking into the room, the sparkling lights, the lively talk, the music. She listed the triggers as she saw them in her mind. "Of course, the martinis and bottles of Chivas . . ." She looked at Ruth. "Talk about triggering a craving."

"Now?"

"When I imagined that Chivas. On the rocks."

"But look," Ruth said. "You're sitting here and you're okay. You can stop the thought before the craving is triggered. What happens next at the party?"

"The main thing is pressure — my bosses, the clients, worrying about the booze."

"Feel what your body's doing," Ruth instructed. "Be aware of what's happening in your head."

Diane interjected, "Can you just go, make an appearance, do what you have to do, and leave?"

Ruth asked, "What do you think, Rosalyn?"

"Maybe I can."

"That's part of the scheduling work we do," Ruth explained. "Scheduling isn't just about getting group to group or lunch to dinner. It's planning how you'll navigate a party or Thanksgiving dinner with relatives or a night when you're on your own at home. If you make a plan and stick to it, you should be fine. You walk into the room, you get yourself a glass of mineral water so you have something familiar in your hand, you speak to the people you have to speak to, pay attention to everything you're thinking and feeling, stop dangerous thoughts, breathe, and get out of there when you can . . ."

Rosalyn shrugged. "We'll see."

"Try it. Let us know how it goes on Monday."

Next the rest of the group focused on their scheduling. Clients wrote down detailed agendas, planning their time until the next group session. The session ended and the clients filed out, and Ruth smiled at Rosalyn. "Good luck," she said.

Contingency Management

CBT helps addicts become conscious of cueing (triggers) or a relapse (that initiates priming), and trains them to stop the thoughts or defuse them. MI helps addicts imagine long-term rewards—they envision life clean—and short-term rewards can be an effective tool too. Found mostly in outpatient programs, contingency-management therapy utilizes rewards that keep an addict from using for a brief period, a few days or a week or possibly from one therapy session to the next. Clinical trials have shown that addicts respond to even modest rewards and that CBT works even better when contingency management is added. It works for adults, and it can be particularly helpful for teens, who may have a hard time envisioning the long-term future. In a clinical trial, patients who earned vouchers (which were exchanged later for gift certificates) for clean urine samples did far better than those without those incentives. "It's hard to believe that a McDonald's gift certificate can outweigh the intense pull of drugs, but it can help," said John Roll, associate dean of the College of Nursing at Washington University, who has studied contingency management. He explained that the reward itself may be less significant than the offer of a specific, short-term, and achievable goal.

Group Therapy

Almost everyone in recovery will encounter group therapy at some point. Research confirms that it can be useful, but not in all cases. Experts say that groups shouldn't substitute for individual sessions—because every patient is dealing with individual issues and progressing at his or her own pace—but many programs have few if any one-on-one sessions. One reason is cost. In an hour, a therapist can see a single patient in individual therapy, or a dozen or more in group therapy. However, individual therapy is a critical component of treatment, especially for patients who feel nervous in groups and are more comfortable opening up in one-on-one therapy. Feedback and encouragement from others in a group can be components of effective therapy, but for some people, especially teenagers, some forms of group work can be harmful. Adolescents may be intimidated in group settings. If they are, they may feel inadequate and retreat farther inside themselves, winding up more depressed or anxious—the opposite feelings from the ones they need at this point in their recovery. Therapists must carefully choose group members who will help rather than threaten or intimidate one another. I've sat in on group sessions where some participants listened passively while addict after addict told horror stories about drug use. Sometimes the descriptions of drug use seemed to do little more than trigger craving. "These kids are sometimes put in groups of other patients who have more serious problems, and there's the risk of contagion," Sharon Levy of Boston Children's Hospital explains. "Take a group of kids who want to be in recovery and introduce a kid who doesn't and is still using, talking about how great it is, and other kids will flip." Similarly, Dr. Onken warns against a sort of gang effect in which the poor attitude or behavior of some kids causes others to think or act the same way.

Other forms of group therapy can backfire with adolescents too. In some, patients are encouraged, or even manipulated, to tell stories about traumatic events or unhealthy relationships in their lives. In individual therapy, revisiting trauma can be therapeutic, but in groups, it can increase an adolescent's stress and anxiety, which can also fuel the desire to use.

The biggest problem with group therapy is that some therapists don't know what they're doing. Their lack of expertise prevents them from recognizing when patients are becoming overwhelmed, depressed, or traumatized anew. In some groups, counselors not only fail to protect patients from others in the group but bully and humiliate patients themselves.

That said, while studies have shown that some forms of group therapy can negatively affect kids, other studies have shown that peer-group therapy or positive peer culture is an effective treatment when it's carefully monitored and directed by a therapist. Jeanne Obert points out that group therapy can be effective for teens when "they bond to the group, and form relationships within the group." In the hands of skilled therapists, groups that use EBTs can create a supportive, therapeutic environment with positive rather than negative peer pressure, a place where kids help and learn from one another. They may respond especially well to praise and affirmation in a group setting. Addicts who have been isolated from friends and family may be driven by a yearning for connection. They desire and are motivated by the acceptance they feel within the group.

I witnessed a therapy session for teenagers when I visited Hazelden's youth facility in Plymouth, an hour away from the main Hazelden campus in Center City, Minnesota. The purpose of the group was to get kids to become conscious of the impact of their drug use on their lives. The style was open, what Jim Steinhagen, executive director of youth and young adult services at Hazelden, described as traditional group therapy, which evolves as patients evolve and their needs change; the goal is to address whatever issues are relevant at the moment. "The power of effective adolescent groups is the interaction among peers," explained Rebecca Keithahn, the counselor who led the group. She took a back seat — she asked questions, guided the patients, but encouraged them to have a dialogue among themselves.

Patients in the adolescent program are between fourteen and twenty-five years old, but the kids in the group I visited were on the younger side of that range. When they introduced themselves, I learned that most were there because of an addiction exclusively to pot — anyone who says marijuana isn't addictive should talk to these kids. Indeed, in spite of a basketball net outside and other recreational facilities, it wasn't summer camp; those kids had all suffered devastating consequences from their pot smoking , and most had tried to stop but couldn't. Steinhagen said, "These kids are pretty well traumatized by the time they get here. They've been through it. They come in stigmatized, but here it's about dignity and respect."

Most of the boys were dressed similarly. One had Kurt Cobain hair falling in a curtain over his eyes. There was a stocky boy with black buzzed hair and a seriousness that made him seem older. Lots of T-shirts, ragged; big jeans on most; big sneakers, some untied.

Keithahn listened closely as the patients spoke about the ways drugs affected their lives. The boys told the kinds of stories you'd expect to hear — experimentation turning to consistent use turning to addiction. Problems in school (some were expelled). Problems at home (one boy was kicked out of his home and now lived with grandparents). Some had been arrested for using or selling. One was arrested because he'd struck his mother ("It just happened. I lost it. I felt real bad").

Some hadn't experienced such dramatic calamities. One said, "I just couldn't stop. No shit. You think, *I'm not an addict. I can quit. I just like it. I'll stop when I feel like it.* But you don't quit. Then you're like smoking every day."

Another boy said, "For me, there was one thing that happened that bothers me. I have no memory." He added, "It's really a drag."

"I know what you mean," another boy said.

"I . . ." A boy wearing a T-shirt with a picture of Bob Dylan jumped in and then paused. Scanned the room to be sure he had an audience. "Ah, fuck . . . I forget."

There was laughter.

It was a freeform discussion, though Keithahn jumped in now and then to keep it focused and encourage quieter kids to participate. A boy said, "Yeah, then there's the breathing thing—I had bronchitis all the time. I know it was related because it's gone now that I'm not smoking."

A boy with long auburn hair parted in the middle said that another result of smoking was burning through money. "I thought, *Aw, it's cheap,* but when you're smoking every day it's not cheap unless you're getting shwag [low-grade pot]. So you run out of money and you have to figure out how to get more, and there was always more in my mom's purse. She never suspected. Even now."

There were nods of assent. He wasn't the only one who had stolen from his parents.

"I never had a problem with money," said a boy in torn jeans and a white T-shirt. "My main thing was just that I stopped caring about shit."

Keithahn said, "Talk more about that. What's that feel like? What does it mean not to care?"

"Pretty bad. I mean . . ."

Another boy said, "Depressed."

"Yeah."

"I cared when I was high, I guess. That's why I kept doing it."

"It wasn't that you cared," the other boy said. "You didn't notice that you didn't care."

"Weed's a depressant," said a boy on the opposite side of the circle. "I'm on like forty antidepressants and I'm smoking a depressant."

The others nodded.

The boys continued talking.

One of the patients took it upon himself to speak to a boy who hadn't said anything. "What about you, man? What happened to you? You've been pretty aloof the whole time you've been here. I mean, not participating."

Keithahn watched closely. The boy who'd been addressed had long, unkempt hair. He fixed a stare at the floor. When he glanced up for a minute, it was clear that below the hair, he was Brad Pitt handsome. But he had an angry glare.

A boy in a V-neck sweater said, "Yeah, you don't really contribute to groups."

Another boy said, "I think you're holding back."

Keithahn seemed to be gauging the situation, deciding if she should intervene.

Clearly the boy didn't like the attention. He looked down again and began rocking back and forth in his chair.

The boy who'd first addressed him said, "But even when we're doing work . . . Like you aren't even here."

"So what is it, man?" another boy asked. "What's said here stays here. I mean, we're all here because of shit we've done."

The boy kept looking down, and now he wasn't just rocking; he was vibrating. He mumbled, almost whispered, "Nothing. I was just sent here. My stepfather didn't want me so here the fuck I am. I'm a bad influence. My little stepsister and brother."

Another said, "I hear that. I have a stepmom. She's on my case. She looks at me like I'm a total fuck-up. And she never says shit to her own kids who are, like, brats, ransacking the house."

The other boy was vibrating more, as if he were freezing to death. He said, "It's just that bitch is why I'm here. My dad's pussy-whipped, never says anything. . . . They're all so fucking paranoid since I tried to kill myself."

There was quiet.

The boy was rocking and vibrating and the other boys were looking down, but then one looked at him and said, "Holy shit, I'm sorry. Why'd you do it?"

He didn't answer.

Keithahn asked the boy, "How're you doing?"

No answer.

A boy said, "Who the fuck hasn't tried to kill themself. I mean, we're here, aren't we? Welcome to the fucking club."

Another said, "I was fucking trying to kill myself. Just the slow way. By using."

He asked, "How'd you do it?"

The boy didn't respond at first, just sat there shaking, and then, still looking downward, he said, "Gonna jump. I was at the bridge. Just ready to go. To fly off."

"What happened?"

"Some girl, just some girl." It was difficult to understand him. He was speaking in a dark monotone. "I didn't know her; she come up and ask me what's going on, and how do I get to some place, and I'm looking at her like *What the fuck,* and she looks like she realizes she's talking to a psycho, and she goes off, and I didn't jump."

He was noticeably relieved when the attention turned away from him. Slowly he shook less. Slowly he stopped rocking. There was a feeling of relief, as if a bomb had been defused.

Soon the meeting ended. The boys had free time until dinner.

As I walked out with Keithahn, I asked her about the research I'd read that said that some forms of group therapy are counterproductive for kids — they influence one another negatively, and some kids are intimidated. I asked if she was worried about the boy who'd confessed that he'd almost taken his own life. She responded, "You have to stay right there with them. You have to protect them. But for kids, there's nothing like peer support. That was hard, but it was the beginning of a bond between [that boy] and the others. Sometimes they seem hard, but they're good kids. There's compassion. They come to care for each another and support each other. Most of them."

Steinhagen explained that these kids are among "safe peer groups, which they'd probably never known. It's not just safe because these kids aren't using. They can be vulnerable with these peers. Many of these kids never have had genuine relationships because they've been high for so long."

Given the research that shows that kids are much more interested in what other kids are saying and thinking than in what adults are saying and thinking, it makes sense that they'd be affected by their peers in group therapy sessions. "They see themselves in each other," Keithahn said. "They learn from each other. They support each other over time and inspire each other."

Part of it may be that they become acclimated to being with peers in settings that encourage their self-reflection and camaraderie — so they aren't running as many yellow lights.

As I left the building, I saw the boy from the group — the one who had tried to kill himself — in a lounge, curled up on a couch, playing a guitar. Another of the boys, this one reading a comic book, sat beside him.

Family Involvement in Treatment

Before it was understood that families contribute to both addiction and recovery, there was an accepted division of responsibility. Addicts were the ones with problems, so it was the addicts who needed to be "fixed." To cope with the stresses of living with an addict, the family may have needed therapy or Al-Anon, but they weren't part of an addict's recovery.

This began to change when practitioners observed that many addicts who did well in programs relapsed when they returned to their home environments. Some reasons for this were obvious. Particularly when they're in early recovery, addicts find it difficult to remain sober when they go home to live with spouses, parents, or other relatives who use and abuse drugs. Triggers are everywhere. But it turned out to be more complicated than that. Stress — whatever form it takes — is a trigger. If a recovering addict returned to a stressful family environment, one that contributed to his addiction in the first place, relapse was likely. If relationships were improved, though, addicts would benefit.

The progress an addict makes in treatment can be hindered or undermined or even reversed if family dynamics don't change too. This is why, when it's possible, family therapy should be part of addiction treatment. It isn't always possible, of course, and it's important to say that family involvement isn't a requirement; addicts who don't have families or whose families won't or can't participate can get well too. It's also important to point out that there's therapeutic value in family therapy for an addict no matter what form a family takes. "Anyone who is instrumental in providing support, maintaining the household, providing financial resources, and with whom there is a strong and enduring emotional bond may be considered family for the purposes of therapy," according to a SAMHSA report on the efficacy of family therapy in addiction treatment.

Addicts with family support may feel less stress than those whose families aren't available. Not only are they less isolated — and isolation can be a trigger — their families encourage them, offering positive reinforcement for their progress. Supported by their loved ones, addicts may be better able to weather times of doubt, fear, or illness that could otherwise cause them to abandon treatment or relapse. Also, addicts can learn about themselves through their families, even when there's dysfunction, which there often is.

In groups, addicts' parents, siblings, spouses, and other family members are educated about the disease of addiction and the ways families unwittingly contribute to it. They're helped to understand and change destructive dynamics. In family therapy, members learn to treat one another and react to one another differently. They work to improve communication — to listen better, express their feelings — and set boundaries. Behavioral therapies are used to train people to anticipate, recognize, acknowledge, and interrupt old patterns that lead to stress, guilt, and other emotions that contribute to drug use.

The family — whatever form and however many members — is a system of interdependent components. It can be almost impossible to change one component if they don't all shift. Family therapy can make that happen. However, while there's almost always a possibility of positive change, some families can't be changed — family members won't participate in treatment, are incapable of changing, are using. Addicts can learn other ways to change their environment. They may need to move; live separately, possibly in sober-living situations; change jobs; or even cut ties to certain family members, if only for a while.

Family Therapy After Divorce

Families can contribute to drug use, and so can the dissolution of families. The increased risk that divorce entails does not mean that parents should stay together for their kids' sake, though it does mean that parents (and society as a whole) can't pretend any longer that what's good for the parents is automatically good for the kids. In some circumstances, contrary to the conventional wisdom, parents *should* stay together for the kids. Of course, it's not always possible or advisable. When it isn't, it's critical that divorcing parents acknowledge the fact that most divorces traumatize kids. Difficult divorces — contentious, angry, volatile ones in which one or both parents fall apart — are even more likely to cause kids the sort of trauma that can lead to drug use.

Divorcing or divorced parents may no longer consider themselves a family, but they must understand they are still their child's family. Doctors have said that unless a patient's therapist or counselor advises against it, both parents should participate in treatment. After their parents' divorce, kids often harbor resentments about the arguments they heard, about being made to take sides, about feeling ignored, abandoned, unsafe, and alone. Problems for children of divorce can be compounded when parents remarry and there are stepparents and stepsiblings in the mix. Kids already reeling from their parents' divorce can be traumatized anew when they're forced into a situation with more complicated family dynamics. Second families can ultimately be strong and nurturing systems for the children, but parents must acknowledge the stress and potential harm — and understand that well after they've settled into their new lives, trauma lingers in their children. No matter how they feel about each other, divorced parents must keep in mind that they have a common goal: to save their child's life.

The Multisystemic Approach

People don't live in vacuums, which is why treatment should, when possible, involve family. But families don't exist in vacuums either. They live in a complex system that includes many people and institutions. What's called a multisystemic approach (or MST, for multisystemic therapy) can be an effective component of addiction treatment, particularly for children. It's used in primary outpatient treatment and outpatient treatment (or aftercare) that follows residential programs.

The theory behind MST is simple. Just as it's hard for a person to stay sober if he returns to a family with dysfunction, it's also hard if he returns to a neighborhood or situation (school, the workplace) where his drug use began and escalated — unless the system is altered; improving it is the goal of the multisystemic approach. In MST, as many people in the child's life as possible are enlisted to help. Teachers, coaches, extended family, friends, neighbors, coworkers, family physicians, and others in the addict's life are informed about a person's drug problem and asked to keep watch, offer support, provide feedback, and be allies in a sort of full-court press of treatment. An MST therapist visits a child at home or school and is on call twenty-four hours a day, seven days a week. The therapist works with parents or other caregivers and trains them to help a child's recovery and handle problems when they arise. He helps a child cope with family, peers, and school or work. The therapist and caregiver work together to encourage and guide a child to get involved with positive and healthy activities and peers. The therapist visits the family regularly, possibly once a week, to work with them. He may check in with teachers or other important figures in a child's life. In one study, kids who were treated with MST had a quarter of the drug use that kids who participated in "treatment as usual" approaches did. It's also been shown that kids who are treated with MST improve their grades, exhibit less "problem behavior," are less likely to get into legal trouble, and have "greater family cohesion."

Therapies in Combination

The above list of treatments is by no means exhaustive. There are dozens of other forms of therapy, including art therapy, trauma therapy, anger management, work with life coaches, and a range of therapies designed to treat co-occurring illnesses. Usually treatments work in concert with one another. "The data show that the best drug addiction treatment approaches attend to the entire individual, combining the use of medications, behavioral therapies, and attention to necessary social services and rehabilitation," Dr. Shoptaw says. Whatever the combination of treatments, the specifics and mix should be monitored and modified over time. Many traditional rehabs and aftercare programs repeat the same schedules for weeks, but they should be adjusted as a patient moves forward (or backward) in his treatment. Clean time predicts more clean time, but there are points during treatment when addicts may regress. A general rule: ramp up what works, and gradually introduce more advanced (that is, cognitively demanding) treatments. Adjust medication and EBTs as needed. And remember, treating addiction isn't like treating other diseases. There's nothing straightforward about it. We try one thing. If it doesn't work, we try another. Steve Shoptaw points out that our brains are "not hydraulic machines. We can't just pull a lever. Sometimes the only way to learn is to do."

13

Treating Drug Problems with Drugs

USING MEDICATION TO TREAT some psychiatric illnesses — schizophrenia, for example — is accepted as standard and essential. Confusion and criticisms are understandable about using medication to treat addiction. First, prescription drugs are the nation's fastest-growing category of abused substances, so there's concern that they'll create, not treat, addicts. In addition, according to many reports, psychiatric medications are overprescribed in general. Pharmaceutical companies cash in on the use and misuse of prescription medication. In fact, they may even benefit from the War on Drugs, because there's no war on their drugs. And even when taken as directed, some medications still have risks. For example, one report linked methadone, a common treatment for opiate addiction, to suicide. Another report discussed a relationship between suicide and SSRIs, a class of antidepressants sometimes used in conjunction with addiction treatment.

Many traditional drug-and-alcohol counselors oppose using medication to treat addiction on principle. They believe, as I've frequently heard rehab counselors say, "You don't treat drug problems with drugs," not only because some addicts abuse some of these medications but because medication itself is anathema in certain interpretations of AA and the Twelve Steps. These people assert that a person on medication isn't sober.

However, none of these objections outweighs the incontrovertible evidence that drugs help treat some addictions. A variety of medications, when prescribed, monitored, and adjusted by a good psychiatrist, in combination with behavioral therapies, dramatically up the odds of successful treatment. For many addicts, the impact of medications can be profound — even lifesaving. And for myriad addicts with concurrent mental illnesses, drugs can be essential.

Some of the same medications that help during detox can be part of primary care. Some inhibit cravings, and some treat the symptoms that come with sobriety following intense and consistent drug use. Some replacement drugs not only reduce cravings but act as deterrents; they block certain drugs from attaching to receptors, thereby preventing the drugs from triggering a high if they're taken. Other medications interact with alcohol and cause people who drink to become violently ill, which can be an effective deterrent. In addition, medications can treat the concurrent and underlying problems, including anxiety, depression, and other disorders, that cause or contribute to addiction. If these problems go untreated, patients will be less able to participate in many therapies.

It's true that pharmaceutical companies fuel the proliferation of addiction medications. The companies are motivated — it's a growing multibillion-dollar business — and they fund research and clinical trials. But Big Pharma's efforts aren't the reason that psychopharmacology has become standard practice when treating some addictions. The reason is: it works. "To become widely practiced, an innovation has to be substantially better than the old practice," Rick Rawson of UCLA said. "Not marginally better, but demonstrably better." Some addiction medications are *profoundly* better.

It's important to emphasize that even the most effective medication isn't treatment in and of itself. If only it were; taking medication is easier than going to therapy. But research confirms that medications are more effective when used in combination with behavioral treatments. The team approach advocated by pediatrician Holmes is an effective model in which psychiatrists providing and monitoring medication work closely with therapists providing CBT and other treatments.

Medication for Opiate Abuse

Methadone was the first medication developed to decrease drug abuse, and it's still one of the most effective. It attaches to the opiate receptors, thereby preventing withdrawal and easing craving in heroin addicts. Tom McLellan explains, "It's extremely inexpensive and produces substantial reductions in opiate use. There are other benefits, such as it's been shown to reduce crime, violence, and self harm. It's a public health benefit because it reduces the number of IV drug users who inject opiates and are at risk of AIDS."

Those who use methadone are five times more likely than those who don't to be sober after a year. "From a clinical perspective, few practitioners experience the satisfaction of participating in a process that restores and enhances quality of life to the extent seen in methadone treatment," J. T. Payte, cochairman of the Committee on Opioid Agonist Treatment, wrote in a review, "Regarding Methadone Treatment." "After more than thirty years, I marvel at the corrective properties of methadone on the human brain as seen in the wonderful changes that occur."

Methadone sometimes causes drowsiness, nausea, and, rarely, serious side effects, including seizures, and using it does entail replacing one addiction with another. But a methadone addiction managed by a doctor is far less harmful than a heroin addiction. For one thing, unlike heroin, methadone rarely causes blackouts, and it doesn't impair cognition and judgment the way heroin does. People can function normally while on methadone. If people have immediate adverse reactions to the drug (they're rare), they're usually in a clinic where they're being monitored. (Most clinics require addicts to stick around for a period of time after they take their daily dose. Doctors say that if they don't, they should.)

Though methadone has received more scientific scrutiny and evaluation than any other medical treatment for addiction, it remains highly controversial, and not only because it's addictive. It can be difficult to wean addicts off it. In a relatively small number of cases, withdrawal from methadone has landed people in ERs, and in extremely rare cases, it's been fatal. Also, addicts can get high on methadone if they take large doses or mix it with medications like Xanax and Valium. It can also be lethal in those combinations or at some doses. Another serious concern are reports of suicide linked to methadone use, but it's rare. Still, those on methadone maintenance should periodically be examined for mental and physical health issues. Generally, according to Dr. Dave McCann, associate director in NIDA's Division of Pharmacotherapies and Medical Consequences of Drug Abuse, "If you compare opiate addicts not in treatment, the mortality rate is unbelievably different, and not just from overdose, but gunshot wounds and other violence. Treatment is related to lower HIV rates; lower mortality; less crime — if you're not trying to get money for drugs all the time, you're much less likely to commit crime. There are lower incarceration rates. If you had a drug that decreased mortality in cancer at the same rate as methadone does with addicts, everyone would say it was a miracle drug."

To get a sense of what's involved in methadone maintenance, I spent a day at the Matrix Institute's clinic on Washington Boulevard in Los Angeles. It's housed in a two-story medical building under a sign with a caduceus. Patients entered and registered at the counter in a waiting room that looked like one in a typical doctor's office. A man wearing a motorcycle jacket rocked nervously on a black leather couch. A woman near him couldn't sit still. She moved from one couch to another, shuddering, pulling at her stringy brown hair. Another guy wore a grimy WIDE LOAD T-shirt, which described him — he filled half of a couch. I learned that some of the patients were employed or in school, and a few appeared to be middle class — including an eighteen-year-old who took up heroin after becoming addicted to the OxyContin he was prescribed for a high-school football injury — but some were clearly indigent. Sitting in the office, a man named Michel, with slicked-back hair and paper-white skin, told me that he was back "in" after a couple days gone "out," when he'd relapsed on junk. He said he relapsed because he was living with a drug dealer who had bags of heroin lying around the house, and sobriety was, he said, "impossible." Then he nodded, stood, and got in line at a window. He could have been queuing up to see a bank teller. This teller, though, was a nurse who handed him a tiny paper cup containing his dose of methadone in a cherry-flavored syrup.

I've indicated that experts say that methadone treatment should be accompanied by therapy, and this program requires its patients to attend sessions. As I learned when the group filed into a small conference room, there can be a downside to mandatory treatment groups. Though some were willing and engaged participants, others clearly weren't. The man in the WIDE LOAD T-shirt slept through most of the session. A few got up and left. One left and returned twice. Later I asked the group's therapist, Kenneth, why that was allowed, and he said, "We're here to help people who need it, when they need it. You can focus on the fact that they left the meeting or the fact that they were present for half of it. Maybe next time, or the next, they'll be in a frame of mind to become engaged, and we can help them more." His optimism is evidence-based. Research has shown that heroin addicts who come to therapy groups while they're on methadone are more likely to stay on the medication and less likely to relapse.

There were a dozen people in this session, four men and eight women. Patients introduced themselves. Kenneth, a veteran psychologist, looked out of place in his white shirt, necktie, gray pants, and loafers. There was a period of checking in — basically, the clients told him how they were doing, a range of reports from "Awright" to "It's been a shitty, fucked-up week." The rest of the meeting was devoted to CBT, a discussion of cues and scheduling. Michel, whom I'd met in the waiting room, seemed bored. He slumped over, looked down. When it was his turn to talk, he just kept looking down, didn't say anything for a while. Finally he told the group about his living situation: that he was living with a dealer. "I go home to a place where there are a couple lines on the coffee table and needles and dope on the kitchen counter."

After explaining his predicament, he seemed slightly more animated, and he listened intently when another member of the group, a thirtyish woman who'd been a nurse before she got addicted to H and lost her job and children, told him to "get the fuck out of there." The therapist didn't respond. Though triggers can be neutralized over time through intensive cognitive-behavioral therapy, it's safer to avoid them. It's obvious that an alcoholic, especially in early recovery, should stay away from bars, especially ones where he drank. And clearly an addict should stay away from an apartment where a roommate is dealing and people are shooting up in the living room. Methadone should help protect Michel — the physical craving should be dampened. But it would be a hazardous situation for any addict.

Kenneth tried to get Michel to reach his own conclusion that he had to move out. He used a kind of MI technique, guiding him with open-ended questions. Michel responded, "I know I gotta get the fuck out of there." There was an impediment, though. Michel said he had no money, nowhere else to go. A girl, Lily, dressed neatly in a blouse and jeans, posed a question that got him thinking. "Do you think maybe it's better to sleep anywhere else, maybe a shelter, than die?"

At first, Michel looked hurt, as if he'd been attacked, but then he seemed fearful. "Yeah, I know," he said. His eyes watered. "I don't know what to do."

Kenneth asked, "What might you do to find a place that's safe for you?"

The man looked dumbfounded — he didn't know. "Maybe someone in the office here" — Kenneth named a colleague — "can help you find a shelter where you can stay for a while. I think she can hook you up with something. There's permanent housing out there — public housing, a halfway house . . . where it's safe."

The group moved on to a discussion about conditioned cues. Other than the man who slept through most of the session, and despite the comings and goings of a few, the group was focused.

"For me, the biggest trigger is anger. I get pissed off, I want to get high."

"Anger's it for me too. I get mad and I want to use. If I just shut up about how I'm feeling, I want to use, or if I blow up, I want to use."

"Does anger get you high? No. Your actions get you high."

"If anger forced you to get high, everyone in the world would be getting high."

"I just have to face facts. Everything's a trigger for me — the street, the smell of weed, a hot summer day, a cold foggy day, a woman who looks like an old girlfriend, beer ads, cigarettes . . . The only reason I don't relapse is coming here. That's the only reason."

"I hear that. I don't feel the triggers now. Because of the methadone — I went off it about a year ago and I was wasted again in a couple days. The craving was right there, like lurking, waiting for a way in. I was instantly back into it — couldn't resist. So then I came here, got my dose, drank it down, and I was back pretty fast, and I haven't missed a day . . . It'll be a year next week."

There was more talk about triggers. Then, as at the West LA Matrix group, the final part of the meeting was devoted to scheduling. Clients were asked about their plans for the rest of the evening and accounted for their time until they returned to the clinic. The first order of business for Michel was clear: He was going to find somewhere to stay. The plan was too vague for the therapist. He pressed him. "What about tonight?" Michel looked up and blinked. Then he looked down at the floor. He shrugged. They made a plan together. He'd come back in the morning, when he could speak to someone about a sober-living house. But there was tonight to get through.

The meeting ended and as the patients were filing out, Kenneth asked Michel to stay for a minute. When the others were gone, he said, "I'll feel better if you sleep tonight at [a shelter]. It'll be easier for you to get back here in the morning. What do you think?"

Michel shook his head no. "I'll be okay."

And then he left.

Methadone has changed the prognosis for opiate addicts, but there are practical barriers to its use. One is that patients can get it only through a licensed methadone treatment center. This hurdle causes some patients to drop out of treatment and explains why there has been so much excitement about a relatively new drug that works similarly to methadone. Rawson calls it "the most important advance in the treatment of opiate addictions in thirty years."

The drug, buprenorphine, works similarly to methadone but has been shown to be less addictive and has fewer and less severe side effects. Another drug, naltrexone, can block heroin too, but it has some negative effects; for example, it has been linked to depression and dysphoria. However, in clinical trials, Suboxone, a combination of buprenorphine and a drug called naloxone, has been shown to be as or more effective than methadone and works similarly. If someone on Suboxone injects heroin, he feels little effect, because the opiate receptor is already occupied. Because the medications mimic the abused drug, a person doesn't experience withdrawal and there's less craving. The value of Suboxone in the treatment of some opiate addictions is so great that Dr. Shoptaw, who's otherwise conservative when it comes to pharmacology for addiction, says, "I won't treat opiate addicts unless they take Suboxone."

In November 2012, Maia Szalavitz reported that Hazelden was beginning to use Suboxone to treat opioid addicts. Hazelden medical director Marvin Seppala acknowledged, "This is a huge shift for our culture and organization." Szalavitz wrote, "Seppala is keenly aware of how dramatic this decision is for the organization, which once debated whether or not coffee was acceptable in its abstinence-based program . . . Driving the need for change is the sobering reality of what happens to patients addicted to prescription pain relievers—a growing segment of those in need of drug recovery—once they leave the Hazelden program. Within days of leaving the residential treatment facility, most were relapsing—and at least half a dozen have died from overdoses in recent years. It was time, Seppala argued, for a radical change."

Unlike methadone, Suboxone can be taken at home or work; it doesn't require daily visits to a clinic, the way methadone does. Another reason behind the growing popularity of Suboxone is the stigma surrounding methadone, which is associated with down-and-out addicts. "Anonymous1234," posting on an online forum, wrote, "I was on methadone maintenance for 5 years this time (clean from other drugs for 4 years) and I just switched to Suboxone . . . I switched off methadone b/c I got sick of going to a clinic all the time, putting up with the bull**** and everyone treating you like you are a worthless junkie, even if you are doing everything right and working the program."

As with any medication, there are risks. Suboxone has less abuse potential than methadone, but people can become addicted to it. When the drug is taken in large doses, it's possible to get high on it. There's also a black market for Suboxone. Still, in spite of these drawbacks, there's no arguing the high rates of sustained recovery for opiate addicts on Suboxone.

Even so, Suboxone and methadone remain controversial; as I've explained, some people feel strongly that an addiction's an addiction, and any drug use will inevitably lead to other drugs. However, the evidence simply doesn't support this, and I've met many people on Suboxone, methadone, and other medications who credit the drugs for the fact that they're living full, normal lives—indeed, for the fact that they're alive. "Do I want to be physically dependent on any drug?" a Suboxone user asked me. "No, but is it better than living on the streets? I function. I work. I'm there for my wife and kids."

Medication for Other Addictions

Methadone and buprenorphine are effective for treating opiate addiction, but there are not yet any medications that have been proven as effective for treating addictions to other drugs. There are, however, a variety of drugs that have been shown to be useful adjuncts to treatment.

Naltrexone is also used to treat alcohol addiction. Often sold under the brand name Vivitrol, it's been shown to reduce an alcoholic's craving. Naltrexone can also prevent minor slips from becoming full-blown binges. A medication called acamprosate (the brand name is Campral) sometimes reduces cravings, though it's not clear why. The drug may help stabilize the chemical imbalance caused by alcohol abuse. In any case, it can reduce the physical and emotional distress that come when alcoholics quit drinking. Another drug, Antabuse, makes patients sick if they drink alcohol; the drug blocks the body's ability to metabolize alcohol. These drugs benefit some, though not all, alcoholics. There are other drugs that have been shown to be promising adjuncts to the treatment of alcoholism. These include an anticonvulsant called topiramate; Baclofen, a muscle relaxant; ondansetron, an antiemetic; and a drug called gabapentin.

No medications have been found that effectively block the cravings or the highs caused by cocaine, marijuana, meth, or other drugs, but there's promising research and clinical trials that may lead to new pharmacological addiction treatments. Some researchers maintain that antidepressants can help recovering addicts, no matter what his or her drug(s) of choice, since depression is so prominent in the early stages of treatment.

Those who categorically reject the notion of taking drugs to treat drug addiction are mired in a misguided and dangerous form of fundamentalism. But it would be similarly misguided to believe that drugs alone can treat drug addiction. There's ample evidence to support what common sense tells us: for a disease that combines chemical and behavioral components, the best treatment for many addicts includes both medication and therapy.

14

Where Does AA Fit In?

In the wake of my spiritual experience there came a vision of a society of alcoholics, each identifying with and transmitting his experience to the next — chain style. If each sufferer were to carry the news of the scientific hopelessness of alcoholism to each new prospect, he might be able to lay every newcomer wide open to a transforming spiritual experience. This concept proved to be the foundation of such success as Alcoholics Anonymous has since achieved.

> — from a letter from Alcoholics Anonymous
> founder Bill Wilson to Carl Jung

So this purports to be a disease, addiction? A disease like a cold? Or like cancer? I have to tell you, I have never heard of anyone being told to pray for relief from cancer . . . So what is this? You're ordering me to pray? Because I allegedly have a disease? I dismantle my life and career and enter . . . treatment for a disease and I'm prescribed prayer?

> — David Foster Wallace, *Infinite Jest*

WHEN PEOPLE INITIALLY WANT HELP for their drug problems, many look to AA. Partly it's because they don't know what else to do; most think it's their only option. And often they're right; those bound for rehab are almost guaranteed to encounter AA and the Twelve Steps, because almost every existing treatment program is based on them. In many rehabs, the Twelve Steps are taught in lectures and reinforced and practiced in one-on-one meetings with counselors and in group therapy where addicts share their stories and offer one another feedback and support. In addition, in most rehabs, addicts are required to attend one or more AA meetings a day. In many programs, patients are educated in and helped to (sometimes forced to) practice the Twelve Steps. Twelve Step–based treatment isn't the only game in town, but it can seem that way, because it's so ubiquitous and because other options are so hard to come by. Almost all accredited or licensed programs — more than 90 percent of them — include AA, at least as an option.

Alcoholics Anonymous and the Twelve Steps were created in the 1930s by Bill Wilson, a failed stockbroker. Setting his sights on becoming a lawyer, he struggled through years of law school, but, as the oft-told story goes, he was too drunk to pick up his diploma. He got to know a physician named Robert Smith whose tales of drunkenness trumped Wilson's. He even admitted to performing surgery while drunk. Both of them had tried to stop drinking but hadn't been able to. They became known to those in the Program — AA — as Bill W. and Dr. Bob.

After a bender, Wilson admitted himself into Towns Hospital in New York, where alcoholics went to detox. This was Wilson's fourth time in the hospital. He was given hourly infusions of a hallucinogenic drug made from belladonna (also called deadly nightshade) combined with extracts of prickly ash and henbane, followed by castor oil. This belladonna cure was one of many unsuccessful attempts by physicians to help alcoholics detoxify. Another was the Keeley cure, which involved administering a "secret substance" that turned out to be a form of chlorine.

A friend of Wilson's, another longtime alcoholic, visited him in the hospital. After decades of unsuccessful attempts at getting sober, the man had stopped drinking and he attributed his success to religious conversion. In the article "Secret of AA" in *Wired* magazine, Brendan I. Koerner reported that Wilson's friend said to him, "Realize you are licked, admit it, and get willing to turn your life over to God." Wilson, an atheist, was miserable and desperate. He later described a night that would lead to the founding of AA. "I said aloud, 'If there is a God, let Him show Himself! I am ready to do anything. *Anything!*'" He wrote that he saw a white light. "It seemed to me, in the mind's eye, that I was on a mountain and that a wind not of air but of spirit was blowing. And then it burst upon me that I was a free man."

Following his religious epiphany, Wilson accompanied his friend to meetings of the Oxford Group, a Christian organization that was defined by the belief that all human suffering was caused by sin and that absolution came from prayer. At these meetings, members shared stories about their lives, and they studied Oxford Group literature that elucidated the group's "assumptions": "Men are sinners." "Men can be changed." "Confession is a prerequisite to change." "The changed soul has direct access to God." "The age of miracles has returned." "Those who have changed must change others." Wilson would later acknowledge, "The early AA got its ideas of self-examination, acknowledgment of character defects, restitution for harm done and working with others straight from the Oxford Group . . . and from nowhere else."

Wilson, now devoted to helping other alcoholics, converted Dr. Bob. Breaking from the Oxford Group, the pair founded Alcoholics Anonymous in 1935, the year Dr. Bob had his last drink. The story continues with Dr. Bob going on to help five thousand men get sober (at the time, women were excluded) while Wilson wrote *Alcoholics Anonymous: The Story of How More Than One Hundred Men Have Recovered from Alcoholism.* Twenty-three million copies of the book, renamed *Alcoholic Anonymous* and usually referred to as just the Big Book, have been sold, and it has been translated into forty-eight languages.

This book, the bible of Alcoholics Anonymous, has been guide and inspiration for countless people. In it, Wilson introduces the concept of AA meetings, incorporating the Oxford Group's support groups and similar meetings that had been held in "reform clubs." In addition to AA meetings, Wilson advocated spirituality and prayer, and he introduced the Twelve Steps, based on the Oxford Group's tenets. Wilson's steps were also inspired by William James's *The Varieties of Religious Experience,* in which James affirmed Wilson's beliefs when he wrote about the necessity of surrender and "letting go" and contended that "the only cure for dipsomania is religiomania." In addition, Wilson was influenced by Carl Jung, who also contended that spirituality was required for alcoholics to stop drinking. Wilson settled on twelve steps because of the twelve apostles.

The steps Wilson devised require anonymity, atonement for actions that have harmed others, commitment to helping other addicts, humility, and prayer. Those who "work the steps," as the process is called, are told that they must accept their powerlessness and turn their lives over to God or to some other higher power.

Every day and night, AA meetings convene in thousands of church basements, schoolrooms, and community centers. Koerner reported, "Some 1.2 million people belong to one of AA's fifty-five thousand meeting groups in the US, while countless others embark on the steps at one of the nation's eleven thousand professional treatment centers." Wilson founded the group to help alcoholics; for decades, addicts of other substances were excluded, but now almost all AA meetings are attended by drug addicts as well; AA adherents recognize that alcohol is one of many drugs of dependence. (Addicts also attend Narcotics Anonymous, Cocaine Anonymous, Marijuana Anonymous, and other spinoffs.)

It's no surprise that AA has survived and spread. "I believe, along with many other people, that perhaps the greatest event of the 20th Century occurred in 1935 in Akron, Ohio, when A.A. was established," said M. Scott Peck, author of *The Road Less Traveled*. Since its founding, the Program has had the best track record of helping addicts. Also, AA meetings are everywhere. It's decentralized; anyone can start a chapter and initiate meetings. No one's in charge, no one can profit, and no licenses are required. It's free, which is no small enticement, especially for those who have little or no money because of their drinking and using. And for some addicts, AA provides a clear path away from the ravages of their disease.

"I'm Anna, and I'm an addict and alcoholic." Introductions like this are spoken countless times every day in AA meetings. Those in this program are offered a way to stop drinking and have happy, productive lives with "new friends, new horizons, and new attitudes," as described in "This Is A.A.," an introduction to the organization. "After years of despair and frustration, many of us feel that we have really begun to live for the first time."

After she lost her job, she felt she was "losing it," the author Anna David recounts. She stayed up all night doing drugs and then took Ambien and slept all day. Her drug use quickly escalated. She was, she says, "a mess," and she told her parents she needed help. She entered rehab, where she was introduced to the Program. "I was in AA before I even realized it," she says. "I was so out of it, and I'm such a rule follower, I just did what I was told. It's what I needed. AA just worked. It never occurred to me to question it."

She was clean for six months, working the steps with an AA sponsor. "I'd get an assignment and I'd do it right away," she says. That's how it works. With a sponsor, you start with Step One: Admit powerlessness. You continue through to Step Twelve. You begin again. "I love the steps," she says. Step Four, "Made a searching and fearless moral inventory of ourselves," had an especially deep effect on Anna. "It was a revelation to sit in a café with my sponsor and read from the list [I'd made] of my resentments. I'd been waiting my whole life to have someone sit with me and listen to the list of who I was mad at. The fact that I could then see how I was in fact responsible for all those resentments was a revelation. It made me see how much I'd been playing the victim. The Fourth Step was like a dream for me."

But when she was six months sober, she relapsed. She took four hits of ecstasy. AA acknowledges that addicts sometimes relapse. The organization strives for "progress, not perfection." Rather than spiraling downward from there, Anna did what the Program had taught her to do — she called her sponsor and went to a meeting. She's been sober ever since.

All AA meetings generally begin the same way. Addicts wander into a nondescript room and take seats that are arranged in rows or a circle. While researching *Clean* and, before that, accompanying my son, I attended many AA meetings. One time I went to one with a group of women living in a homeless shelter.

The shelter, with plate-glass windows covered in newspaper, was located in what appeared to be a former car dealership. Now dilapidated, the building had scarred walls and dingy shag carpeting. Lighting came from dim fluorescent tubes held up by twisted wire. Many of the women wore clothes that didn't fit — dirty T-shirts and baggy pants — and most had old ripped tennis shoes.

The women filed out of the shelter and trudged down the block as passersby stared. They stopped in front of a brick building, a small church, and entered through a wooden door.

The room was airy with high ceilings, and there were semicircles of molded plastic chairs. It was presided over by Jesus on the cross carved in wood. The chairs faced a white front wall with a pair of banners, one headed THE TWELVE STEPS and one THE TWELVE TRADITIONS. Atop a card table in the back corner were pamphlets and books.

The women from the shelter chose chairs close together on one side of the room. The other chairs filled with people dressed in suits, skirts, jeans. From the looks of them, most were professional people. This was probably the only place in the world where these two groups could be found sitting together with a common purpose. Outside, if they came in contact, one would probably be asking the other for money.

There are a several kinds of AA meetings, including step study; speaker meetings, where AA veterans tell their stories of dissolution and redemption; and meetings at which sections of the Big Book are read and discussed. Some meetings are open (anyone can come), some closed (only the addicted are welcome).

The meeting in the church was an open speaker meeting. A man in his thirties, dressed in shirtsleeves, jeans, and loafers, was the secretary. (Secretaries, usually elected by the group, generally serve for six months or a year. Organization guidelines note, "Our leaders are but trusted servants; they do not govern.")

His light brown hair was longish, sort of wild, and he pushed it to the side with one hand.

"I'm Rick and I'm an alcoholic-addict," he said.

The room responded, "Hi, Rick."

He repeated it: "Yes, I'm Rick and I'm an addict and alcoholic back from hell."

Resounding applause. One of the women from the shelter called out, as if in church, "I hear you, Rick. We've all been there."

"This is the regular meeting of the weekly Thursday-afternoon group of Alcoholics Anonymous," he went on. "As an introduction for anyone who doesn't know the details, I'll read the Alcoholics Anonymous preamble about what we're doing here and who we are." He read: "'Alcoholics Anonymous is a fellowship of men and women who share their experience, strength and hope with each other that they may solve their common problem and help others to recover from alcoholism. The only requirement for membership is a desire to stop drinking. There are no dues or fees for A.A. membership; we are self-supporting through our own contributions. A.A. is not allied with any sect, denomination, politics, organization or institution; does not wish to engage in any controversy; neither endorses nor opposes any causes. Our primary purpose is to stay sober and help other alcoholics to achieve sobriety.'"

He asked if someone in the room would volunteer to read from the Big Book, a section called "How It Works." A woman in the front row nodded. Rick found the page he wanted and handed the open book to her. "I'm Julie and I'm an alcoholic-addict," she said. The group replied, "Hi, Julie."

She read the passage and then recited the Twelve Steps. She began, "'We admitted we were powerless over alcohol — that our lives had become unmanageable.'" She read the other eleven.

When Julie finished, Rick made some announcements and then turned the floor over to a woman in her late thirties. After introducing herself as Rita, she told her story about growing up with an alcoholic mother, a "functioning alcoholic" who kept her drinking hidden. The speaker said she began smoking weed at fourteen. "My friends smoked and I didn't think twice about joining them. Soon I was buying bags and smoking on my own in the woods near my house. I smoked all the time. Loved it. Started drinking. Loved that. Tried coke and X. Loved them.

"Like it did for everyone in this room, my life became hell. It's hard for me to remember everything I did while I was high, but it's a story you know, right? Stealing from my parents. Lying to everyone. I'd be high and swearing I'd never used drugs, and my parents believed me. My mom was drinking and I don't even think she noticed what I was doing. My dad was clueless.

"I think a lot of my using was about growing up feeling like a toad, ugly, lame, unlovable. So I'd get high and go to parties or hang out in the mall or wherever and I didn't have trouble finding guys who made me feel like I was the most beautiful . . . desirable thing in the world. And I loved that. Maybe more than the feeling of being high. Of course, almost all the guys were assholes . . ."

There were laughs from the crowd. The same woman from before yelled out, "We've been there, sister!"

More laughter.

Rita continued her story. She'd gone down, she said. "So far down." She described losing her job after repeatedly showing up at work reeking of alcohol. She said, "Did that make me stop? No, it made me go out and get high." She'd continued using for more than a year. "First I was like my mom — functioning, though barely. Soon, functioning involved living in a squalid room in a friend's basement, getting out of bed long enough to score, and getting high again. To me that was functioning. I'd sit there high, resenting everybody for my problems. It never occurred to me that I'd become a lush and an addict."

She said that one night she was in a grocery store stocking up on booze when she ran into a guy she'd known from work. Rita said that he saved her. "He was in the Program, recognized me for what I was. I denied it, but he said I was an addict and he dragged me to a meeting.

"I came to my first meeting with a bag of dope in my pocket and thinking the whole thing was lame and it was something to do for an hour. That was four years ago. I think about that song, 'Amazing Grace,' and that was me: I once was lost and now I'm found. And it's good to be back."

Applause.

"And every day I thank God for AA, and I thank God for all of you."

Rita returned to her seat, and Rick asked the group if anyone was celebrating an anniversary. A boy stood and said, "I've got seven days again. I had thirty but then I slipped. But seven days." Another member was applauded when he announced that he was ninety days clean.

The meeting leader asked if there were newcomers and said that if they felt comfortable, they should introduce themselves to the group.

A young girl with a white button-down shirt and blue eyes — by appearance, the mostly unlikely person here — stood. "I'm Sarah," she said. "And I guess I wouldn't be here if I wasn't an addict." The group welcomed her. "You're in the right place," someone said. "Keep coming back."

She briefly spoke about her drug use, which began when she was a child sneaking drinks at her parents' cocktail parties. When she sat down, Rick passed a basket around the room. Most people put in a dollar or two, even a couple of the women from the shelter.

Then, without being instructed to do so, everyone stood and gathered at the front of the room in a long, lopsided circle. They held hands, bowed their heads, closed their eyes, and in unison chanted the Serenity Prayer: "God, grant me the serenity to accept the things I cannot change; courage to change the things I can; and wisdom to know the difference."

Then they opened their eyes, swung their hands back and forth, and chanted, "Keep coming back. It works if you work it."

The Program

AA's growth was aided by its liberal interpretation of "religiosity" at the core of the Program. Wilson's original draft of the Big Book was intensely religious. Without alterations, it might have alienated many people. Wilson anticipated the problem and revised the book. Until 2010, when the original Big Book was published by the Hazelden organization, the extent of editorial modifications to the first drafts of the Big Book, broadening its conceptualization of God and traditional prayer, wasn't known. In an article in the *Washington Post* that appeared when the original Big Book manuscript was made public, Nick Motu, senior vice president of Hazelden Publishing, acknowledged, "If it had been a Christian-based book, a religious book, it wouldn't have succeeded as it has."

In addition to revising the Big Book, Wilson emphasized in speeches that AA didn't require belief in God at all, that it could help those who "cannot accept a belief in God and His grace as a means of recovery." He emphasized, "Happily [non-belief] does not prove to be an impossible dilemma at all." However, the steps still insisted on submission to a "higher power," "a power greater than ourselves," and God "as we understood Him." That is, some form of God was required, though practitioners were allowed to conceptualize whatever deity worked for them. I've heard people describe their higher power as nature, art, surfing, Buddha, Earth, and "the still small voice inside me."

In spite of Wilson's modifications, religion is still key to almost every AA principle. "In many ways, Alcoholics Anonymous is a religious program," Susan Cheever wrote, "although this statement would no doubt provoke howls of protest from most group members." Lennard Davis, author of *Obsession: A History*, says, "The God thing . . . If you read the literature, it doesn't matter what you believe in — you can believe in a horse or a tree — but it's so clearly about believing in God."

"The only condition [required for a person to recover] is that he trust in God and clean house," wrote Wilson in the Big Book. "To get well, we had to have God's help," he said in an interview. And, in spite of Wilson's alterations, seven of the steps still require an acceptance of, prayer to, and surrender to God "as we understood Him."

This emphasis on God isn't relegated to the tenets and writings of the Program. At most meetings I've attended, speakers and participants talked about the grace of God, being saved by Him, and praying to Him. The nonreligious aren't turned away, but people have told me about the shame and guilt they've felt while sitting in meetings because they didn't or couldn't believe. Some nonbelievers said they felt uncomfortable or even dishonest in AA meetings. Some became angry, and many left, never to return.

Fake It till You Make It?

AA abounds with well-known slogans — "One day at a time," "Let go and let God," "Keep it simple, stupid" — including one directed at non-believers and others who struggle with the Program. The slogan "Fake it till you make it" is a suggestion that those who don't initially understand or believe in AA's principles or prescriptions act as if they do. Newcomers are told that they should practice the steps and participate in meetings even if it feels disingenuous; eventually, they'll no longer have to fake it. I've also heard patients in rehabs, including a rehab Nic was in, instructed to "fake it till you make it" when they claimed they didn't or couldn't believe in a higher power. Counselors said to pretend to believe in God and pray to Him. They said to fake it and promised that a conversion would come.

Sometimes it did. I've heard testimonials of addicts who said they were desperate for help with their addiction and did what counselors, sponsors, and others in AA told them to do — they faked it — and epiphanies came. Eventually, they no longer had to fake it; the transformation was genuine. However, I've also met people who faked it and never made it. They remained discouraged and alienated, ultimately leaving the Program. Some of them became fatalistic. Unable or unwilling to act as if they believed, because they couldn't or wouldn't turn their lives over to God or some other higher power, they assumed they were hopeless cases.

In AA, there are as many varieties of teachings and practices as there are in churches, from conservative and evangelical to liberal and temperate. Many AA groups and participants accept doubt about and even rejection of a higher power. In some Twelve Step–based rehabs, though, believing and praying isn't just an option; patients are ordered to do it. Those who can't or who choose not to pray are told that they'll never recover. People have written to me about being admonished, warned, and threatened. I sat in the audience for a speech by a judge who presides over a drug court in which he offers drug offenders the opportunity to choose rehab rather than prison. He said that when addicts come into his court he tells them, "If you don't believe in God, you're like a bug on a windshield."

This warning — and the insistence that there's only one way to get and stay sober — is not only wrong but harmful. Most addicts who wind up in rehab are initially belligerent, angry, uncooperative, and unwilling or unable to embrace the steps, because they're detoxing and miserable. Sometimes, after being exhorted — sometimes ordered — to pray, or after persistent badgering and threats, they acquiesce and at least try to turn their lives over to God, as the steps require them to do. Some conversions last, but many don't. Desperate to get well, they try to embrace and work the Program, but their successes are short-lived. Pressed by rehab counselors, they try to trust God, but ultimately they can't.

The danger comes not from AA but from rehab counselors who impart a message, sometimes hidden and sometimes explicit, that those addicts who won't acquiesce to the Program are weak, narcissistic, and obstinate. These are exactly the judgments that stigmatize addicts in the first place and stop some from pursuing treatment. In "The Drunk's

Club," an essay in *Harper's,* the novelist and essayist Clancy Martin writes, "To its credit, AA insists that the alcoholic who cannot recover should not be blamed for her failure. But listen to the language." He quotes from the Big Book:

> Rarely have we seen a person fail who has thoroughly followed our path. Those who do not recover are people who cannot or will not completely give themselves to this simple program, usually men and women who are constitutionally incapable of being honest with themselves. There are such unfortunates. They are not at fault; they seem to have been born that way. They are naturally incapable of grasping and developing a manner of living which demands rigorous honesty.

Blaming the Victim

It's understandable that many addicts are fiercely protective of a system that has helped keep them alive, especially if their sobriety is fragile and they retain it primarily through their devotion to AA. But the original form of AA itself doesn't condemn addicts who reject the steps. Bill Wilson said, "The Twelve Steps are but suggestions." However, as Stanford's Dr. Humphreys says, "You often don't hear that from people, especially in the rehabs." Humphreys adds that it's important to differentiate AA and rigid my-way-or-the-highway programs that are based on AA. "The ones that say you have to do it my way have nothing to do with AA," Humphreys says. However, he does admit that many people don't know what's part of the core of AA and what's distorted or misused.

There are rehabs that employ less confrontational or nonconfrontational styles. In these programs, addicts resistant to AA are encouraged to participate but not attacked. However, in many programs, addicts are told that their "defiance" — as it's viewed by some counselors — will kill them. When addicts remained recalcitrant and left treatment on their own or were ejected from treatment — even if they left and relapsed or even if they left and died — they were blamed because they wouldn't embrace the Program.

• • •

" You aren't sick '

In His Disease

Blaming the victim is convenient for those who treated the victim, including counselors and rehabs, because it absolves them of accountability. They can take credit when a person gets well, but they take no responsibility when he doesn't. Similarly, many rehab counselors try to have it both ways. They rail against the notion that addicts are weak, but when their own patients don't follow the Program, they label them as weak. Sometimes, as many practitioners will say, it's just a matter of time before a person embraces AA. But what about the many people who don't?

I understand the impulse to blame addicts when they continue using or resist the advice they get in treatment. I've heard counselors in groups tell people that their resistance is their "disease talking"; I've heard therapists speak about someone who resists as being "in his disease." In a way, it's true. As I've explained, often addicts' refusal to accept that they're ill or their inability to participate in treatment *is* a result of their illness. "This is an illness that convinces the individual, 'You aren't sick,'" says Joseph Lee, the medical director of Hazelden's adolescent programs. "Other than a few other mental illnesses, addiction is the only disease that has that." It's especially problematic because the Twelve Step program, like many other mental health treatments, requires that patients participate willingly in order for them to succeed. People who can't see that they're ill will resist treatment for an illness they don't believe they have.

Another symptom of addiction is narcissism; addicts, their go system unregulated, think they know better than the people trying to help them. Addicts can be paranoid, convinced that counselors and doctors want to manipulate or control them. All of these symptoms are the result of biological changes that impair rational thinking. Therefore, resistance, belligerence, and denial may indeed be "the disease talking." But any treatment of addiction must address these symptoms, not use them as an excuse when treatment fails.

Again and again, people told me that their addicted loved ones heard that unless they surrendered to the steps, turned their lives over to God, atoned, prayed, and made amends, they'd die. And again and again, people told me that their loved ones did die.

Was it their fault? Blaming an addict for relapse is like blaming a cancer patient when radiation and chemotherapy don't work. It wasn't his fault. It was the fault of a crippling disease and a treatment system that failed him.

The Peril of Anonymity

Another reason AA has proliferated is the second *A* in its name. In the Program's early days, anonymity was essential. Without the promise of privacy, many people would have stayed away. "Doctors and other professionals wouldn't attend meetings if their privacy wasn't protected," an AA old-timer told me. "The stigma against addiction was even worse then than now."

This aspect of AA, which is extolled as one of the organization's main virtues and which has served many of its members well, can have unintended negative consequences, for people in the Program and for the culture at large. It was and is important for many people to participate in AA without revealing their identities; otherwise, they wouldn't show up. As the research I cited shows, society still judges addicts harshly. And people have a right to their privacy. No one who attends AA should fear that he or she will be outed; that should always be an individual's choice.

Also, AA requires anonymity not only to protect members' privacy but to buttress a more subtle principle of the program: the need to embrace humility and a sense of one's own powerlessness. The organization professes that the ego, the part of a person that makes him feel as if he's in control, is deluded and must be repressed. When one is anonymous, he is better able to put his ego aside. Shorn of his ego, he can humbly ask for help.

From the outside, addicts may appear to be impervious to others' opinions and influence, may seem to have no conscience, but they aren't, and they do. Most of them are tormented by shame. The Program's insistence on anonymity reinforces that shame by contributing to the stigma and isolation that addiction inflicts on those who suffer it. Anonymity can also deprive an addict of the comfort of knowing that even when she isn't in a meeting, she isn't alone — that the person in the next cubicle or sitting beside her in class also attends AA — and it prevents all of us from appreciating the magnitude of this disease and the urgent need to treat it properly. When addicts are told that they must keep people's involvement in AA secret, the implicit message is that there's something to hide.

The history of other diseases shows dramatically how closely linked openness and health are. Perhaps the most notable example in the last half a century is cancer. "The Big C" was once spoken of in hushed tones; those who suffered from it were often shunned. But now cancer is discussed freely by those who have it and by society at large. It is no coincidence that this trend tracks closely with markedly higher cancer treatment rates (and funding) since the 1970s. Another example is from the late 1980s, when a handful of AIDS activists (who later started ACT UP) fought effectively to make that disease impossible to ignore with their Silence = Death campaign. At the time, AIDS was dismissed by many as the "gay plague," and those who suffered from it were ignored if not loathed by mainstream America. ACT UP's and others' efforts to push HIV into the spotlight were instrumental in drumming up the funding and research that has since made it a disease one can live with rather than die from. Silence = Death when it comes to addiction too. Openness will help destigmatize addiction, which will make addicts' lives easier, because they won't have to hide their affliction, and lead to increased support for combating the disease. Perhaps most important, people who don't feel the need for anonymity might be quicker to admit they're addicted and to get help.

Another problem with the Program's insistence on anonymity is that few people talk about successful treatment, and few people advertise abstinence. Drug users have no such requirement. Boastful tales of using are common. At parties, socialites and business executives never hide their martini drinking, but a person who nurses a glass of mineral water all night often has to explain quietly, sometimes with embarrassment: "I'm an addict. I'm in recovery." While conducting interviews, I've spoken to actors, musicians, writers, and businesspeople about their involvement in AA, but off the record, not for publication. One said, "It violates the principle." It would be far more useful to many if people in the Program said, "I'm in AA, and I'm proud of it."

In 2011, Susan Cheever, whose father, John, died of alcoholism and who is herself in recovery, wrote that it might be time to reject the second *A* of AA. In the *New York Times,* David Colman quoted novelist Molly Jong-Fast, who had gotten sober in AA thirteen years earlier: "It seems crazy that we can't just be out with it, in this day and age. I don't want to have to hide my sobriety; it's the best thing about me." In the *Times* article, Rick Ohrstrom, the chairman of C4 Recovery Solutions, a consulting firm, said, "I violate my anonymity daily. I am twenty-five years in recovery, and have been out there fighting for the rights of people in recovery, and I'm sick and tired of people in A.A. meetings not lifting a finger to do anything about it. They hide behind anonymity — if you don't tell anyone else that recovery works, that's what you're doing."

"We can let those around us know that we're addicts, that we're doing our best to stop our compulsive behavior, and that we want them to hold us accountable," wrote Adi Jaffe in *Psychology Today.* "If we slip, we can get back up because we don't compound the shame of a relapse with lies we tell, and those around us know that even a relapse can be overcome because they've seen those examples over and over in all the other 'confessed' addicts around. It's time to leave the addiction 'closet' and start living."

Counting Days Sober

There are other common AA traditions that are useful for some people but hurt others. In many meetings and some rehabs, addicts are awarded chips in celebration of having arrived at some milestone of sobriety — a month, six months, five years, twenty years. The chips, which look like poker chips, are handed out amid applause and congratulations. Intuitively, this practice makes sense: people are justifiably proud of their sober time, and they deserve recognition for it. However, the practice can backfire; as one addict told me, after relapsing, "the prospect of starting over can be so discouraging that we give up." He said, "I had three hundred and twenty days, almost a year, and went out [relapsed]. I felt like hell. I wanted to come in, and went to a meeting. I left, though. I couldn't bring myself to go back and start over. It was too depressing. I left and got high."

"In A.A. people feel that if they slip and have a drink they're lost entirely, back to day one," said Howard J. Shaffer, an associate professor of psychiatry at Harvard Medical School, to the *New York Times*. "That attitude in itself can sometimes be enough to turn a slip into a full relapse, since it can lead to the attitude that if you've had one drink, you're off the wagon, so you may as well keep drinking."

Moral Inventories

When addicts reach Step Four of the Program, they're instructed to make a "moral inventory"; in Step Nine, they are to make amends to those they've harmed. Obviously, it's positive for any of us to soul-search, acknowledge faults and work to remedy them, and strive to repair damaged relationships. However, these actions aren't requisites for a person to get and stay sober. A step that requires a form of atonement implies that addiction is a sin and injects morality into treatment.

AA and Adolescents

Earlier I described the ways that some forms of group therapy endanger some teenagers. It can be similar for impressionable adolescents in AA meetings. I've been told by some that they were so intrigued by AA speakers' stories about ecstasy and meth that they later tried those drugs. Addicts whose drug of choice was marijuana described feeling like lightweights when they heard the colorful, sometimes hilarious, war stories from other addicts about heroin, dealing, drug-fueled crime, and taking combinations of drugs. Recently a boy wrote and told me that he'd never considered taking OxyContin before he attended an NA meeting, but "it sounded amazing." He actually scored some at the meeting, took it, loved it, and became addicted to it on top of his addiction to marijuana.

Another tenet of AA that can backfire when it comes to adolescents is the admonition that they "keep coming back" for the rest of their lives. Many addicts may need to continue treatment, and they remain susceptible to relapse. However, most teenagers are disinclined to view their drug problem as chronic — and in some cases, it may not be. A teenager's serious drug problem may be confused with addiction, and there's evidence that some teens grow out of their tendency to abuse drugs.

Finally, AA can clash with adolescents on the most existential level.

Teenagers, by definition (partly owing to the lagging development of the stop center of the brain), feel the opposite of powerless. They are adamant that they won't turn their lives over to anyone — their parents, authority figures, a higher power. The step that requires addicts to accept that they're powerless and to surrender their will to a higher force can foster a feeling of defeat in teens. "You hear over and over again that you have this disease and this is the only way out," a boy told me. "You're told you're doomed unless you pray and believe in God."

Michael Pantalon says that adolescents "seem to be particularly resistant to the Twelve Step idea of powerlessness, perhaps because it is developmentally appropriate for them to feel powerful, even invulnerable, which makes it difficult for them to comply with [treatment] programs, most of which are heavily Twelve Step–based." He continues, "Further, in many programs, punitive measures are used to promote acceptance of Twelve Step principles (e.g., additional writing assignments, withdrawal of privileges, extra meetings and groups), which only seem to engender greater resistance among adolescents and in turn a greater chance of relapse post-treatment."

Parents have claimed that by forcing their kids to attend AA — to "surrender" to the Program — rehabs have missed opportunities to help. Having been told that accepting the tenets of AA was the only way to recover, children decided they'd never be able to stay sober — and their drug use escalated. I received a letter from an addict's father who said his son "just couldn't do Step 1, 'give himself over to a higher power.' He didn't want to do it, he couldn't do it, he hated that they kept hammering in that he had to do it. Now he's incarcerated. His crime was using drugs, but his real crime was that he wouldn't give himself over to a higher power. Those people are the ones who put my son in prison. Then in prison, guess what, they have a so-called drug rehabilitation program, and it's run by a guy who screams at [my son] and tells him he has to give himself over to a higher power. [My son] just can't do it and so he feels angry and doomed."

"You Don't Treat Drug Problems with Drugs"

Another serious problem applies to only some interpretations and implementations of the Program, ones practiced in meetings and treatment centers that forbid all drug use, including the use of prescription medication. Whereas AA-approved literature emphasizes that it's "wrong to deprive any alcoholic of medication which can alleviate or control other disabling physical and or emotional problems," the message espoused in many meetings and AA-based inpatient and outpatient rehabs is very different. I personally witnessed instances and heard of many other instances of people being told to stop taking prescribed psychiatric medication because they "weren't really sober," or "weren't AA sober." In rehabs, I spoke to people who were forbidden to take their psychiatric medications — counselors confiscated them. Some of these patients had been clinically depressed; some had other psychiatric conditions; and some had attempted suicide.

As shown in the previous chapter, there's irrefutable evidence supporting the use of pharmaceuticals in treating some addictions. In addition, if someone with a dual diagnosis is not treated for his mental illness as well as his addiction, there's a good chance he won't be effectively treated at all, so Twelve Step–based programs that forbid medications may be setting up people to fail. In his *Harper's* article, Clancy Martin described an AA meeting at which he spoke about his sustained sobriety, which he attributed to the Program paired with the antidepressant Celexa. His disclosure was greeted with "embarrassed silence," he wrote. However, after the meeting, several younger members came up and thanked him. "Everyone said the same thing: 'I'm on' — fill in your drug, these days the fashion is Lamictal or Seroquel, plus something else — 'but I've always been afraid to talk about it. My sponsor doesn't even know.'" Clancy concluded, "As much as AA, my psychiatrist . . . saved my life."

AA *Is* an Evidence-Based Treatment

Clearly, several key aspects of AA are problematic — even dangerous — for some people, and these problems help explain why the Program succeeds in helping only a minority of addicts. But the main problem isn't with AA itself. The most serious problems have to do with how some of its adherents apply its principles, as well as how those principles have monopolized addiction treatment and perpetuated the widespread, persistent, and deadly misunderstanding that addiction is a moral failing.

However, none of these criticisms negates the fact that AA has saved millions of lives. So it's well worth asking why the Program works so well for many people, and researchers have begun to do just that.

It would seem that AA, devised by laymen and based on spirituality, would be rejected by a science-based approach to addiction treatment. It wasn't developed through the usual medical model of hypothesis, research, and then clinical trials. AA's development reversed the process. It was created by a businessman and put into practice, and only recently has it become the subject of scientific inquiry, as researchers and doctors attempt to understand why it works. By breaking the Program down into its components, researchers discovered that Bill Wilson unwittingly designed and implemented contingency-management, CBT, and group therapies that would prove to be valid evidence-based treatments.

As I said, AA is replete with slogans. The most famous, "One Day at a Time," is, Dr. Rawson says, "one of the most brilliant pieces of cognitive behavioral therapy ever developed." Rawson explains, "CBT reframes what may seem impossible into what seems possible. One day at a time seems doable."

The one-day-at-a-time concept anticipated time-planning and scheduling, important EBTs that are used in outpatient programs and by patients when they leave primary inpatient care. Addicts aren't told to do something they may not be able to imagine: "Never have a drink/smoke/use for the rest of your life." Instead, they're taught to make a plan to get through the next day or two. Staying sober for just one day at a time isn't overwhelming.

Other well-known AA slogans point to other aspects of the Program that research has shown to be effective. When most AA meetings end, the attendees chant, "Keep coming back," a concept that acknowledges that retention in treatment is the most important component of success. I described the problem with the slogan "Fake it till you make it" — some people fake it but don't make it — but it works well for some, and it's a simple way of describing the end result of cognitive-behavioral therapy, when behaviors that initially required effort (anticipating and noticing triggers, interrupting them, accepting them, choosing alternative behaviors) become, over time and repetition, automatic.

CBT teaches addicts about cueing so they can recognize and stop a process that might lead to relapse. Similarly, AA warns addicts about the people, places, and things that trigger drinking. Clearly, Bill Wilson understood condition cues long before scientists named them. The Program also notes that triggers need not be external. HALT is an acronym often repeated in meetings; it stands for "hungry, angry, lonely, tired" — states that can lead to relapse. Science has confirmed that those and other emotions cue craving too.

Even the chips that can be discouraging for some addicts can be effective for many others. The concept of chips prefigured contingency-management techniques. "Working toward those chips can be a meaningful endeavor," Dr. Humphreys says. "It's motivation. It's a tangible symbol of a substantial accomplishment that's rewarded in meetings when people cheer and congratulate you." As I said, there's some evidence that the way chips are awarded — for a month, three months, six months, or a year sober — can hurt in some cases. Six months until the next chip can seem daunting. Moreover, a single slip can be discouraging. But chips act as rewards, and rewarding abstinence is generally a sound evidence-based practice.

Finally, some researchers have speculated that AA works for many people by changing their environment. At AA meetings, addicts are in a setting that celebrates and reinforces abstinence. It's easy to imagine that part of AA's success, similar to the success of the positive-peer-culture model of treatment, is connection to the group, positive reinforcement from the group, and emotional rewards for those who "keep coming back" (praise, applause, hugs, friendships that develop over time). Addicts may be walking themselves through a kind of motivational interviewing when they recount their stories and describe the consequences — and especially the benefits of not using. Also, others' stories may make change seem possible, which is another goal of MI.

How Effective Is AA?

Some AA adherents will bristle at the idea that the Program can be deconstructed in ways that make it fit in with science-based treatments, and it's true that the parallels aren't exact. In addition, no one would deny that some aspects of AA don't fit the model. Maybe that doesn't matter, at least to those for whom it works. When AA does work, it may or may not be because of components that mirror EBTs. Or the whole may be bigger than its components. Regardless, the test of whether AA belongs in the category of evidence-based treatment comes down to whether or not it works in clinical trials.

The fact is, there's no scientific evidence that answers definitively how often AA and the steps succeed. In my research, I've found claims that AA helps just 5 percent of the people who try it, as well as claims that it helps 90 percent of them. I examined many of the studies and meta-analyses of studies to tease out an accurate number. I looked into AA's own surveys and an internal report by the AA General Service Office. I read studies conducted by Stanford's Drs. Humphreys and Rudolf Moos that looked at whether patients who landed in emergency rooms did better if doctors encouraged them to go to AA, and another by Dr. Moos that tracked hundreds of alcoholics over a sixteen-year period to determine if those who "merely dabbled" in AA were less likely to stay sober than those who attended meetings frequently. A study called Project Match and one conducted by the medical journal of the National Council on Alcoholism compared AA to other therapies. And I considered meta-analyses of studies conducted by Marica Ferri of the Italian Agency for Public Health in Rome and by J. Scott Tonigan, research professor at the University of New Mexico's Center on Alcoholism, Substance Abuse, and Addictions. In an effort to distill the research, I also spoke at length with Humphreys and Tonigan and communicated by e-mail with Moos and Ferri.

I wanted a hard number, but with addiction we don't even know how to measure success. Does it mean to sustain recovery for six months? A year? Five? What if there are relapses along the way? Is it fair to judge AA by the number of people who try it and don't continue? What does it mean to commit to AA or to be a member — daily attendance? Weekly attendance? For a month? A year? How do we verify clean time? Are subjects drug tested, or do they self-report? Can you trust them? How do researchers count treatment failures in a program as porous as AA? People leave for a while. They come back. Some must fall off researchers' maps because they relapse and disappear, and some must die.

What I learned from the studies is that no one really knows how often AA works and for whom. But some facts did emerge that allow me to draw some conclusions: retention in AA is low, attrition is high, but one AA slogan is true for many people: "It works if you work it." This means that AA lowers drug use for those who actively engage in the Program, though that's a self-selecting group of people, and even they aren't guaranteed to stay sober; relapse is common even among ardent AA participants. Do they relapse less often or less severely because they're in AA? No one knows.

It's also impossible to know if the AA attendees who don't drink or who use less do so because of the Program itself — that is, because of the steps, the sharing that takes place in meetings, and the camaraderie. The results of a number of studies suggest that AA may work simply because people show up, not for any scientific or mystical reason. That is, there's evidence supporting the contention that any treatment is better than no treatment. People who show up are motivated to stop. Motivation isn't enough for most addicts, but it's been shown to be a factor that improves the odds of successful treatment.

Or maybe it comes down to personal taste. If you go to AA and like it, you'll respond to it. If you don't, you may respond to one of the alternatives. The Project Match study found that when AA meetings were led by a therapist (an addition that would seem to invalidate the research, because in the real world, they aren't), AA worked as well or slightly better than the behavioral and motivational treatments it was compared to (at least, as the treatments were practiced twenty-five years ago). Reviewing this and other studies he analysed, Ferri concludes that compared to other treatments, AA is "no better, no worse."

How much is no better, no worse? Tonigan's research led him to sum up: "The general conclusion is that thirty percent of people who go through AA are sober a year later." The figure seems to jibe with the findings in a number of other studies. Still, this doesn't answer several questions. Did some members of this 30 percent relapse along the way? Did they drift in and out of AA? (A strength of AA is that addicts can come and go as they please.) Did they undergo other treatment? "Even defining the outcome requires making choices," says Gantt Galloway of the Addiction and Pharmacology Research Laboratory at the California Pacific Medical Center. "Abstinence from the day of admission through one year would yield minuscule numbers and also isn't a very useful measure, as treatment may take a bit of time to work. Is the heroin addict who hasn't used opioids for six months but is smoking marijuana once a week without problems a success? Using cocaine once or twice a month without problems? Once a day with problems?"

The 30 percent statistic also sheds light on the treatment system as a whole — and demonstrates why more and better options are needed. If 30 percent of those in AA stay sober for a year, then seven out of ten don't, proving that the Program treats many, but still only a minority of those who stick with it. But these figures ignore those who don't stick with it. According to *Scientific American*, 40 percent of those who try AA drop out within the first year (the article notes that some may return). If *Scientific American*'s and Tonigan's figures are accurate and represent the number of people who both remain in AA and stay sober for a year, AA's success rate for addicts who try it is, at the one-year mark, 18 percent.

There's More Than One Way

However many people AA helps, the fact is that it doesn't work for many, and there is a dire need for alternatives. As I've pointed out, the AA organization itself recognizes this, even if some of its advocates don't. "We do not think we are the only people who have the answer to problem drinking," according to "This Is A.A." There's more than one way to get and stay sober, and people don't have to turn their lives over to God or another higher power to get well. Most addicts, no matter who they are and what they believe, can be treated. The many reasons people use drugs in the first place belies the notion that there's a one-size-fits-all solution.

Some people embrace AA immediately and passionately; some embrace it over time; some embrace various aspects of it; some never embrace it; and some initially embrace it and then find later that it's no longer effective (or solely effective or as effective). "It's important to respect the patient," Dr. Rawson says. "Doctors may recommend chemotherapy or radiation to a cancer patient. They list the pros and cons, the statistics supporting the various choices, and the risks and side effects. It should be the same with addiction treatment."

Earlier I described what I consider the most useful view of AA as it applies to an EBT regime, Stanford's Humphreys advice that people try it. By his own admission, he's an AA advocate: the first thing he recommends for people with drug or alcohol problems is that they go to meetings. If it works, great. If it doesn't, they should pursue other treatments, because, as Ferri says, AA has never been shown to be better than other forms of EBTs.

But though there must be alternatives, one thing is undeniable. AA can be profound and transformative for those who embrace it. It was for Luke Gsell.

The rehab Luke's parents found, the Camp in Santa Cruz, California, had a bed that would be available in a week. Luke had committed but was unsure about going, though he felt he had no choice at that point. Everyone knew about his drug problem. There weren't many options. Suddenly, being homeless in San Francisco didn't sound so great. Waiting, Luke used up whatever drugs he had left, and then his parents drove him to the Camp and he checked in.

Luke was fourteen. His birthday was in three days. When he arrived at the Camp, he was anemic and emaciated — he was six feet tall and weighed 115 pounds — and he was put in detox. His roommate was in rehab because of a court order. The boy had figured out how to sneak out at night. He'd go to a grocery store and steal alcohol. The night before Luke's birthday, this roommate snuck out and returned with alcohol and boxes of stolen Dramamine, the seasickness medication. "If you take enough of those, you get really high," Luke says. "It was for my birthday. He stole me some." That's how Luke celebrated his fifteenth birthday: He took Dramamine and drank beer.

"I remember waking up in the morning and just looking at myself in the mirror and thinking, *This is your fifteenth birthday. You just used drugs in rehab.*

"Everything snapped," Luke said. "I thought, *This is my one shot and*

I'm getting high. I was tripping on seasickness pills in rehab. Coming down from it, you're just [feeling] shitty, so I felt really bad all that day. I recognized that I was an addict. I said, 'I'm done with this.'"

If he needed confirmation that his decision was a smart one, he got it: his roommate OD'd later that day after taking thirty-six Dramamine pills. Luke found him foaming at the mouth and watched an ambulance take him away.

The program at the Camp was based on the Twelve Steps. Besides working the steps, Luke says, the program's counselors focused on teaching kids that they could have fun without drugs, which was something he didn't think was possible. "We did a lot of beach trips. They had a ropes course. We'd go to the boardwalk. And it *was* fun. There were these young counselors who were in recovery. I didn't know that it was possible to have a life without being stoned, but I saw kids who [were doing it]." In addition to outings at the beach and boardwalk, there were daily AA and NA meetings. Luke completed his freshman year in the rehab's continuation school.

It was a relief being away from drugs and his friends who used. And he found strength in the one-day-at-a-time principle. "I still have kind of bad anger problems, so I'd get pissed off at kids at rehab or mad at something," Luke says. "The counselors would say, 'Look, do whatever you can to keep your sobriety this minute. You don't have to think of it as the whole day. Stay cool.' That's really how I got through it."

By the program's end, as Luke finished his freshman year of high school, he was determined to stay sober, though he had no plans to stop dealing. "I was so addicted to the money and the power and the popularity of being a drug dealer that I thought, *Oh, I'll be home and I'll be sober, but I'm definitely still going to sell drugs.* That was my attitude, almost to the last day." But then it changed. "I wanted to live a different life."

Luke was scared about coming home. But once there he did what he'd been instructed to do. He went to one or two AA or NA meetings every day. He got a sponsor to help him work the Twelve Steps. As they'd been instructed by counselors at the rehab, Luke's parents took the door off his bedroom — he needed to be watched and to know that he was being watched.

In spite of the precautions, after a particularly stressful day, Luke was on the verge of relapsing. "I ran to the park, and I tried my sponsor three times. I tried a friend, but she was out of town. I tried my sponsor again — nothing. I dialed my dealer."

Luke was about to press the send button, but then the phone rang. It was his sponsor. "Hey, what's up, Luke? I was at band practice, sorry I didn't pick up."

Luke says, "I told him everything, and he goes, 'Okay, where are you?' My dad was looking for me. I called him and he came to pick me up. We met at a diner with my sponsor. My sponsor and I went through my phone and deleted all the contacts that needed to be deleted."

The new school year began. Luke was a sophomore. He joined the lacrosse team.

"My first year of sobriety was tough, to say the least. I'm surprised I got through it, but I just did what was suggested and what my sponsor kept saying. I went to meetings every day."

I met Luke again about two and a half years later. He was eighteen and had been sober for just over three years. His hair was short — swept up and to the side — and he had clear emerald eyes. He was handsome; some high-school girls walking by Peet's, where we'd met for coffee, checked him out. It was almost impossible to connect him with the gaunt, emaciated, sick, wasted kid he'd been.

Luke was graduating from high school that week and would begin college in the fall. He told me that people often asked him if he was going to drink in college. "I'm not thinking that far ahead," he said. "I take things one day at a time."

VI

Treating a
Chronic Illness

15

Treating Dual Diagnosis

MANY ADDICTS WHO RELAPSE, particularly those who relapse more than once — what they call serial relapsers — have what's termed a dual diagnosis. I've mentioned dual diagnosis previously — it's the presence of addiction plus one or more co-occurring psychiatric disorders. Everyone who faces addiction suffers, but those with dual diagnoses, and their families, suffer more. And as flawed as the treatment system is for addicts, it's worse for those suffering dual diagnoses. It was for Brian Mendell.

Brian was in his sixth rehab when he was caught taking a Vicodin and immediately kicked out of the Fellowship Club, the halfway house he was in. As I've said, that zero-tolerance policy isn't unusual in rehabs. One strike and he was out. His father, Gary, was called and told that Brian had to leave the next day. There was no offer to help Brian transition into a new program.

Gary told Brian he'd pay for a hotel room for a few days to give them both time to investigate options. By then, Gary had learned about dual diagnosis, and he believed that Brian fit the description. He called Brian's psychiatrist and therapists at Hazelden and asked if they could recommend an appropriate program for someone with Brian's history. They suggested the Menninger Clinic, an inpatient psychiatric hospital. Gary called the clinic and spoke to a doctor; he was told that Brian's problems weren't severe enough for their program. Gary says that Hazelden had no other useful suggestions, and in the meantime, Brian was languishing in a hotel. Gary had to do something. He connected with an interventionist, who recommended that Brian be sent to a well-known program in Boca Raton, Florida, called Caron Renaissance, that treated patients with dual diagnoses. Gary made arrangements for Brian to go there, but Brian refused, and he disappeared.

Other than a few phone calls every five or six days, there was no word from Brian. Soon, Gary hired a detective, and he eventually found Brian living in a house with two others in the middle of Minnesota, strung out on heroin. Gary wanted to intervene right away, but the interventionist counseled him to wait until Brian "hit bottom." Gary remembers asking, "What if hitting bottom for Brian is dying?"

A week later, guided by the interventionist, Brian was convinced to come to a hotel where his father had booked a room. His parents, grand-mother, a cousin, and a close family friend were there. They all read him letters expressing their deep love for him and telling him that if he didn't return to treatment, they'd be left with no choice but to change their phone numbers and sever contact with him. After a several-hour session that went late into the night, Brian finally agreed to go to Caron Renaissance.

After four months there, Brian transitioned into what Caron called phase two. He remained in the program but also got a job and attended classes at Palm Beach Community College. Gary says that after eight more months, the program director and Brian's therapist said that Brian was ready to graduate from Caron. He moved into an apartment and continued with his job and school. But he soon relapsed again.

Gary heard that Sierra Tucson, a rehab in Tucson, Arizona, was one of the few treatment centers in America that employed full-time psychiatrists as well as psychologists and other therapists trained in both addiction medicine and dual diagnosis. Soon after arriving there, Brian called from the program. Gary was thrilled by the optimism in his son's voice. "This is the only place I've ever gone to that gets it," Brian said. "The therapists are great. For the first time in my life someone actually cares about the underlying causes of my drug use. They're really help-ing me." After a month, Brian called Gary and asked to stay an extra six weeks. A psychiatrist assessed him and wrote in Brian's chart, "[Because the patient is] amenable and motivated for treatment and given the support of his extended family, his prognosis is extremely favorable."

Brian was put on Suboxone for his opiate addiction, and Lexapro for anxiety and depression. After two and a half months, his doctors concluded that he was ready to be discharged. His psychiatrist wrote, "By the time of discharge, the patient was feeling more optimistic — symptoms have been quiet for several weeks. The patient was hopeful. Discharge medications: Suboxone 8 mg a day, Lexapro 10 mg a day. No suicidal ideation intent or plan. No psychosis."

According to Gary, Sierra Tucson recommended two halfway houses for Brian's next step. Gary researched them and decided on one in Los Angeles called Transcend. He also chose an outpatient program recommended by the interventionist. On its website, PCH Treatment Center (Psychological Care and Healing) advertises itself as "advanced mental health treatment for depression, bipolar disorder, anxiety, personality disorders, self-injury and psychological trauma." It proclaims, "Your loved one will be safe."

Brian moved into Transcend halfway house and enrolled at PCH, where he attended therapy sessions Monday through Friday. At first, Brian seemed to do well, living in the halfway house and working with a Twelve Step sponsor and a sober coach — someone assigned to help an addict retain his sobriety. Brian started working out at a gym. Gary once again felt guardedly optimistic. Soon thereafter, Brian got an internship writing about recovery on the website of the company that provided the sober coach. Following the advice of his case manager at PCH, Brian dropped to four days a week at PCH, then three, and then two. A few months later, he enrolled in a program at Sober College — he had decided to become certified as a drug and alcohol counselor.

It was March of 2011. Gary and his brother Steve flew out and spent a day playing golf with Brian and had "a super day," Gary says. "It was the old happy and smiling Brian." But by midsummer, Brian was doing worse. He told his therapists at PCH that he was feeling hopeless that there would ever be relief from his anxiety, and on several occasions he mentioned suicide. His parents weren't informed about this.

In September, Brian was a year clean — a remarkable accomplishment for anyone addicted to drugs. Gary flew in to celebrate. In spite of the anniversary, rather than feeling hopeful, Brian was "down," Gary says. In addition, Gary learned that Brian's support system in LA was unraveling. He explains that Brian's sober coach, with whom Brian had become close, had been called away on anther assignment, and Brian hadn't yet made much of a connection with the replacement. Brian's AA sponsor was also away for four weeks.

According to Gary, two weeks later, Brian was informed that he was being terminated from the sober-coaching program. In contrast to what the original sober coach had been reporting to Gary, that Brian was making good progress, the replacement said Brian wasn't following the suggestions for a sustained recovery. Brian's internship writing articles was tied to working with the sober coach, so the next day, even though he'd been frequently commended on his writing, he was told he'd lost that too.

A few days later, PCH recommended that Brian move out of the half-way house into a house with yet another sober coach. His father says that Brian felt betrayed, and he resisted, but PCH advised Gary to give Brian an ultimatum: to move in or be cut off from his family's support. Gary questioned this on two separate occasions — "Given that Brian had stayed clean for a year, and everything he'd been going through in the past few weeks, giving him an ultimatum felt really wrong," Gary says — but the PCH recommendation didn't change and Gary followed it. Brian grudgingly agreed and moved in with the new sober coach on October 15, 2011. Gary reports he later learned that when Brian moved into the home, he mentioned suicide twice, once with a description of how he was going to do it. Again, his parents were not told — in fact, they were never informed that their son had mentioned suicide.

On October 19, Brian spent time writing a résumé and cover letters for internships for alcohol and drug counseling programs. He set up an interview for the following Monday. Later that day, ostensibly because he was rude to his case manager, Brian was, as Gary recounts, "terminated on the spot" by PCH. In the treatment records, there is no indication that the independent therapist Brian was seeing was told or consulted in advance. Neither were his parents. There was no next-step support plan in place.

On October 20, Brian arranged to meet a friend for lunch the following day. A short time later, his new sober coach asked Brian to sign a release that gave the coach permission to speak to Brian's therapist and have him drug tested. Brian was angry. The coach would later say that he calmed Brian down and went out to run some errands, leaving Brian home alone — even though Brian had mentioned killing himself.

The history on Brian's computer browser shows that he spent the next hour researching suicide notes. The first one he read was Kurt Cobain's. He read other notes and then wrote his own. It wasn't like Cobain's, which was confused and bitter and angry. Brian's was coherent and conveyed sadness and tired resignation. He wrote lovingly to his family. In the note he indicted the treatment system that had failed him.

Then Brian hanged himself.

Over the course of his life, Brian had been diagnosed with attention deficit hyperactivity disorder, pervasive developmental disorder, bipolar disorder, bipolar II disorder, generalized anxiety disorder, depression, and posttraumatic stress disorder. Brian had been given over a dozen different psychiatric medications; had seen over three dozen psychiatrists, psychologists, and addiction counselors; and had been in seven inpatient and outpatient treatment centers — plus wilderness programs, hospitals, and sober-living houses.

Despite the fact that every trained addiction expert I've spoken to insists that those with dual diagnoses must be treated for both conditions if they are ever to stay sober, very few doctors are trained to treat it, and few treatment programs are equipped to help the afflicted — which doesn't mean they don't pretend they can, often misrepresenting themselves to vulnerable people who call asking for help. Other than the ten weeks at Sierra Tucson, Brian received almost none of the intensive treatment he clearly needed for the psychological disorders that accompanied his addiction. Once, when Brian was at Caron, Gary asked a therapist why she thought his son had become addicted to drugs, and she answered, "It doesn't matter. He feels entitled. . . . He must be forced to stop using. Period."

Brian seemed to have had more insight into his own problems than most or all of the professionals who cared for him. Writing Gary from one of the wilderness programs, Brian said, "One thing that I have been thinking about here in the woods is the true nature and origin of my problems. At previous programs I went to, whether you were there for pot, painkillers or cocaine, you were designated an addict. Although it was mentioned that drug [use] was a symptom and not the core issue, we were only treated for addiction. This was a mistake in these programs. . . ." At times Brian knew that he needed treatment for his dual diagnosis. During those last months of his young life, his pain was such that he'd spoken of suicide on several different occasions, but his calls for help were ignored by those his parents had entrusted with their son's care.

Mental Illness

Each year almost fifty million people in America suffer from one or more mental illnesses. More than eleven million have "serious" mental illness that results in "serious functional impairment" that "substantially interferes with or limits one or more major life activities." According to the American Academy of Child and Adolescent Psychiatry, fifteen million children and teens in the United States suffer from some kind of psychiatric disorder (and about 80 percent of them never get help, by the way) and SAMHSA reports that almost 30 percent of those between eighteen and twenty-five have episodes of mental illness. The World Health Organization says that mental-health disorders are responsible for more disability in developed nations than any other health problem, including cancer and cardiovascular disease.

The correlation between mental illness and drug use has been clearly established. According to the Dual Diagnosis Fact Sheet, published by Dartmouth-Hitchcock Behavioral Healthcare, "about one-third of those with a psychiatric disorder also develop a drug or alcohol abuse problem at some point in their lives. About half of those with a drug or alcohol abuse problem show signs of psychiatric disorders." The study breaks the numbers down by disorder: Of those with bipolar disorder, 56 percent abuse drugs, and 46 percent of schizophrenics and 32 percent of those suffering depression abuse drugs or are addicted. Other sources offer similar statistics. A study published in the *Journal of the American Medical Association* said that 50 percent of those with mental disorders are affected by substance abuse; 37 percent of alcohol abusers and 53 percent of drug abusers also have at least one mental illness; and of those diagnosed with any mental illness (mild to serious), 29 percent abuse drugs. Dr. Volkow at NIDA said that six out of ten addicts have at least one other mental disorder. Some other researchers have deemed even that estimate too low. Dr. Ruben Baler at NIDA points out, "It's impossible to know the exact number of people with psychiatric disorders who become addicted, because many people who abuse drugs may have undiagnosed or subclinical mental illness." Hazelden's Marvin Seppala told me that of the patients that arrive at Hazelden for treatment, as many as 75 percent of adults and more than 90 percent of adolescents are dual diagnosis patients.

Sometimes people are diagnosed with psychiatric disorders — depression, anxiety disorder, bipolar disorder — before they become addicts. However, more often those disorders aren't diagnosed, and then drug use begins, and drugs take center stage. It can be impossible to know if an addict has underlying depression when he's high on pain pills. Bipolar disorder can be characterized by extreme mania followed by dark depression — but so can using crystal meth.

If it hasn't been diagnosed in advance, an addict's co-occurring mental illness must be identified in primary treatment, and treatment of both problems should begin. However, this rarely happens. I've explained that many rehab programs simply have no psychiatrists on staff who regularly see patients. Addicts can spend months in rehabs and never see a single doctor qualified to assess them for dual diagnosis. Even seeing a doctor doesn't guarantee the patient a proper diagnosis. My son Nic saw psychiatrists and psychologists — a dozen of them in all — and attended half a dozen rehabs. One doctor detected depression and prescribed an antidepressant, but Nic's descent continued. When Nic was nineteen, I brought him to a new psychiatrist, who asked for Nic's psychological tests. I'd never heard the expression and asked, "What psychological tests?" This doctor was appalled that none of the other experts Nic had seen had ordered any. The doctor ordered the tests, but then Nic relapsed and disappeared. Finally, when he was twenty-four, Nic was tested by a psychiatrist who diagnosed him with bipolar disorder and depression. Nic believes that the recognition of his dual diagnosis and treatment with therapy and psychiatric medication are central to his ongoing sobriety. At the time of this writing, he's been sober more than five years.

Some traditional rehabs insist that depression and other problems are

symptoms of addiction and that they'll go away when an addict is in recovery. That's often wrong. Dual diagnosis treatment is critical; experts I
interviewed said that untreated dual diagnosis correlates with high rates
of relapse after primary treatment. In one study, 86 percent of patients
with dual diagnosis (compared to 40 to 60 percent of those without it)
relapsed at least once within six months of treatment.

Diagnosis

The high rate of comorbidity (more than one illness) means that it's essential that assessment includes the *assumption* of dual diagnosis for
patients with severe addiction or multiple relapses until it's ruled out.
If a patient's already been diagnosed and is being treated, it's a critical
time to reevaluate the diagnosis and treatment. Psychological testing is
only one tool used to diagnose problems. Case histories, information
from families, and observation by doctors and nurses also help isolate a
psychiatric disorder that accompanies addiction. Sometimes these tests
and other assessments show that an initial diagnosis was wrong, or that
treatments for it were ineffective and should be replaced.

It can take time for a doctor to correctly diagnose a co-occurring
mental disorder. There can be trial and error. Symptoms of a mental
illness may emerge over time. But whenever co-occurring illnesses are
identified, treatment for them must begin at once. If a patient requires
treatment that's beyond the capabilities of a particular doctor or treatment program, he should be transferred to one equipped to treat dual
diagnosis.

A diagnosis of psychiatric comorbidity can overwhelm an addict and
his family; the words *mental illness* can induce fear. By contrast, I've
also heard from addicts and their loved ones that a diagnosis of mental
illness came as a great relief. An addict in treatment for bipolar disorder told me, "It was like, 'Thank God. I'm not imagining it.'" Other addicts have told me that dual diagnosis explained their lifelong feelings
of despair and suffering. "It always felt as if life was harder for me," said
Lara, a twenty-five-year-old from Chicago whose addiction was accompanied by clinical depression. "I could never do what people told me I
should do. I couldn't just 'buck up.' I couldn't feel better by recognizing
how lucky I was compared to others. I'd think I was crazy, and ironi-

cally it was a relief to know that I wasn't crazy to think I was crazy." A psychiatric diagnosis can explain why a person turned to drugs in the first place, became addicted, and repeatedly relapsed. Addicts, baffled by their continual relapses, can now understand that their recidivism isn't a reflection of their lack of willpower or character. In any case, an accurate diagnosis can change a life, because it can lead to appropriate treatment.

Treating Dual Diagnosis

As more people are being educated about dual diagnosis, and as the demand for treatment is increasing, more rehab programs are claiming they treat it. Online, there are hundreds of programs that advertise that they treat dual diagnosis. Some programs do, but some justify the claim because they have a relationship with a local psychiatrist they can call to see a patient (for an added charge, of course). Or a program may have a token one who sees patients for fifteen minutes a week at most.

Some traditional rehabs have evolved enough to offer genuine dual diagnosis treatment that's appropriate for patients with less severe or complex disorders. Hazelden, for example, still focuses primarily on addiction treatment, but it has a growing dual diagnosis track. While its approach is firmly Twelve Step–based, Hazelden also offers a range of EBT to all of its patients. The patients work with a team of therapists, including psychiatrists who assess and treat them and, when appropriate, prescribe medication. The dual diagnosis focus of Hazelden is relatively new. Its current medical director, Marty Seppala, is a renowned addiction psychiatrist skilled at working with dual diagnosis patients. Joseph Lee, another psychiatrist on staff (he's medical director of the adolescent program), explains that Hazelden treats many forms of dual diagnosis but acknowledges the program's limits. Patients "must be functional," he says. Patients with severe psychiatric problems that co-occur with addiction are referred elsewhere.

I asked a number of experts for the names of reputable dual diagnosis programs. The ones mentioned most often were McLean Hospital, affiliated with Harvard University, in Belmont, Massachusetts; the Menninger Clinic in Houston; the Austen Riggs Center in Stockbridge, Massachusetts; Sierra Tucson in Tucson, Arizona; Sheppard Pratt in Baltimore; and Silver Hill Hospital in New Canaan, Connecticut. (Only some of these have adolescent programs.) This is by no means a list of "best" dual diagnosis programs, only ones that were recommended by psychiatrists and researchers I spoke with. Nor is it an exhaustive list. It's critical that patients consult doctors and get second opinions before selecting one of these or another program.

I visited the Menninger Clinic, which was founded in 1919 in Topeka, Kansas, and was moved to Houston in 2003. It's located on a newly built fifty-acre campus. Its amenities include a state-of-the-art gym, a saltwater swimming pool, two cafeterias (one for adults, one for adolescents), and an indoor basketball court.

Dr. Jim Flack, a psychiatrist and professor at Baylor University, is assistant medical director at Menninger. He explained that 60 percent of patients who come to Menninger are dual diagnosis. (When he receives calls from patients who need primarily addiction care, he sends them to Hazelden, Caron, or similar programs that focus on drug dependency.) The Menninger adult inpatient program lasts for six to eight weeks. (There's a shorter-term psychiatric assessment and stabilization program that's two to three weeks.) The clinic has separate programs for adolescents from twelve to seventeen years old; young adults from eighteen to thirty years old; and older adults. There's also an intensive outpatient program that lasts for three or more months. The residential adult program costs $1,300 a day; the programs for adolescents are each $1,200 a day. Menninger doesn't accept insurance. Here, state-of-the-art dual diagnosis care could cost more than $50,000 for an average stay, and that might be just the beginning of treatment.

The saltwater swimming pool and comfortable accommodations are frills (though healthful eating and exercise are interwoven into treatment for some patients), but mostly what $50,000 buys is intensive treatment by a team of top doctors and other professionals. Every patient is assigned at least six specialists. Each team's leader is a primary psychiatrist (there are fifteen psychiatrists on staff); other team members include a psychologist, social worker, individual therapist, nurse, and addiction counselor. When necessary, treatment begins with medical detox. After that, Flack says, "We do what's needed. Everyone has different needs — a patient with a formal thought disorder [like schizophrenia] has different treatment needs than a patient with severe depression." Sometimes, following detox, patients who have been self-medicating with drugs are, he says, "psychotic after withdrawal." Bipolar patients may be manic.

Diagnoses are based on physical and psychiatric exams, psychological testing, the patient's self-reported history, nurses' notes (nurses monitor patients twenty-four hours a day), consultations with family members, and whatever medical records are available from previous treatments. The team consults on the diagnosis and forms a treatment plan. (And it meets regularly to monitor a patient's progress and adjust diagnosis and treatment as needed.) According to many addiction specialists, this comprehensive approach is required for patients with dual diagnosis and especially "treatment-resistant patients," including those who haven't been helped by multiple attempts at rehab.

Menninger employs a wide range of therapies — CBT for psychiatric issues such as depression or anxiety; DBT for emotional regulation issues such as anger; and psychopharmacology. The social worker works with patients on developing skills such as family communication. In addition, the clinic uses therapies geared toward patients with specific co-occurring disorders (there are tracks for those with eating disorders, for example). Toward the end of the six- or eight-week treatment program, doctors consult with the patient's social worker to plan next-step treatment, which may include a period in the Menninger outpatient program. As Dr. Flack says, "Eight weeks is enough to properly diagnose dual diagnosis and begin treatment, but for these diseases you don't leave a hospital with a clean bill of health — no more than a diabetic, treated for a crisis, leaves the hospital cured."

For those who can't write $50,000 checks or whose insurance policies won't cover treatment at other programs, there are options. Some dual diagnosis patients don't require the level of care available at the top psychiatric hospitals, but they do require programs staffed by professionals trained to treat them. There are other reputable dual diagnosis programs, some of them less expensive and some covered by insurance (McLean, Sierra Tucson, Austen Riggs, Silver Hills, and Sheppard Pratt do accept some insurance). Some patients with mild cases of dual diagnosis can be treated in outpatient programs while seeing a psychiatrist.

The treatment of addiction and another mental illness is a lot harder than the treatment of either alone. One reason is that the two illnesses undermine each other. "Patients who have both a drug-use disorder and another mental illness often exhibit symptoms that are more persistent, severe, and resistant to treatment compared with patients who have either disorder alone," says Dr. Seppala.

Many of the same EBTs that treat primary addiction also treat mental illness. To be effective, they must be tailored to patients according to their specific diagnoses and other factors (a patient's age, the severity of the addiction, the level of family support). The goal of behavioral therapies for both addiction and mental illness is similar. Just as addicts can learn to recognize the mechanisms that lead to relapse and stop them, the mentally ill can learn to intervene at the onset of a new episode of their illness. Patients learn to monitor their moods and behaviors. They learn how to pay attention to their internal monologues and interrupt negative and destructive thoughts. They learn how to recognize triggers and interrupt the cueing mechanism.

Some of the integrated therapies that have proven successful for both addiction and mental illness focus on the similarities between them — their similar triggers and behavior. If an addict is prone to denial, add mental illness to the mix and it's immeasurably harder for him to understand that he's ill. There's an old saw about the Catch-22 inherent in mental illness: If you understand you're insane, you're thinking properly and therefore aren't insane. You're psychotic if you don't know it. It's critical to break through denial of this sort, and MI can help. Patients treated with MI's gentle approach are more likely to accept input from others, grasp that they're ill, and participate willingly in behavioral treatments.

It's as critical for the mentally ill to trust their doctors and therapists as it is for addicts. This trust serves as a motivator as patients undergo MI, CBT, DBT, positive-coping-skills counseling, social support therapies, and, in many cases, family therapies.

Medication for Dual Diagnosis

I've explained that psychopharmacology is an important addition to some addiction treatments. It can also be critical to the outcome of patients suffering from many versions of dual diagnosis. But medication isn't enough. Effective treatment combines both. For example, both CBT and SSRIs like Prozac are used to treat addicts with depression. CBT along with such medications as lithium and Lamictal are used to treat some addicts with bipolar disorder. In early trials, bupropion (known as both Wellbutrin and Zyban) has been used to treat depression, bipolar disorder, and methamphetamine addiction. Medications haven't been shown to treat borderline personality disorder, but some can help minimize symptoms even as patients are treated with DBT and other therapy. Another advantage of medications that lower anxiety levels and treat depression is that they can help keep patients in treatment through periods when they might otherwise relapse. Of course, these are generalizations. Treatments for psychological disorders depend on many complex factors, which is why patients must be treated by psychiatrists and psychologists who specialize in dual diagnosis.

Medications are used to treat children as well as adults, but, as always, there are special risks with kids. It's understandable that parents and others are reluctant to medicate kids. Besides having concerns about stigmatizing their children, parents reasonably worry that medication might cause serious problems. For example, the media has reported that antidepressants have led to suicides in adolescents. However, there hasn't been as much attention paid to reports on the overwhelming evidence that when judiciously prescribed and monitored, antidepressants can prevent suicides, improve children's performance in school, and allow them to have better relationships. Another reason parents may resist medicating their kids is that they're afraid powerful psychoactive medications could damage their adolescents' developing nervous systems — and there are risks and side effects to consider. But depression and bipolar disorder can damage nervous systems too, whereas proper treatment can repair damage. It's also important to understand that, like addiction, mental illness that goes untreated can worsen and become even more difficult to treat. For example, untreated depression and bipolar disorder are associated with brain disorganization and nerve-cell atrophy. Like addiction, mental illnesses are often progressive — the longer the episode, the greater the anatomical disorder that results. When the episodes are treated, the disorganization lessens and cells heal. However, when a dual diagnosis isn't effectively treated, both problems — addiction and the other disorder — progress. Behavior associated with them worsens. As a result, drug use may increase, and the vicious cycle begins anew.

It's important for those experiencing the opposite — a virtuous cycle of sobriety and improving mental health — to remember that they may not be ready to stop treatment just because they're doing so well. Maybe they're doing so well because of the treatments. Adjusting treatment should be done only in consultation with a psychiatrist or psychologist.

It's essential to keep in mind that despite CBTs and/or medication, sometimes relapses recur and worsen. There can be signs that concurrent mental disorders aren't improving or are getting worse. In such cases, more intensive treatment is called for. But even in such serious situations, the vicious cycle can be stopped. For almost everyone, treatment can lead from mental illness to mental health.

16

Relapse Prevention

ON A THURSDAY MORNING in June of 2010, Steven Garfield awoke early, slipped his MacBook into a shoulder bag, and grabbed his overnight bag. He kissed his wife and kids goodbye and left for the airport.

Steven was vice president of sales for a division of an international IT company, and he was on his way to a biannual sales conference in Atlanta. A full schedule awaited. Day one was jam-packed with meetings, followed by a banquet. More meetings the next day. Another dinner. Golf, paintball, and other "fun" events on Sunday. "Team building," they called it.

The first night's dinner was held in a conference center banquet room. First there was a cocktail hour. In recovery for five years, Steven clung to a glass of cranberry juice. After drinks and schmoozing, he and the others found their way to their tables. Over dinner, others drank wine, but Steven was fine with water. He didn't miss drinking at all. He liked being alert. Liked waking up in the morning not feeling like hell. Liked having his life back.

He'd entered rehab five years earlier because of his wife's fretting and pleading after he'd spent a night in jail for failing a sobriety test. He'd had only a couple beers, that was true, but he'd used them to chase down some Vicodin. The cop who stopped him wanted Steven to get out of the car and walk a straight line, but standing up was difficult enough.

And so he checked in. He didn't really need it, he insisted. He checked in for his wife. Rehab was fine, and he'd been good since then. That's the way he thought about it. He'd been good. For a while he did as he'd been told, attended AA meetings, but then he tapered off, and finally he stopped altogether.

Over dinner were the requisite toasts and speeches, and then coffee, after which Steven and a few of the other bosses sat in the poolside lounge. His colleagues were drinking hard stuff. Steven complained about being tired because of the time change and having to wake up so early and announced he was calling it a night. A guy from Frankfurt said he was turning in too and walked with Steven toward their rooms in the wing of the hotel opposite the pool. The German lit up a joint and offered it to Steven, who shook his head no, but then accepted it — to be sociable.

Later he told me: "That was all it took."

Back in his hotel room, stoned, he couldn't enjoy the high; he felt too nervous and guilty. There was no way he would sleep. He watched some late-night TV. At two in the morning, he was still awake. He knew he had breakfast and the first conference session in five and a half hours. He needed a sleeping pill, but where the hell could he get one at that hour? There was the minibar, which wasn't a sleeping pill, but one drink would help him sleep. One couldn't hurt.

He had one and then another. It was soon four in the morning, and it wasn't worth trying to sleep any longer. He'd feel like shit anyway, so he decided he'd stay awake. He drank another little bottle, and finally it was 6:30, and he took a shower and dressed, knowing it was going to be a hellish day. He would have skipped out, except he was on a panel and had to sit with some of the bosses at lunch, and at 3:00 there was a workshop he couldn't miss. He'd tough it out, he thought.

That night, dinner was outside. An ersatz luau. He planned to eat something, pay his respects, and duck out early. But there was the guy with the pot. Steve approached him and smiled.

Sunday night Steven flew home and then picked up his car in the airport parking lot. *I pulled it off,* he thought. He'd survived the weekend. He felt pretty bad about smoking and drinking but it wasn't much, not an official relapse. No pills. No hard stuff. He'd managed fine on the panel and done the required socializing. Playing while stoned, he thought his golf game wasn't half bad. He hung out by the pool. No one knew he was buzzed.

He knew he had to make himself look bright and alert—not hung over—before he saw his wife. She was a hawk and would know. His heart was thumping. A Vicodin would even him out. Maybe Rick, who worked in his office and was known to deal pot and pills, would have some. Steven called.

Rick had Vicodin, and Steven took a detour to his apartment complex. It had been built in the 1950s and looked like a motel.

In the small kitchen Rick found a large bottle in a cabinet and asked Steve, "How many?" Steven thought he should probably have a couple, just in case, and so he bought a dozen. And swallowed one.

The next morning at 7:00, the alarm blasted. April said, "They should give you Monday off after they make you work all weekend." Steve said, "They don't consider it working. They think they're giving us a vacation."

He'd come home the previous night, peeked in at the kids, who were sleeping, and watched TV with his wife; they had sex, and then he went to sleep, but not before he got up and took another pill. To sleep. In the morning he dressed again, a blazer and tie. No breakfast, only coffee. He kissed his wife.

On the drive to work, he took just a half, swallowed it without water.

It's often noted that relapse can be part of recovery, because addiction is a chronic disease with relapse as a symptom. But just as a recurrence of cancer can be fatal, so can a relapse with drugs. A mother wrote, "[In your book] you said that relapse is part of recovery. I had not known that with heroin, relapse often equals death." It's sadly accurate, which is why relapse prevention is an essential component of treatment. It can help addicts remain sober or help them stop a slip from becoming catastrophic. Ultimately it's what helps addicts build lives that are no longer characterized by drug use.

Doctors agree that primary treatment alone isn't enough for most addicts; that is, a patient who completes a treatment program of whatever length still isn't cured. With all chronic illnesses, there's always a chance of recurrence. With addiction, there's always a chance of relapse.

Scans, chemical tests, and addicts' behavior suggest that most brains eventually return to relatively normal when the drug use stops. But the neurological and psychological aftereffects of drug use persist, and they make relapse a significant possibility for months, years, or even decades after one stops using. Genetic predisposition doesn't disappear. And as Dr. Rawson said, once the "addiction switch" in an addict's system is activated, it cannot be deactivated.

Milder addictions can cause damage that lasts months, whereas more serious addictions can cause damage that persists for years, and some damage is probably permanent. The potential for full recovery depends on the kind, volume, duration, and combinations of drugs that were used, the way they were administered, and the number and severity of relapses. For example, people who have used ecstasy at least twenty-five times have low serotonin levels for up to a year after quitting. Long-term methamphetamine use can cause measurable deficits in dopamine for even longer. One study measured the dopamine levels in meth-addicted monkeys and tracked how long it took the receptors to function normally. At one month, the monkeys' dopamine activity was mostly gone. Six months later, there was still scant evidence of dopamine. After a year, however, it began to come back. At two years, it appeared to be normal. In *Beautiful Boy,* I described brain scans and chemical tests of meth addicts that showed normal functioning after two years of abstinence. A study conducted by Nora Volkow showed that after meth addicts had been sober for fourteen months, there was some evidence of growth in the damaged dopamine receptors, but their cognitive functioning wasn't back to normal. Even for those who suffer some permanent brain damage, memory deficiencies and cognitive impairments do improve gradually, in most cases.

It's important for addicts to realize that it can take months or years for their brains to recuperate so they can understand why recovery is so hard to sustain over the first months, the first year, and beyond. This knowledge can console and motivate them. The intense cravings, muddled thinking, depression, and other symptoms that come and go can be normal reactions to the neurological deficits and should abate as the brain continues to repair itself. For therapists working with addicts over the long term, "The goal is to keep going with appropriate levels of treatment until the addict isn't working against his brain," UCLA's Rawson explains. "There's no rushing it. We must let the brain heal."

Eventually, whatever damage remains can be negligible, functioning may appear normal, and cravings may disappear. However, recovering addicts are still vulnerable. "The support structure remains fragile the way a broken arm, though healed, may break again in the same spot," researcher Ulrike Heberlein explained. The addiction pathways may be dormant, but they remain highly susceptible and can be turned on again by triggers or — of course — drugs. I've heard from addicts who told me that after years of clean time, they decided it was okay to "just" smoke a joint or have a beer. That single act switched on the priming mechanism. One hit led to more, and more led to a full-blown relapse. Studies have shown that when mice in "recovery" are given a tiny dose of the drug to which they were addicted, they begin drug-seeking behavior. Their bodies' autonomic and neurological systems respond just like they did when the mice were hooked. To use again is to pour gasoline on a fire you thought was extinguished but has been smoldering.

Aftercare

Addiction is a web of physiological and psychological cause and effect. As the brain improves, so too may emotional problems and psychological disorders, but they may not. Formerly hidden medical conditions as well as personal problems can emerge or worsen. Sobriety by itself doesn't make relationships possible or repair damaged ones. It doesn't solve financial or career difficulties. Sometimes drugs served a psychological purpose: they assuaged trauma, loneliness, or insecurity. Now the addict must find other ways to cope with those challenges. Time heals some problems, but some, if they aren't addressed, escalate.

CBT, DBT, and other relapse-prevention therapies continue through primary treatment to the next stage of recovery. There are numerous forms of aftercare. Patients should work with their doctors and therapists to decide what's appropriate.

After the completion of treatment as inpatients, most addicts should transition to continuing care in residential programs or outpatient programs. Outpatient programs are usually tapered off. They too should be followed up by ongoing relapse-prevention work that can take the form of therapy, AA meetings, and medication.

Upon completing residential primary programs, some patients can return home, but they must have a continuing treatment plan in place. However, many addicts need a slower and more structured transition.

What's appropriate depends on the level of care that's required. Some patients need another residential treatment program, though one that offers a lower, or step-down, level of care. Other addicts, like some in outpatient programs, should go to halfway or sober-living houses.

Paul Anderson, supervisor of the adolescent male primary treatment unit at Hazelden Plymouth, says that the average stay in the initial intensive program is twenty-one to forty-five days. After that period, 90 percent of patients are referred to "structured continuing care" for at least three but normally twelve months. One such program is Gray Wolf Ranch in Port Townsend, Washington. I visited the ranch, which was founded and is run by a Hazelden alum. It's an impressive AA-rooted program for boys from fifteen to twenty-five years old who stay an average of five months. At Gray Wolf and similar continuing or aftercare facilities, along with their relapse-prevention work, patients are taught practical skills — how to write a résumé, participate in an interview, and balance a checkbook, for example — so they'll be prepared when they transition to the post-inpatient stage of treatment. Some work, and some begin or continue school. In a supportive peer community, working with therapists, they also learn to establish and build relationships while being sober — something they may never have done before. "The goal is to learn how to build healthy relationships in recovery and apply sober living skills so they continue to build a solid foundation in early recovery," says Gray Wolf founder Peter Boeschenstein.

Sober Living

Another option that can follow primary treatment (or follow extended care or be combined with outpatient treatment) is sober-living housing. Traditional halfway houses, as they were sometimes called, didn't include much more than substance-free housing, but many programs now also have communal meals and host AA meetings, and some offer activities — bowling nights or movies. Some provide group therapy. Some have behavioral treatments led by therapists. Some have groups structured to help addicts learn how to build relationships and address conflict. Most require drug testing and enforce curfews. These protected surroundings can offer addicts a safe haven. Of course, not all sober-living homes are well run. Some exploit addicts and their families. As with rehabs, sober-living homes should be researched. They should include close supervision, monitoring, and support as addicts follow a comprehensive relapse-prevention plan.

There's a broad range of sober-living environments. Some are free or low cost; others charge thousands of dollars a month. An example of the latter is Loft 107, in Brooklyn, located on the fourth floor of a former warehouse that's on a street lined with yoga studios, boutiques, cafés, and galleries.

The loft has a large, high-ceilinged communal area with an open restaurant-style kitchen, a long dining table, and a lounge with plush couches, leather armchairs, and a Jasper Johns–like painting of an American flag hanging on the wall. Wandering about are the resident dogs: Churchill, a bulldog, and Luci, an enormous mastiff rescued from a local shelter, where she was to have been put to sleep. "Somehow it seems very appropriate, given her near-death experience, [that Luci is now] the most loved dog in our program," says Melissa Burton, executive director of Core, the company that owns Loft 107. (Besides running the sober house, the company also stages interventions and provides sober companions.)

Loft 107's gourmet food, maid service (no chores required here), and beds with down comforters draw a well-heeled clientele (or clientele whose parents are well heeled), most of them referred by high-end rehabs, including Sierra Tucson and Betty Ford. The cost is $9,000 a month for a double room, $15,000 for a suite. (The company does have scholarships available.)

The place is posh, but the most important offering of the facility is not its hotel-like amenities but the aftercare it provides. Its residents stay a minimum of a month, and most stay for ninety days or more — and some more than a year. After prescreening, a patient arrives at the house and is assigned a room. He or she (the house is co-ed) is required to sign a release so the program's directors can have access to a resident's treatment records and discharge notes and so they talk with doctors and family members, if necessary. "We want the ability to consult with their doctors, because we view our program as a continuation of treatment, not just sober housing," says Joe Schrank, a social worker who founded Loft 107 in 2008.

Some patients arrive with full treatment plans, but given the haphazard discharge process at many rehabs, often there's nothing in place. Loft 107's staff members require residents to be in treatment—for most, that means an intensive outpatient program—and when it's needed, they help put a plan together. Schrank and Burton consult psychiatrists and psychologists when helping patients select appropriate outpatient programs. Those who aren't in outpatient programs must be under a doctor's care. "They have to have some clinical supervision," Burton says. Residents are also helped with their other needs: career or financial counseling, referrals to dentists, relationship counseling.

Residents must work or be in school. They're required to attend five Twelve Step meetings each week, including two AA meetings at the home. The program has an all-night staff that monitors patients. Drug testing is part of the regimen. Unlike at many sober homes, if a test comes back positive, residents aren't ejected. "Ultimately they have to want to be sober," Schrank says. "Sometimes they're here to placate their wife. If they're not able to stay sober, we help them transition into another level of care. But you don't realistically live with ten addicts and not expect stuff to happen." Addicts who relapse are helped to stabilize, if it's possible for them to do it in the sober-living setting. If it isn't, or if the relapsing addicts are in any way threatening to other residents, they're transitioned into alternative programs. Some must return to residential treatment.

Wednesday night at 7:30, current residents and alumni gather in the Loft 107 lounge for an AA meeting. One I attended was a speaker's meeting with a dozen people. As at most AA meetings, it began with a participant reading from the Big Book, though in this case, he read from an electronic version of the book that he pulled up on his iPhone. The speaker, Clark, talked about his recovery as Churchill, asleep on the couch, snored loudly.

Clark, tall and wiry, wearing an untucked white shirt and a loosened thin necktie, described the isolation and depression that characterized his childhood. He said he didn't begin using until he was twenty-one, but once he started, he used "around the clock." He said that his using was driven by self-loathing disguised as misanthropy. "I hated everybody," he said. "'Poor me.' I blamed everybody for the sad state of my life. I'd think, *If you had my life, you'd drink too.*" He spoke about an "itching" he had — a physical itching — "because I was so uncomfortable in my own skin." He then described his recovery in rehabs and AA. He said, "I've only been sober for two years. I struggle every day. I'm fine in meetings, but I know that a test of your sobriety is how you handle yourself outside these rooms, something I'm learning slowly."

Next was a round robin in which attendees responded to the speaker for four minutes apiece. The man with the iPhone volunteered to be the timer.

First a young boy — probably nineteen (the program is for people eighteen and older) — with sunflower tattoos up and down his arm responded to Clark. "When you talked about the itching," he said, "I get that. As an opiate addict, I had the itching too. The itching on my skin was like bug bites, but that's not the bad part. That was the itching inside me that I could never scratch." He said that he was doing all right but admitted that he had a difficult time with AA. "I'm not religious. I have no higher power. I just don't. But I'm trying."

Another boy, addressing Clark, said, "Like you, I'd get sober and relapse, get sober and relapse. I figured out I was trying to run before I hadn't ever learned to walk. So that's why I'm living here — a day at a time, a step forward at a time. I know I'm just not ready to be out there on my own."

The next boy, another heroin addict, had a 1950s-type haircut and wore a T-shirt and jeans. "I couldn't get to the grocery store without heroin," he said. He told Clark: "You say you have only two years. I *pray* that I'll have two years."

Another: "I'm grateful to you for telling the truth. That's what I hear in these rooms. I haven't heard a lot of truth in my life."

The iPhone's timer sounded. Next.

"Holy fuck," a boy said. "People can get through life without booze and drugs and be okay? I didn't know it was possible. I'm working day to day to stop behaving in a dysfunctional way. Forget day to day. I take it hour to hour sometimes, just getting through an hour at a time knowing that soon I'll be back here at this house where it's safe among my people. I'm trying to envision something better . . ."

Next in the circle was a twentyish girl with wavy dark hair. She said, "Thanks for sharing, Clark. I related. Like you said, usually I'm thinking about myself. My favorite sport is to read people's minds — what they're thinking of me. I'm narcissistic and pessimistic. And angry. I'm dealing with anger. I always thought I was a bad person. Maybe I'm learning I'm not so bad . . ." The timer went off. She concluded, "Sorry to go on. I just had a bad day. Work is hard. I don't want to grow up. I never want to leave here." She laughed — she was joking. Sort of.

Mike, next in the circle, said he'd been in six rehabs. "I'm living here because I just couldn't do it on my own. I couldn't go home to an empty house. I couldn't stay away from my using friends. I'd get high. I'd go back to lying to everybody. So I'm grateful for this place and all of you."

The iPhone's timer sounded, and the meeting ended with the Serenity Prayer. Residents headed to their rooms. Some stopped at the dessert bar for miniature cupcakes. Churchill still snored on the couch.

How long should patients stay in sober-living houses or continuing-care treatment? There's no single answer that applies to every patient. For some, a month to a few months in a transitional program is enough, but some stay for much longer. Outpatient programs can continue for months or years, though the frequency of individual or group therapy sessions usually is decreased over time. The intensive outpatient program at Freedom Institute in New York serves as primary treatment for some patients and for others as an aftercare program following residential treatment. The program begins with three group and one individual therapy session a week for twelve weeks, followed by a period of twice-weekly group and once-a-week individual therapy. The initial intensive phase of the Matrix outpatient program runs for twelve to sixteen weeks. There are three sessions a week for the first four weeks devoted to early recovery. These are followed by four to twelve weeks of relapse prevention. Afterward, patients attend weekly and, eventually, monthly group support sessions. Some patients continue for months, some for a year or more, and all are encouraged to return whenever they're struggling and need help. On days that sessions aren't scheduled, clients are encouraged, though not required, to attend AA meetings.

Outpatient programs can be supplemented by individual therapy and support groups, particularly AA. There are now online AA meetings, though I have never found research that measures their effectiveness.

RMC
recovery
management

checkup

Many people find it helpful, or necessary, to attend AA meetings for decades — and many for a lifetime.

Wellness Checkups

Relapse prevention should include monitoring any aspect of an addict's life that could threaten his sobriety, whether psychological, physical, social, or environmental. Michael L. Dennis and Christy K. Scott, doctors at Chestnut Health Systems, developed what they call Recovery Management Checkups (RMCs), which Dennis compares to quarterly checkups for other chronic conditions like diabetes or asthma. "Given the high risk of relapse, we need ongoing monitoring and early re-intervention for addiction," he says.

Addicts schedule quarterly checkups with professionals trained in the RMC process. The managers ask how things have gone over the previous few months: whether they've had any relapses, whether they've remained in treatment, and whether they've attended AA or other recovery or support groups. Patients who are doing well are encouraged to keep up their recovery regimen. If an addict is using or at high risk of relapse, however, the RMC-trained manager uses motivational interviewing to help convince him of the value of returning to treatment. The manager and patient review barriers to going back to treatment and talk about what did and didn't work last time. Then they make a plan. If the patient agrees to return to treatment, the manager will schedule and actually go with him to the initial treatment session and then stay in contact for two weeks to make sure the patient engages in treatment. If the patient isn't willing to go to treatment, he'll be encouraged to go to AA or other recovery support. If he's not willing to do that, he's encouraged to modify the way he's using (to reduce use; to use in safer ways).

For a study of RMC, Scott and Dennis followed addicts in the program for four years. Dennis reports, "Participants in the RMC condition were significantly more likely than participants in the control group to return to treatment sooner (13 vs. 45 months), to return at all (70% vs. 51%), to return more times (1.9 vs. 1.0 readmissions), and to receive more total days of treatment (112 vs. 79 days). They subsequently had significantly fewer quarters in need of treatment, fewer substance re-

C BT
Cognitive
Behavior
Therapy

lated problems per month (89 vs. 129), and more total days of abstinence (1026 vs. 932 days)."

How long must a patient monitor his condition? Just as long as a diabetic has to monitor his glucose levels; as long as a schizophrenic has to take his medication; as long as a heart patient has to have regular EKGs. That is to say, a long time, perhaps forever. After the success of initial cancer treatment, patients in remission may be instructed to watch for warning signs of the disease's return. With their cancer in remission, most patients are advised to visit their oncologists for periodic checkups. Early on, they may be told to come in for exams or tests every three months. Depending on how things go, eventually the doctor may see them every six months. Then every year. As with cancer patients, depending on how things go, addicts may get checkups less frequently over time.

Added Therapies and Crisis Intervention

Some addicts' problems — emotional ones, psychological ones, ones related to their living situations, careers, finances, and so on — are identified while they are in the primary program. Often, though, new problems — and potential triggers — can emerge. For example, people can't be protected from life events. Loved ones get sick and die. Relationships end. These can be triggers too.

Relapse prevention means intensifying the interventions when needed. Or starting new ones. New problems must be treated with whatever is appropriate — new kinds of therapy (psychotherapy, anger management, assertiveness training; CBT for impulse control; counseling or coaching to help addicts cope with trauma or stressful changes in their lives). Addicts may learn that they must avoid certain social situations or escape a toxic environment. They may need more training to anticipate and handle stressful events that might threaten their sobriety — the holidays, a family reunion.

Therapy may need to focus on a common experience that comes after the first stage of treatment: some addicts in recovery, especially early on, describe their sober lives as boring, devoid of meaning, and hopeless. Anhedonia — lack of pleasure — is common. Food, companionship, sex, walks in nature — whatever — may not provide much joy, at least for a while. Raymond Chandler's Philip Marlowe observes in *The Long Goodbye* that alcoholics who quit drinking can find "a different world. You have to get used to a paler set of colors, a quieter lot of sounds."

Through therapy, addicts can learn to tolerate this anhedonia until it dissipates. They can redefine what is most meaningful to them and appreciate subtler and healthier pleasure, whether in a sunset, a walk on a beach, or a relationship characterized by friendship and love rather than the intense but fleeting high from their drug of choice. In therapy that includes MI, they can further analyze their lives, envision positive futures, and assess and, if necessary, modify their course. Addicts frequently say that profound life lessons come with sobriety. Crises almost always pass. Pleasure returns; one can feel more deeply than ever.

Addicts may begin to address dysfunctional relationships in primary treatment, but the work should continue. Sometimes things worsen when an addict isn't using because drugs numbed him, and now he's experiencing a fuller range of emotions — the good as well as the bad. For some addicts, family therapy or marriage counseling in primary treatment has helped. In many cases, these therapies should continue. Or it may be necessary to begin them. Some addicts' families who participated in the early stages of treatment won't continue in therapy, but often they should. Some family dynamics can't, or won't, change, but family therapy and marriage counseling can help people relearn intimacy, change destructive family dynamics, and rebuild trust. Some addicts have never been in healthy relationships, but individual psychotherapy, CBT, or group therapy can help them understand what's gone wrong in the past and how to do better in the future.

As they continue in recovery, many addicts also need to learn how to function in the real world. They may have no experience with the basic skills it takes to hold down a job — being on time, taking direction and criticism, being organized, and so on. Some life skills training may begin in primary treatment, but it's usually not enough. If they're going to function and thrive, recovering addicts must build these skills.

A person's poor physical health can contribute to relapse too, so relapse prevention must include treatment for medical problems that preceded addiction and/or were caused by it. Pain can lead to relapse, so doctors must work with addicts to manage it, using methods that don't rely on addictive drugs.

Relapse Prevention for Adolescents

As always, teenagers face particular challenges. Those who leave primary treatment and return to the communities, schools, and friends that surrounded them when they were using are especially vulnerable. Those emerging from the relatively safe confines of residential treatment may return to a world where triggers are everywhere and drugs are plentiful. Temptations to relapse take many forms. Compared to what's available for adults, sober communities and social activities for kids are hard to find — sober teenage parties are few and far between. Some kids thrive sober, even in environments that would be dangerous to others, but many struggle. They face intense challenges, which can lead to stress, and stress can lead to relapse.

Many kids heading home should continue in outpatient programs, therapy, and/or attend AA meetings or other support groups. After kids leave residential treatment, outpatient programs help them integrate recovery into their lives and continue their therapies. In addition, they provide a sober community that can help kids as they navigate stressful high-school years. After an evening therapy session or AA meeting, kids can go out together to the movies or dinner. Friendships can develop.

Students returning to or entering college can be especially likely to relapse. College students face a welter of triggers and stress: being away from home, challenging academic work, social tensions, and, often, a culture of extreme use: binge drinking, pill parties, performance-enhancing drugs for athletes, performance-enhancing drugs for studying and test taking. Increasingly, colleges offer substance-free dorms, which help kids connect with other sober students. (However, sober dorms are not always monitored to ensure they're actually sober.) Most colleges have an array of health services, including counseling. Adolescents in recovery should meet with counselors or others to help plan an ongoing program. Don't wait for crisis. Students in crisis, or those who need support, should have a place to go for help immediately — a health clinic, treatment center, or on-call psychologist or psychiatrist. Even while they attend school, some students should continue in outpatient programs. There are AA meetings on and around most college campuses. Meetings, as well as relationships with others in AA, like a sponsor, help prevent relapse in adolescents, as in adults. There's moral support, plus an addict in danger of relapsing or who's relapsed has someone to call — a sponsor or other AA member.

Some teens require protected environments and intense therapy to continue after primary treatment — for a year, maybe two. Hopefully these kids are identified in early treatment. Some examples are kids with co-occurring psychiatric and behavioral disorders. Kids too young for most sober-living homes but who need structure and support and for whom going home is ill-advised may be good candidates for therapeutic boarding schools that combine addiction treatment, therapy, and high school. Some kids may have completed primary treatment in these schools and are ready to come home, but many need time measured not in months but a year or more. There are also post-treatment programs in some cities that include a combination of sober high school and regular participation in an APG: an adolescent peer group. Kids meet with counselors and attend Twelve Step meetings and social events together. For example, Houston's Archway Academy is a sober high school that requires its students to participate in one of four local APG programs.

The most effective relapse-prevention strategies for teenagers are the multisystemic ones I described for primary care — continuing work with a therapist that involves an adolescent's parents and other family members, physician, and, if possible, teachers, coaches, and other adults in his life. And as with adults, teenagers should continue to see professionals, at least for the kinds of recovery checkups I described. There may be intensely stressful times when a teenager or young adult must return to more intensive levels of care — more frequent sessions with a therapist, more AA meetings, new forms of therapy, or outpatient or even residential treatment. In fact, there may be times when addicts of any age must return to intensive treatment.

The morning after he returned from the company conference, Steven Garfield popped another Vicodin on his way to work. Midmorning he took another. The little plastic bag was feeling light — a familiar anxiety. He thought he'd call Rick to arrange to buy another half a dozen. Maybe a dozen. "That was the moment," he said later. "To live or to die." He called his wife and told her what had happened. She packed a suitcase and, as he'd asked her to do, met him at a residential treatment center he'd called. She stood with him as he signed himself in.

They cried together. She said, "I'm so proud of you," and then she left him there. Looking back, he says, "I could have tried to stop on my own, and maybe I would have. But there was too much at stake to risk sliding backward. My wife. My kids."

Nip Relapse in the Bud

Relapse-prevention strategies work, but, of course, not always. As I said, depending on the statistics you trust (and none are exact), more than half of all addicts relapse within a year of treatment, and though the risk of relapse declines over time, it doesn't go away — ever. It's not uncommon to hear stories of addicts who relapsed after years, even decades, of being clean. But researchers have found that if a person makes it to two years, his likelihood of relapse diminishes dramatically, and after five years, most addicts will continue to stay sober.

A relapse might seem to indicate that previous treatments failed, but it doesn't. First, the treatment worked for however many days, months, or years that person stayed sober. Second, addiction treatments are cumulative, part of what I've heard doctors describe as a "treatment trajectory." There are forward steps, followed by backward ones, followed by more forward ones.

The heartening fact is that most addicts who relapse return to recovery. Relapses can be progressively less severe. Using the techniques they've learned in CBT and elsewhere, addicts can interrupt the priming mechanism and halt the relapse. They can reframe a relapse and think through the implications. *I can't believe I had a drink. This is it. If I don't do something I'll be shooting heroin in a day or two. Everything I've worked for will be gone again.* Sometimes that awareness is enough. Sometimes a learned behavioral intervention is necessary. Again, a person should do whatever has already worked for him: leave the party and go see sober friends, go to the gym, call an AA sponsor, go to a meeting, call a therapist, return to an outpatient program. Whatever the cause, relapse requires a return to treatment, a redoubling of efforts.

Minor relapses can require minor interventions — a return to therapy or AA or more sessions or meetings. Some addicts may need to return to outpatient programs. Some attend "refresher courses" — Hazelden in Minnesota has a renewal center for addicts who have relapsed, though they have to be clean when they come. After a severe relapse, an addict might have to go through detox again.

As I pointed out above, relapse doesn't mean that one should abandon the treatment that preceded it. But it does mean that an addict should work with a psychologist or psychiatrist to reevaluate ongoing treatment. Something isn't working. Since relapse is often related to stress, anxiety, depression, frustration, and similar factors, addicts must be guided to determine what event or aspect of their lives led them to use. What were they frustrated about? Why were they more anxious than usual? Were they bored? Were there problems with family, friends, coworkers, or others? Was there a crisis — a death in the family, the loss of a job? Often, serious or multiple relapses are a sign that a patient has an undiagnosed co-occurring psychiatric disorder. He should be evaluated, whether for the first time or again, for comorbidity. Assessment, or reassessment, is critical, because patients with unidentified and untreated dual diagnoses are at high risk for relapse.

Rebuilding a Life, Living with Addiction

Traditional Twelve Step programs promise more than sobriety. They hold out the prospect of spiritual awakening and redemption for those who work the Program. As part of the process, the Twelve Steps require addicts to make amends to people they've harmed. Addicts work to be forgiven, and they aspire to forgive. To stay sober and improve their lives, addicts are instructed to become involved in service to others — to help other alcoholics and addicts.

The fact is, treatment doesn't require people to seek forgiveness for harm they've caused others. Redemption of one kind or another isn't needed to treat an illness. Those who can't or won't heal damaged relationships can still stop using. And the reality is that getting sober doesn't necessarily make a person wiser, kinder, or more selfless. However, many people who stop using do describe profound changes in their lives beyond physical well-being that can come with sobriety. It's often possible for people who've never had meaningful relationships because of their addictions and other psychological problems to develop ones that are deep, trusting, and nurturing.

Often, the addict has betrayed, lied to, stolen from, and otherwise tormented his loved ones. It may be impossible to repair some relationships that were harmed by these actions, but most can be mended. Just as it takes time for an addict's nervous system to heal, it takes time for relationships to heal — but most can.

Meanwhile, as addicts work to earn others' forgiveness, they should work to forgive themselves. For many addicts, it may be the most elusive and challenging step of all. No, self-forgiveness is not a requirement either, but self-doubt or — worse — self-hatred can lead back to drug use. Forgiving oneself can be at once a means to and a measure of repair of the damage caused by addiction. Forgiving oneself may come from a deep understanding of one's illness. Understanding and accepting the past and its consequences can bring a kind of peace. Therapy helps people heal and change. Often self-blame and a lack of self-worth predate drug use. Targeted therapies, including DBT and CBT, can be especially helpful in this regard. Addicts can work to replace their self-defeating negative self-talk. Addicts who feel better about themselves are less likely to relapse.

Although a spiritual awakening isn't a necessary component or result of getting sober, almost all addicts who get treatment will live better lives. Their lives also improve as they treat psychological disorders that underlie and accompany addiction. People can simply have an easier time, fewer or more contained lows, more frequent and sustained feelings of contentment and joy. Desperation, denial, and suffering make way for measured optimism, wisdom, and in some cases even a kind of enlightenment — the hard-earned rewards of freedom from a disease that had controlled one's entire life.

VII

Ending Addiction

17

The Future of Prevention
and Treatment

A BARBER-POLE-SIZED CYLINDER filled with what looks like coffee filters sits on a shelf in Ulrike Heberlein's lab. She invented the device, which she calls an inebriometer, to measure the amount of alcohol it takes to get fruit flies wasted.

Heberlein pours a test tube full of flies into an opening at the top of the inebriometer and clicks shut the tiny door. Next she twirls a dial, releasing a flow of alcohol mist, brewed from straight ethanol in evaporators — jugs labeled TIPPLE, DELIVERANCE, and DEAN MARTINI.

As I soon see, when fruit flies get drunk, they act sort of like drunk people. They wobble and buzz erratically, crash into one another and the walls. After a while, they lapse into a sort of stupor and fall to the floor. If they're really drunk, Heberlein tells me, they black out. It takes twenty or so minutes before they recover, a bit worse for wear. They're hung over, I'm guessing.

Heberlein, who's from Chile, has clear, light blue eyes and shoulder length blond-brown hair. She's dressed not in a lab coat but in a black knit sweater and a string of pearls. She speaks quickly and seriously, though a grin appears for a moment when she talks about her barflies and, in another laboratory, her cocaine-addicted mice.

Heberlein's research wing occupies a suite of adjoining laboratories at the UCSF Medical Center's Mission Bay campus (since I visited her, Dr. Heberlein has moved her laboratory to the Howard Hughes Medical Institute's Janelia Farm Research Campus). On one wall is pinned a pencil sketch of a fly smoking either a cigarette or a spliff and holding a martini. Heberlein oversees a dozen postdoctoral fellows, including one who was just then hunched over a desk, staring into the lens of a microscope. He had stripped the exoskeleton off a fly and was preparing to separate its brain and spinal cord. I looked into the eyepiece and saw that the fly's brain — bulbous, lobed, and sort of white-gray-cream-colored — looked a lot like ours.

Heberlein studies fruit flies (genus *Drosophila*) because they and humans display many of the same vulnerabilities and behavioral responses to alcohol and cocaine. "Genetically speaking, people and fruit flies are surprisingly alike," she explains. "Three-quarter of the genes are the same, or nearly the same." Her discoveries about the genetic makeup of fruit flies are then tested on mice, which, gene-wise, are even more like humans.

Obviously, flies don't get addicted in the exact way humans do — presumably there's no psychological component the way there is in people. However, revelations from her research come because, as she says, "we deconstruct a very complex problem into its primary components. We can't ask a fly, do you have a hangover? What we try to measure is tolerance, in various circumstances, how much a fly will take in on its own, and levels of reward from different drugs and amounts. All we know is that we get flies into that state of intoxication. We have no idea what they're feeling."

In one experiment, Heberlein exposes one group of flies to the odor of rotting apples, another group to the odor of vinegar. The apple smell is accompanied by an intoxicating mist of alcohol; the vinegar smell isn't. After three ten-minute sessions of exposure, the flies are put into a Y-shaped maze. At the end of one branch is the odor of apple. This time, there's no alcohol. At the end of the other, more vinegar. Almost all of the flies that were trained to associate the apple odor with a burst of alcohol mist choose it. When Dr. Heberlein reverses it and spikes the vinegar, flies choose vinegar. "Whichever odor is delivered at the same time as a mist of ethanol is preferred," Heberlein explains. "Flies 'remember' that they prefer that odor. The implication is that they find ethanol intoxication rewarding. They like it." And they want more.

How much more? A lot. In a separate experiment, an electrified grille is placed on the path that leads to the odor associated with getting high. This time, to get to the source of the odor, flies have to cross the grid. When they do, they're blasted with 100 to 120 volts of electricity.

It doesn't stop them. These flies will endure electric shock to get to the odor that they remember was associated with alcohol. They've become addicted, or at least the fly equivalent of addiction; their drive to procure drugs is greater than the self-preservation instincts that make them avoid pain. There's no way to know if they "like" the feeling, but they seek it, even if they're electrocuted along the way. "Addicted" flies will do whatever it takes to get high. Similarly, addicted humans will do whatever it takes to get high. They'll steal, lie, become violent, and endure great pain.

In her experiments, Heberlein has learned that not all flies are created equal when it comes to drug-seeking behavior. "Like in humans, we know that dopamine is the neurotransmitter associated with rewards in flies," Heberlein explains. "Like in humans, some flies appear to be more slave to their reward system than others." That is, in their pursuit of drugs, some flies will endure more pain than others. Why the difference? It's likely that gene variations are responsible for the fact that some flies, like some people, become addicted and some don't. Heberlein says, "We have found genes that regulate how rewarding ethanol is to flies."

In yet another series of experiments, Heberlein studies the link between stress and drug taking. As I've reported, there's ample evidence of a connection, and in surveys, teenagers have acknowledged that stress is the number one reason they use drugs. Heberlein is attempting to understand the connection between stress and drugs beyond the obvious — that, when one is high, stress can seem to melt away. And her research is also helping to uncover why stress can lead to not only drug use but addiction. "We're exploring a pathway that links alcohol tolerance and stress in flies that also exists in humans," she says. "This finding may explain why people who have been in a stressful situation often have a blunted response to alcohol and may need to drink more to feel inebriated, putting them at greater risk of becoming addicted."

She adds, "There is growing recognition that stress, at both cellular and systemic levels, contributes to drug- and addiction-related behaviors in mammals. Our studies suggest that this role may be conserved across evolution." Understanding the link between stress and drug use could be a key to effective prevention and treatment. If it's true that stress is connected to addiction, that's more evidence that if you find ways to lessen stress, you may be able to prevent addiction or relapse.

I can't resist asking Heberlein how she stresses flies. She says that she shakes them up, heats them, overcrowds them, isolates them. She can also, as she describes it, "suppress courtship and mating."

How does one sexually frustrate flies? "There's a very sophisticated courtship when male fruit flies are presented with virgin females," Dr. Heberlein explains. "But if males are presented with a previously mated female" — not a virgin — "she rejects them pretty vehemently." In one experiment, the males are set up to be rejected for three days in a row, three one-hour sessions a day, and then they are allowed to choose food with or without alcohol. The more sexually frustrated they are, the more they drink.

Further experiments helped isolate the connection between sexual frustration and drug use. Some rejected males were moved to a different environment, where groups of males mingled with receptive females. Those who then had sex were less interested in alcohol. Researchers also paired thousands of other male flies with dead virgin females, so that they didn't experience rejection but didn't have sex either. They also drank or used heavily.

Heberlein's pioneering research with flies and mice has shown that some animals, like some humans, are genetically predisposed to addiction. She has had some success isolating genes that appear to be linked to some addictions. She's shown that flies with specific genetic mutations are more likely than others to seek drugs; compared to "normal" flies', their drug-seeking drive overrides even their survival instinct. She has also shown that flies with a particular genetic makeup are more affected by stress than others. This suggests that people with certain gene combinations are more vulnerable when they're stressed than others are. But what's possibly most significant is her discovery of a gene mutation in fruit flies that alters their sensitivity to crack cocaine, and she's identified a gene that helps flies develop tolerance to alcohol and cocaine. These discoveries could lead to medications that would make people more resistant to, or would even cure, some addictions. (Besides the potential to lead to treatments, Heberlein's research is more proof that addiction is a disease, not a choice, putting the lie to the view that some people choose to get high no matter the price. As with flies, it's not a choice. We can assume that the flies who become addicted aren't succumbing to peer pressure. It's doubtful that they're weak, selfish hedonists choosing to party.)

Hope for the Future

Dr. Heberlein is one of many researchers working to further our understanding of addiction and to develop and test new prevention strategies and treatments. They're making progress, but it's slowed by problems we've already seen: the stigma of addiction; the roots of treatment in superstition and religion rather than science; the tendency to approach drug use as a criminal versus a health problem; a paucity of money for research and treatment; too few researchers and doctors, given the need; and more.

Researchers in the field I've spoken with share my view that addiction medicine is at least forty years behind where it could and should be. And, as inadequate as the best prevention strategies and treatments are, the system for disseminating them is even worse. Few people know about evidence-based prevention and fewer still are able to access evidence-based treatment. As I've explained, most physicians haven't been trained in addiction prevention, diagnosis, and intervention, whether that involves treatment or referral to treatment. A CASA study published in 2012 concludes, "Addiction treatment is largely disconnected from mainstream medical practice. While a wide range of evidence-based screening, intervention, treatment and disease management tools and practices exist, they rarely are employed." Stanford's Dr. Humphreys said, "One of the fundamental barriers to providing effective treatment is the fact that addiction is not integrated into medical practice." Worse, Humphreys added, "A lot of medical people like and want it that way; they do not want to deal with addiction; they do not like to deal with the people and they do not feel effective addressing the problem."

I've recommended that those who are worried that they or loved ones might be addicted contact AAAP- or ASAM-certified doctors, but at the end of 2011, there were only 2,500 of them in the United States, compared to an estimated 12,500 oncologists and 20,000 cardiologists.

If those in need do find doctors trained in addiction medicine, their next-step options can be limited. A doctor may determine that an addict needs treatment in an outpatient or inpatient program, but as we've seen, few of these programs offer evidence-based treatments. Also, even if the programs are certified or accredited and claim they use evidence-based practices, unless doctors visit and monitor treatment programs, which isn't practical, there's no way to know if centers actually do use EBTs or, if they do, if they're practiced effectively. We need a system to help people who need treatment find it (and a system to help doctors find it for their patients).

Such a system would require three components. First, researchers must identify what in medicine is called best practices — a standardized, evidence-based treatment protocol that includes the way the treatments are administered, who administers them, and how they're combined and adjusted over time depending on a patient's individual needs. Next, there must be a universally accepted accreditation system for treatment programs so consumers will know that patients receive care from qualified physicians, therapists, and counselors who correctly administer the evidence-based practices. Finally, there must be an online guide that points people to programs that use EBTs and are appropriate for a particular person depending on his age, drug or drugs of choice, severity of addiction, presence of co-occurring psychological disorders, and other factors. Listed programs must be continually monitored so addicts will be assured that they're getting the treatment they need. There's now promise of such a guide supported by funding from NIDA and being developed by Tom McLellan's Treatment Research Institute. TRI is creating this guide in stages, initially focusing on Philadelphia. If it's successful, McLellan hopes to roll it out nationally.

Breakthroughs in Treatment

We need a system for finding state-of-the art treatment, but there also must be more and better treatments, and some are coming. I mentioned earlier that several medical schools are pioneering accredited residency programs in addiction medicine, treating it as it should be treated, as a specialty like pediatrics, gynecology, and cardiology. ASAM membership is growing too. In addition, whether they join ASAM or not, more physicians (internists, family practice doctors, and specialists) are learning to assess patients and treat (or refer for treatment) addicts. Also, more therapists are being trained to effectively treat patients with potential or full-blown drug problems.

These efforts will bear more fruit as new treatments are developed and put into practice. Researchers have hundreds of promising ideas for new interventions, medications, cognitive and behavioral therapies, and combination therapies. At the moment, most are untested. These scientists aren't working in a vacuum, however. Their research is being advanced by breakthroughs in other fields of medicine and related sciences — in genetics, pharmacology, and psychology. Research designed to study the actions of various drugs on dopamine and the nervous system is continuing, because there's promise that they'll lead to new and better medications, including, potentially, vaccines.

Vaccines and Other Preventive Approaches

It's hard to imagine a time when children might be routinely vaccinated to protect them from addiction, but many researchers insist that it's possible. Vaccines may never prevent all addiction — according to researchers, it's doubtful — but there's a high likelihood that they'll prevent dependence on some drugs. Because vaccinations show such promise, they're a high priority at NIDA.

By stimulating production of antibodies that bind to cocaine and hold it in the bloodstream, cocaine vaccines under development have successfully stopped the drug from reaching the brain and other organs. One promising vaccine combines components of the common cold virus with a particle that mimics cocaine. According to a study of the vaccine, it produced a lasting anti-cocaine immunity in mice. This vaccine is an advance over previous efforts in that it requires only a single dose. The researchers hope to begin human trials within the next few years. There's been limited success in human trials of other potential cocaine vaccines. One created enough of an immune response in some test subjects that they cut their drug use by half. "It's not a very good vaccine," Dr. Charles O'Brien, professor of psychiatry and director of the addiction studies center at the University of Pennsylvania, told the *New York Times*. "It doesn't raise enough antibodies." Nonetheless, he points out, "It's very important because it shows the feasibility of the approach."

Scientists funded by NIDA are also working on vaccines for other stimulants, including meth, and there have been promising animal studies of a vaccine for heroin that's being tested on humans. Alcohol may be the drug most resistant to vaccination, because it affects so many different body systems. This hasn't stopped researchers from trying to develop one.

Vaccines have great potential, but they're not a panacea. If an addict is vaccinated for opiates, for example, he might well gravitate to another class of drug if the genetic, psychological, and environmental factors that underlie his drug use aren't addressed early and effectively. For this reason, another area of research is exploring if it is possible to identify people who are at high risk of developing addiction, possibly through genetic testing or brain scanning. NIDA's David Shurtleff says, "Someday we hope to test a child with genetic vulnerability measures." It's possible that by using brain imaging or other technology, doctors could one day identify addiction before it manifests. Using scanning technology, scientists have already successfully identified people who are more likely to relapse. Shurtleff describes one research project focused on meth addicts. Based on scans, a researcher accurately predicted who would relapse within a year. Yale researchers conducted a similar study on alcoholics that had similar results. If tests can identify patients whose brain functions show that they're at high risk of relapsing, doctors can intervene before it happens.

Medication

Many of the emerging treatments are psychopharmacological. There are a number of reasons for this. "Addiction is a medical condition," Dr. Volkow said in *Time* magazine. "We have to recognize that medications can compensate or even reverse the pathology of this disease." When medications work, they have a relatively quick and dramatic effect — methadone and buprenorphine are the obvious examples. In addition, the development of medication isn't dependent on government grants. Pharmaceutical companies support research on drugs that are likely to bring sizable returns on their investments.

New medications are under development. Some control dopamine. Some increase the effectiveness of the brain's own inhibitory systems. In addicts, the mechanism of the natural tamping neurotransmitter GABA appears to be faulty, which means the brain can't control the flood of neurotransmitters. Vigabatrin, a GABA booster, is being studied as a possible treatment for methamphetamine and cocaine users — in theory, it could stop the dangerous flood of dopamine. There are currently no replacement drugs for stimulants, so treatments that block amphetamine cravings and prevent a high, similar to the ways buprenorphine affects opiate addicts, would be a significant step forward. In early trials, the Parkinson's drug L-dopa has been used to help cocaine addicts taper off their drug and has been shown to lead to higher rates of successful detox.

Future Behavioral Treatments

Another reason for the focus on pharmacology is that it's easier to prove the effectiveness of drugs than it is to prove the effectiveness of therapy. Clinical trials of drugs are simpler and more conclusive; it's easy enough to compare groups of addicts who are on a medication with control groups who aren't. In contrast, behavioral and psychosocial treatments depend on factors that are difficult to manage. For those that are carried out by therapists, it's difficult to control for adherence to protocols and individual therapists' personalities that affect their relationship with patients. Similar factors are spurring research into computer-based treatments — for example, CBT administered online. Early studies have shown that they're effective at both the prevention and relapse-prevention stages. Like medications, these programs aren't affected by individual practitioners' personalities. That said, we should never minimize the impact of people on other people; the relationship between therapist and patient is and probably will always be an indispensable component of therapy, and promising new approaches are on the horizon.

The Matrix program, which I've described, is one model for standardizing behavioral treatment — standardizing it by having therapists undergo the same intensive training and follow a single manual. Before he went to UCLA, Dr. Rawson, in conjunction with Jeanne Obert and Michael McCann, who are still with the program, sought to replace the invent-as-you-go treatment programs offered at many rehabs with a replicable regimen that's built on evidence-based therapies. They created just that in the Matrix Model, which has been tested and found effective in randomized clinical trials sponsored by the Center for Substance Abuse Treatment (CSAT). It's only one model for standardizing and implementing existing and new evidence-based practices.

Even as some therapies are being standardized, new ones are being explored. Exposure and reconsolidation therapy desensitizes a person to a cue so it loses its power and no longer triggers craving. Treatments based on them have been shown to help people with PTSD and other trauma. Experiments are now under way that explore whether addicts can become inured to triggers through repeated exposure in safe, therapeutic environments. Animal studies have shown that it's possible to retrain a subject's response to cues by repeated contact with them. Currently, exposure therapy isn't an evidence-based addiction treatment (because there isn't enough research to prove its effectiveness), but it may become one. There are ongoing trials, including ones that are investigating whether virtual (that is, computer-generated) cues could be used to reduce the effect of triggers. Even if it's perfected, exposure therapy would not be a panacea for recovering addicts, because it mostly addresses only external cues, but many triggers reside within an addict's mind. Nonetheless, there would be great benefit to disarming external triggers.

At Emory University in Atlanta and a nearby company called Virtually Better, virtual-reality exposure therapy is being used to treat everything from PTSD to the fear of public speaking, and it's being adapted to addiction treatment. Josh Spitalnick, director of research and clinical services at Virtually Better, explains that patients can be put into a virtual environment in which they experience visual, aural, and olfactory cues that trigger intense craving. It's impractical, let alone dangerous, to bring an addict to a real bar or crack house so they can practice CBT in context, but it can be therapeutic to immerse them in those environments — controlled and safe — in a virtual world. The virtual-reality experience I tried, a program for those with a fear of public speaking, was at first disorienting, but it became strangely real. I was in an auditorium filled with a virtual audience that, as I gave a prepared talk, fidgeted and whispered to one another. A cell phone sounded. I didn't venture into a virtual apartment where people were sitting on couches smoking pot (as the smell of marijuana permeated the space), but it's not hard to imagine the intense reaction of an addict. Addicts' cravings can be stimulated by a photograph alone, never mind the experience of being in a virtual bar that looks like a real bar, sounds like a real bar (conversations and clinking glasses), and smells like a real bar (bourbon and margaritas.) At a similar laboratory at UCLA, researchers have even come up with a virtual crack house, as well as a video-based virtual apartment where people are snorting and shooting methamphetamine (the drug in the film that's part of the virtual reality experience is actually baby powder). "Can we get people to jones by exposing them to cues in virtual reality?" Spitalnick asks. Apparently they can.

The VR technology has been shown to be effective in triggering intense craving in addicts, but it hasn't yet been used to attempt to inure them to cueing. In theory it could add an important component of treatment. "All the CBT you've learned in treatment can be hampered by context," Spitalnick says. "The question is whether you can leave treatment with confidence that you can use the CBT skills you've learned in a bar or at a party where people are drinking or smoking pot. If we can get the patient to crave in the office while teaching them CBT skills in the context of craving, they might be more able to use these skills in a real situation that triggers the craving and continue to use them when craving is intense."

Elsewhere in the world, researchers are exploring even more radical treatments. In China, scientists are experimenting with a kind of finely targeted brain surgery that destroys the circuits that make up the primary reward system. The published findings show promise for some heavy abusers, though it causes severe depressive bouts in others. The prospect of surgery conjures images of forced lobotomies to treat the mentally ill, leaving people in almost vegetative states, but the goal of this research is much more selective ablations, as UCLA's Chris Evans describes them. "A part of the brain called the insula that if disrupted may disable the craving mechanism has promise as a target area for surgery for severely addicted patients." He describes a methadone and amphetamine addict who, after developing a bilateral lesion in the part of the brain called the globus pallidus, lost all desire for drugs and food.

Evans acknowledges that these are interesting observations, but he isn't advocating brain surgery for addicts. "Because the insula and reward circuits are so critical to other brain functions — appreciation of natural rewards, perceiving danger, and anticipating threats, damaging this area isn't something you would ever want to do intentionally. With so many of the brain's systems entangled with one another, it could prove impossible to adjust just one without throwing the others into imbalance." However, these findings suggest promising routes for pharmacology: we may hope for the development of drugs that precisely target some pathways that govern addictive cravings.

The Future of Prevention

Of course a main component of tackling America's drug problem is preventing use and abuse in the first place. Because people use drugs for so many reasons, it's tremendously challenging. Finding ways to prevent addiction may be even harder than finding ways to treat it. "Prevention is very different from medication development, where something is developed, tested and rolled out," says Amelia Arria, senior scientist at the Treatment Research Institute and the director of the Center on Young Adult Health and Development at the University of Maryland. "It's about processes that can be ignited that shift the way we think about problems — like learning that eating lard every day isn't a good idea. Another example is traffic injuries. We didn't develop a vaccine to prevent car accidents — we convinced drivers to wear seat belts and governments to help get messages out."

In *Clean,* I've described some evidence-based prevention strategies, and these must be refined, adapted for various populations, and widely applied. There's great promise in in-school prevention programs like Life Skills Training and the Wellness Centers at San Francisco public schools, and there's much more. For example, research suggests that training all physicians in SBIRT could prevent a significant number of drug problems from beginning or escalating. Whether with SBIRT or a similar program, the goal is to have everyone who goes in for a checkup — children as well as adults — screened for drug problems and, if there's a need, treated with a brief or more intensive intervention.

Ultimately, if we're going to change the course we're on, doctors, nurses, teachers, child-care providers, and other professionals must be trained to identify and intervene at the first signs of problems in the people they care for. There must be available interventions for social, emotional, and medical problems that could lead to drug use.

Our prevention strategies must take into account individual risk factors — for example, trauma, mental illness, or a family history of addiction — so people understand their increased vulnerability. Parents and caregivers must be taught about these risk factors too — how to look for signs of emerging problems in their families, and what to do if they see them.

Another more long-range strategy would be parenting courses for people who plan to have children (and current parents who need to improve these skills), because effective parenting is preventive while ineffective parenting raises the risks of drug problems. The exemplary Nurse Family Partnership focuses on teenage mothers, but other parents would benefit from similar programs. Bolstering all families with social services — health care, child care, family therapy — that decrease stress and dysfunction would also lower drug use. Prevention must include improving community services, such as afterschool and weekend programs for school-age children and high-quality child care for younger ones. There should be mentoring programs. Kids with learning disabilities should be helped to surmount them. Those with attention problems, depression, anxiety, and other disorders must be treated. A goal is to replace high-risk with protective factors for all people, especially children. Imagine if we treated young kids' depression before they treated it themselves with marijuana. Imagine if we helped kids with learning disabilities before they checked out and found solace in drinking. Imagine if we could identify a child experiencing his parents' difficult divorce, bullying, abuse, or other trauma in his life and get him effective counseling before drugs appear as a solution, and before use leads to abuse and abuse leads to addiction. Imagine the lives that could be saved. Imagine the suffering that could be prevented.

18

Fighting the Right War

CLEAN DESCRIBES AMERICA'S DRUG problem — its scope, its casualties — but it also chronicles advances being made. The progress is encouraging, but it comes slowly and there are frequent setbacks. Forward momentum is hindered by the complexity of the problem (its social, psychological, environmental, and physiological roots), but also by archaic attitudes that are behind the stigmatization of drug users — the view that good kids abstain, bad kids use — and a basic misunderstanding of addiction (the belief that it's a choice, whereas we know it's a disease). But though these assumptions are outdated and fallacious, America's overarching drug policy is based on them. The sooner we change it — roundly *reject* it — the sooner we'll speed dramatic advances in our ability to prevent drug use and treat the addicted.

The policy that's defined the country's attitudes and responses to drug problems for more than forty years was initiated in 1971. President Richard Nixon is mostly remembered for the progress he made in U.S.-China relations, the Watergate burglary and cover-up, and his role in the Vietnam War. Few remember that he also declared war on drugs. "America's public enemy number one is drug abuse," he said. "In order to fight and defeat this enemy, it is necessary to wage a new, all-out offensive."

Though the war now focuses on interdiction and arrest, it was originally designed to emphasize treatment and rehabilitation of addicts at a time when thousands of Vietnam vets returned home addicted to heroin. In 1974, the National Institutes of Health launched the National

Institute on Drug Abuse (NIDA). Its mission was to improve prevention and treatment of addiction.

The federal government's relatively forward-thinking tack continued through Jimmy Carter's presidency but was radically and disastrously altered by President Reagan, who made law enforcement a priority. Nancy Reagan preached the message of Just Say No, even as her husband cut into the federal budget for prevention and treatment. Research dollars dried up, and treatment centers closed. Since then the War on Drugs has become a literal war fought with arms, soldiers, and police, targeting manufacturers, dealers, and, most disastrously, users — often our children. The War on Drugs has become a war on the American people.

The War on Drugs has failed. We've lost.

The money spent on the war is unconscionable. For almost a decade, America has been in an economic downturn that has led to a decline in the availability and quality of health care, education, social services, and child care. Meanwhile, every year the government adds to the trillion dollars it's already spent on the War on Drugs. In 2011, the federal budget included another $25 billion. And these numbers don't count the billions more spent on courts and imprisonment or the costs of health care and lost productivity due to drugs. What have we gotten for that investment? There are now more drugs, more kinds of drugs, and more toxic drugs used at younger ages; more debilitation; more secondary and tertiary accidents and illness; more suffering and death. The war hasn't altered the fact that people who want drugs will find them — or the fact that people want them.

What else have we gotten for that trillion dollars? Currently, 2,300,000 Americans are incarcerated. We have more people locked up than any other country in the world; Russia is a distant second. As I reported, 85 percent of the U.S. jail and prison population is incarcerated because of crimes committed on or related to drugs. In 2006, alcohol and other drugs were involved in 78 percent of violent crimes; 83 percent of property crimes; and 77 percent of "public order, immigration or weapon offenses; and probation/parole violations." Though drugs are responsible for eight out of ten crimes, only a small fraction of those in prison are cartel kingpins; almost all are users, smalltime dealers, and addicts. In the *National Review,* Veronique de Rugy tracked America's skyrocketing prison population, concluding, "This increase didn't have anything to do with a rise in crime . . . In particular, it had very much to do with the war on drugs."

If this isn't bad enough, this war even targets children. Kids are treated as criminals if they succumb to curiosity — which, as we've seen, many kids will. They're criminals if they bow to pressure from their friends. They're criminals if they try to ease the stress in their lives. They're criminals if they use drugs because they're poor, have been subjected to physical violence, or are mentally ill. They're criminals if they're addicted. That is, they're criminals if they're ill.

Children caught with drugs are arrested, kicked out of school, or incarcerated in juvenile detention centers and jails — all experiences likely to cause them to use more drugs. Because they're committing illegal acts by using, they keep their drug taking secret, making it more likely to escalate to the point that some users will become criminals, and more likely that they'll become addicted. In this way, the War on Drugs doesn't only increase drug use and fill our prisons; it also increases crime. (It also causes inner-city and international crime related to the illegal drug trade.) Pediatrician Fred Homes reminds us: "These aren't bad kids. They're *our* kids."

The War on Drugs further harms our society by breaking up families: 52 to 63 percent of inmates in state prisons and 63 percent in federal prisons are parents. Almost two million kids are growing up with their parents in jail because of the crime of using or for crimes committed on drugs or related to drugs. A report by Justice Strategies, a nonprofit research organization, notes, "Although the pain of losing a parent to prison is tantamount in many respects to losing a parent to death or divorce, the children who remain 'on the outside' appear to suffer a special stigma. Unlike children of the deceased or divorced who tend to benefit from society's familiarity with and acceptance of their loss, children of the incarcerated too often grow up and grieve under a cloud of low expectations and amidst a swirling set of assumptions that they will fail, that they will themselves resort to a life of crime or that they too will succumb to a life of drug addiction." This toxic phenomenon disproportionately affects communities of color, particularly African Americans. According to research by Human Rights Watch, whites and African Americans use and sell drugs at about the same rates, but blacks are arrested at a rate that's three to six times higher than for whites. As a result, though 12 percent of Americans are black, they represent more than 60 percent of those imprisoned for drug offenses. One in three drug arrestees is African American.

End the War on the American People

People at all points of the political spectrum criticize the War on Drugs, and many have called for a ceasefire. I call for its termination.

As employees of a governmental agency, NIDA staffers, unsurprisingly, generally toe the government's line, but a number of the organization's scientists told me, though not for attribution, that they agree the War on Drugs should end. As a NIDA senior researcher said, "If it were effective, I'd opt to keep the status quo, but it isn't. The drug trade is fueled by demand, and the War on Drugs has no impact on demand." Another said, "The War on Drugs is the major stumbling block to turning the tide on addiction in America because it criminalizes drug users instead of addressing the reasons they use."

Voices from a range of political and cultural perspectives have urged an end to the war. In June of 2011, the Global Commission on Drug Policy — members of which include economists, policy experts, and several former world leaders, including former secretary of state George Shultz and former chairman of the U.S. Federal Reserve Paul Volcker — announced its conclusion that "the global war on drugs has failed, with devastating consequences for individuals and societies around the world." In an op-ed they coauthored in the *Wall Street Journal,* Shultz and Volcker wrote, "The costs of the drug war have become astronomical. Inmates arrested for consuming drugs and for possessing small quantities of them now crowd our prisons, where too often they learn how to become real criminals. The dollar costs are huge, but they pale in comparison to the lives being lost in our neighborhoods and throughout the world."

Calls for an end to the war have come from doctors, politicians, economists, law enforcement officers, and business leaders. Drug Policy Alliance (DPA), an organization supported by prominent doctors and treatment professionals, was founded "to ensure that our nation's drug policies no longer arrest, incarcerate, disenfranchise and otherwise harm millions — particularly young people and people of color who are disproportionately affected by the war on drugs." In *Forbes,* economist Art Carden wrote, "Without meaning to, the drug warriors have turned American cities into war zones and eroded the very freedoms we hold dear." Speaking at the Brookings Institution in 2012, New Jersey governor Chris Christie said, "The war on drugs, while well-intentioned, has been a failure. We're warehousing addicted people every day in state prisons in New Jersey, giving them no treatment." President Jimmy Carter, writing in the *New York Times,* said, "The single greatest cause of prison population growth has been the war on drugs, with the number of people incarcerated for nonviolent drug offenses increasing more than twelvefold since 1980. . . . Not only has this excessive punishment destroyed the lives of millions of young people and their families (disproportionately minorities), but it is wreaking havoc on state and local budgets."

Back in 1990, Nobel Prize–winning economist Milton Friedman wrote about the War on Drugs: "Of course the problem is demand, but it is not only demand, it is demand that must operate through repressed and illegal channels. Illegality creates obscene profits that finance the murderous tactics of the drug lords; illegality leads to the corruption of law enforcement officials; illegality monopolizes the efforts of honest law forces so that they are starved for resources to fight the simpler crimes of robbery, theft and assault. Drugs are a tragedy for addicts. But criminalizing their use converts that tragedy into a disaster for society, for users and non-users alike."

The voices calling for an end to the war are getting louder — and they now include a majority of the American people. In a recent poll, only 10 percent of Americans considered the War on Drugs a success. Two-thirds, including majorities of both Democrats and Republicans, said it was a failure.

The Right War

In *Beautiful Boy* I recounted that the War on Drugs wasn't the only one Nixon declared in 1971. In his State of the Union address that year, he also declared war on cancer. "I will also ask for an appropriation . . . to launch an intensive campaign to find a cure for cancer," he announced.

"The time has come in America when the same kind of concentrated effort that split the atom and took man to the moon should be turned toward conquering this dreaded disease. Let us make a total national commitment to achieve this goal." By the end of that year, he had signed into law the National Cancer Act, declaring, "I hope that in the years ahead we will look back on this day and this action as being the most significant action taken during this Administration."

Cancer hasn't been eradicated, of course, but a diagnosis that was once a death sentence often isn't anymore. As I noted, the overall death rate from cancer began dropping in 1990 and has continued to fall every year since then. *USA Today* reports, "From 1990 through 2008, death rates plunged almost 23 percent for men and just over 15 percent for women."

Researcher Amelia Arria sums it up: "Have we solved the problem? No. Are there fewer people dying of cancer? Yes. Do we understand more about the variety of environmental and behavioral risk factors that contribute to cancer? Yes. Have we shifted our cultural biases against talking about cancer in a relative, and getting exams that might detect cancer earlier? Yes."

The war on cancer has been a multitiered assault that has focused on education and prevention, changing public policy, and improving treatment — all toward the goal of decreasing the number of cases of cancer and saving the lives of the afflicted. The War on Drugs has focused on interdiction, arrest, prosecution, and eradication (which has been largely ineffective — America spent a record $100 million to eradicate poppies in Afghanistan in 2008, but it was still a banner year for heroin production there). And most relevant, anybody who wants drugs can easily find them. The war must be ended.

A Cure

If we're finally going to effectively take on America's drug problem, we must end the war on drugs and declare an all-out offensive — against addiction. Like cancer, addiction is a disease that must be conquered. We must work to cure addiction in the ways we have worked to cure cancer. Addiction isn't a criminal problem, but a health problem — a health *crisis*.

When the War on Drugs is ended, resources, including those tens of billions of dollars a year misspent on interdiction, law enforcement, and incarceration, will be freed to support the development and implementation of prevention strategies and treatment, including many of the ones cited in this book. The more money that's redirected from the war to prevention and treatment, the more the prognosis of patients will change. We've seen it with other diseases. The National Cancer Institute's 2011 budget is more than $5 billion, and NCI pays for only about 43 percent of research-project grants. Other federal agencies, the Centers for Disease Control and Prevention, the National Institutes of Health, and the Department of Defense spend millions of dollars more on cancer research. In addition, state and local governments, voluntary organizations, private institutions, and corporations spend an estimated $15 billion every year. In contrast, the 2011 budget of the National Institute on Drug Abuse, which includes most drug-related research and development in America, is just over $1 billion. Of that, about $300 million is earmarked for research related to the connection between illegal drugs and AIDS, so in reality NIDA has only $700 million in discretionary spending for non-AIDS-related drug research. More funding trickles into the field from other sources, but it's trivial compared to the need. There are 1.2 million Americans with AIDS. The total spent on AIDS research is $3 billion — or $3,000 per infected person. We spend $29 per addict.

With a new focus on addiction as a health crisis would come a new national dialogue about this disease: what it is, what causes it, how it manifests, how we should treat it, and how to prevent it. Yes, research would be expensive. Getting effective prevention into the hands of parents, teachers, schools, and communities would be expensive. After they're developed and tested, getting effective treatments, training practitioners, and disseminating treatments throughout the health-care system would be expensive.

But there will be a significant return on these investments. There's a direct correlation between spending and progress in the treatment of many of the most pernicious diseases — again, think of cancer. Think of AIDS, heart disease, and diabetes. Take breast cancer, for example. As funding for the disease increased, the death rate from the disease decreased. War was waged on AIDS in the 1980s and 1990s, and though it's still a devastating illness, far fewer people die from it today (at least, among those that have access to state-of-the-art treatments). Money now spent on interdiction and arresting and incarcerating users could not only support the underfunded projects under way now but allow researchers to explore limitless new potential treatments. Money funds new research, more research opportunities attract an influx of researchers into the field, better treatments are developed and made available to those who need them. There'll be an ever higher return on any investment. We know that a drop in drug use means fewer accidents, less crime, lower hospital and other health-care costs, and fewer deaths. A UCLA study found that, in California, for every dollar spent on treatment, taxpayers saved more than seven dollars in other services, largely through "reduced costs of crime and increased employment earnings."

A Call to Arms

A national focus on addiction would do more than increase spending for improved prevention and treatment. It would also change government policy to focus on making prevention and treatment accessible to everyone who needs it — from early prevention programs that target new mothers to adult addicts. When I met Patrick Kennedy in a Capitol Hill conference room while he was still in Congress, he said that few legislators in Washington even wanted to talk about addiction. One reason is that there's no significant lobby that's pushing for money for prevention and drug treatment; addicts don't have much clout. Those in the advanced stages of the disease have fallen off the grid altogether — many are homeless or institutionalized. And many are estranged from their families, people who would be advocating for their loved ones' treatment if they had any other disease. And the more able-bodied addicts are prevented from lobbying for their own welfare by factors both external (the stigma) and internal (the cognitive and psychological harm their disease has done to them). Most important, legislators share society's general prejudice against drug users and are unlikely to focus on what they and their constituents view as a choice rather than a disease. However, once the nation sets its priorities on ending the disease of addiction, policymakers will no longer be able to ignore America's worst domestic problem. And over time, the cultural prejudices against drug users and addicts will disappear. Indeed, just as the war on cancer successfully led to the destigmatization of that disease, a national focus on addiction would do the same for this one.

Every American has a stake in ending addiction: everyone who cares about safer streets, government spending, and quality health care; everyone who's concerned about poverty, child and spousal abuse, homelessness, and the productivity of this country's citizens. Law enforcement officers don't have to be convinced of the enormity of this problem, because a large part of their jobs involves dealing with addiction and its consequences. Nurses and doctors, especially those who work in emergency departments, have described their frustration with a system that has them patching up addicts after overdoses or accidents and discharging them, rather than admitting them for treatment. Small and large businesses have a stake in this issue too. The costs of insuring employees and their families is astronomical, even if the companies don't offer adequate coverage for drug problems themselves, because they're paying for the consequences of drug use that isn't detected and treated early.

Also, those concerned about American success in the increasingly competitive world economy should think through the impact of drug use on people's ability to contribute to society. "One message that might motivate individuals to change their behavior and parents to take note is that drug use interferes with human capital," says Dr. Arria. "For too long, the public has been fed 'We need to reduce drug use and underage drinking because these are bad behaviors.' Rather than that, we need to explain that reducing drug use and underage drinking will increase the chance that our children will be competitive in the world."

Politicians, of course, have many reasons to take this issue on, but they must be convinced, and they're convinced by money, media attention, and, especially, by votes. There should be marches on Washington. Letter-writing campaigns. Some people think activism is futile, but there's evidence that it can successfully bring change when it comes to health-care priorities. "In the early 1980s, [AIDS] sufferers received neither media attention nor research funding—President Reagan could not even bring himself to utter the word 'AIDS' in public," wrote Vicki Brower in the *European Molecular Biology Organization Reports*. "This changed when a critical mass of patients, friends and families, and celebrity spokespeople made their presence known on Capitol Hill and in the White House." In the article "The Squeaky Wheel Gets the Grease," Brower showed that, by 1989, spending on AIDS reached more than $2 billion, compared to $74.5 million on breast cancer, although breast cancer killed more than 40,000 women that year, compared with 22,000 deaths due to AIDS. Then, using some of the same grass-roots techniques used by AIDS activists, breast cancer advocates successfully pushed for an increase in federal funding for breast cancer research and were "instrumental in getting legislation passed for health coverage of mammograms and outlawing outpatient mastectomies."

Addiction must become the squeakiest wheel out there. As Tom McLellan told TheFix.com, "Typically, a segregated illness moves into the mainstream only when there's been political pressure or scientific discovery. New funding usually follows." Money is hugely relevant in the fight against any illness. New funding will lead to new scientific break-throughs, and as addiction follows other diseases into the mainstream, the current cycle of stagnation and regression will be replaced by one of progress.

Insurance Reform

New government money isn't the only source of funding to target addiction. When insurance policies fully cover this illness, not only will there be more practitioners and treatment programs (they follow the money), but ineffective treatment of the insured won't be tolerated. That is, the insurance industry will bring in another sorely needed component to the field of treating addiction — accountability. Insurers want bang for their bucks, which is shown in positive outcomes.

By failing to pay adequately for addiction treatment, businesses and the insurance companies they contract with — and taxpayers — end up paying dearly for the consequences of addiction. It happens at every hospital in the nation. Insurers and the federal and state governments readily pay for damaged hearts and livers and lungs but not for the disease that caused them. And early treatment of drug problems does more than save health-care costs down the line. Tom McLellan cites a study the state of Washington did of Medicaid-insured patients who went to ERs — "not some fancy private care for affluent people." The study evaluated one of the least expensive interventions possible. In one group, patients were screened for substance-use problems and then given brief advice by physicians. In the control group, patients were screened but weren't given advice. Within one year, those in the treated group had used $3,500 per person less in medical care than those in the control group. Almost all savings came from lower utilization of ERs.

I've explained some of the inadequacies in coverage for addiction. Roberta Lojak and her daughter Ashley paid the highest possible price for the gap that exists between the care of addiction and the care of other diseases. Currently, insurance companies often refuse to pay (or pay at a lower rate) for illnesses or injuries caused by drugs or alcohol. Thirty-two states still enforce statutes — the Uniform Accident and Sickness Policy Provision Laws, enacted in 1947 — that allow insurance companies to refuse to pay for treatment if alcohol or drugs were involved in the problem that brought the patient to be treated. Focusing on addiction treatment requires reform that will force employers and their insurance companies to pay for addiction care (and mental-health care) for anyone who needs it, even if effective treatment can take months or years, which, as we know, it can. One can't imagine an insurance company being allowed to tell a cancer patient it would pay for a week or month of treatment and then leave her on her own.

Insurance companies are often portrayed as the bad guys who don't offer adequate coverage, but it's important to remember that insurance companies are businesses that respond to their customers. Individuals may not have much clout with the insurance companies, but the big customers do. The big customers are America's employers — your employer — who decide what coverage they'll offer. Employees should tell the companies they work for, large and small, that they want insurance that covers addiction just like any other disease.

There's been some progress in insurance reform over the past half a decade. Earlier I mentioned the Mental Health and Addiction Equity Act signed into law in 2008. The act requires insurance companies to cover addiction treatment at the same rates that they cover other treat-ments — *if* the companies cover addiction in the first place. The fact that companies can opt out is the act's major flaw. Building on the parity bill, the Patient Protection and Affordable Care Act (PPACA), signed into law in March of 2010 by President Obama, requires insurance com-panies to include substance-abuse coverage in their plans, though they can exclude and limit individual treatments. Still, addiction treatment is advanced by the PPACA because it provides access to health coverage for an estimated thirty-two million Americans who are now uninsured. A disproportionate number of people with addiction are uninsured, and 60 percent of the uninsured forgo medical care. When they don't seek treatment because they can't afford it, their addiction and related health problems worsen. As we've seen, addiction treatment has focused pri-marily on acute cases — people who end up in the emergency rooms or in treatment for full-blown addiction, usually after suffering physi-cal and mental catastrophes. The PPACA potentially improves access to addiction care in specific provisions too. If they'll be reimbursed by insurance, more medical providers will train to screen, conduct brief interventions, and refer treatments as necessary (using a system like SBIRT). Another provision of the PPACA that could be transformative is the coverage of prenatal and infant care, including home visits such as those provided by the Nurse Family Partnership. There are also provi-sions to expand education and community prevention campaigns, and there will be grants available so school-based health centers can offer mental-health and addiction services (possibly ones like those available at the Wellness Centers in San Francisco high schools).

In addition to those, there are other significant benefits of the Afford-able Care Act that may affect addiction coverage. Companies can't refuse coverage to those with preexisting conditions (many people are now denied coverage if they've been in treatment for addiction); they can't place annual or lifetime caps on coverage; and they can't drop people from coverage if their treatments become expensive. Finally, the PPACA will allow parents to keep their children on their insurance plans until they're twenty-six years old, which means adolescents and young adults will be covered throughout the time they'll most likely need treatment and when it will be the most beneficial.

How much of an impact the PPACA will have remains to be seen. It's still uncertain if all of its components will be implemented. Addiction-care provisions could be eliminated or sidelined if a movement to focus on addiction care doesn't prevent that. Another potential problem that must be monitored is the exclusion of specific procedures, which the PPACA allows the companies to do. A flaw in the PPACA is that in the past, many insurance companies had low deductibles for mental-health care relative to medical care. Many companies are now switching so there'll be one combined deductible that must be reached before insurance will kick in — in many cases, $1,000 or more. If that's the case, people who need mental-health care may be less inclined to see therapists if the first thousand dollars — say, ten or twelve therapy sessions — must be paid out of pocket.

Positive Versus Negative Intervention

One intervention opportunity directly leads to less crime, safer cities, and lower law enforcement and incarceration costs. Along with SBIRT-like interventions when drug users enter the criminal justice system, drug courts have successfully lowered use and crime by changing the trajectory of kids who are arrested for crimes committed on or related to drugs. Drug courts are available in some jurisdictions, but they should be offered everywhere. In some, judges give addicts a choice between incarceration or a drug-treatment program. In others, they're sentenced to treatment — there's no choice.

Most research on drug courts shows that they bring about a decline in drug use and recidivism. One study, sponsored by the National Institute of Justice, examined two drug courts set up in separate counties. Within two years of the drug courts' being established, the felony re-arrest rate decreased from 40 percent to 12 percent in one county, and from 50 percent to 35 percent in the other. According to the National Association of Drug Court Professionals, "Seventy-five percent of drug court graduates remain arrest-free at least two years after leaving the program." In addition to reducing crime, "Drug courts are six times more likely to keep offenders in treatment long enough for them to get better."

Legalize Marijuana

As we dismantle the War on Drugs, we must also address another policy: whether the war on marijuana users should end. After years of analyzing the research into the health and social impact of marijuana, I've determined that it should — that marijuana should be legalized, though in a controlled, cautious way.

Attitudes about marijuana are changing. According to a Gallup poll, about half of Americans support legalization, a dramatic increase over the past decades (only 12 percent did in 1969). Nineteen U.S. states have laws allowing some form of legal marijuana use. In some states, marijuana remains illegal, but the penalties are minor — a citation, for example (in some other states, however, marijuana users are still arrested, prosecuted, and sent to prison). In California, the medical-marijuana business is booming; it's a billion-dollar industry. There are standing-room-only classes in the science of growing marijuana.

Most people seem to accept that medical marijuana is in part a sham, and not because it isn't legitimately used by some people. Cancer patients are one thing, but anyone who wants a prescription can get one. Their illnesses can include, as in the case of *Mother Jones* writer Josh Harkinson, "periodic pain from typing a lot." Harkinson paid ninety dollars for a prescription and a wallet-sized patient-identification card that would allow him to buy pot from any of California's one thousand dispensaries.

While public attitudes about pot are changing, many in the medical community haven't signed on. Many doctors and medical associations support medical marijuana — at least, they support research to prove its efficacy — but fewer advocate for the legalization of pot, because research doesn't support the popular view that marijuana is harmless; as I've shown, it isn't. One exception is the Advisory Committee to Recommend Policy on Marijuana Legalization and Appropriate Regulation and Education of the California Medical Association (CMA), which concluded that marijuana should be made legal for medical research, regulated and taxed for recreational use (similar to alcohol and tobacco taxes), and that legalization should be accompanied by an education campaign so people understand the "risks and benefits" of using.

Former U.S. surgeon general Joycelyn Elders supports legalization. "What I think is horrible about all of this is that we criminalize young people," she stated on CNN. "We have the highest number of people in the world being criminalized, many for non-violent crimes related to marijuana. We can use our resources so much better." In 2002, police officers and members of criminal justice communities formed a national organization called LEAP that endorsed legalization because, its mission statement read, "the policies have failed, and continue to fail, to effectively address the problems of drug abuse, especially the problems of juvenile drug use, the problems of addiction, and the problems of crime caused by the existence of a criminal black market in drugs." Still another reason to end the war is in the findings of a study by the National Council on Crime and Delinquency, which noted that, rather than lowering use, the prohibition against drugs may increase it: "Children . . . are sometimes attracted to drugs because they are illegal."

The issues related to any drug policy are complicated, and facts can be inconvenient. It would be easier for parents and educators if — as has been claimed by some anti-pot crusaders — any and all drug use led to calamity and addiction. Evidence that marijuana was a gateway drug and was addictive would serve their anti-pot campaigns. Some argue — whether to validate their own use or to advocate for decriminalizing or legalizing it — that marijuana is harmless. If pot were unconditionally safe, it would help them justify their use and arm them in their advocacy, especially if research proved that marijuana *didn't* cause structural and functional changes in the brain and *wasn't* addictive. However, when it comes to any drug, including marijuana, there are no absolutes, because everyone responds differently, based on genetics and circumstances.

Many proponents of legalization do both themselves and their cause a disservice by ignoring facts about the effects of marijuana. It's too simple to say that marijuana isn't a gateway drug, because it often *is*. Those who claim that marijuana isn't addictive are wrong; some people do become addicted — about 5 percent of those who smoke it. Those who claim that no one's died from marijuana use ignore the fact that pot is linked to fatal car accidents. While some decry as ludicrous and sensational the claim that marijuana causes brain damage, it does. Many researchers have proved this. Earlier I described the work of researcher Susan Tapert at the University of California at San Diego who demonstrate̶d̶ caused by marijuana on the white and gray matter of adolescen̶ She's only one of the researchers who have used scans and chem̶ to document changes in parts of the brain associated with memory and cognition. There's also evidence that pot can trigger depression, schizophrenia, and other serious mental illness; cause earlier onset of these or other psychiatric illnesses; and impede emotional as well as physical brain development in children at precisely the time when they're supposed to be maturing.

Because of the harms and potential harms associated with pot, my main concern about legalization is that it will send the inaccurate and dangerous message, especially to children, that pot is safe. A comprehensive report by the Rand Corporation explains that legalization could, at least in the short term, cause a spike in marijuana use — potentially even doubling it. However, the illegal status of marijuana doesn't stop millions of people, including children, from smoking it every day, and it may stop many of them from telling anyone and seeking help.

Also, the claim that legalizing pot would cause more people to use fails to account for countermeasures that could and should be implemented before and after legalization. My support for legalization is contingent on a broader policy shift that would pair legalization with education campaigns — evidence-based prevention designed to not only lower use but change the conversation about drugs. Indeed, the billions we will save each year when we stop funding our ineffectual efforts to prohibit growing, trafficking, and using pot should go to prevention and treatment. Adding to this, marijuana, if taxed, would bring in additional billions that should be earmarked for research into treatment — a model that's been successful in reducing cigarette smoking. More than three hundred economists, including three Nobel laureates, have signed an online open letter addressed to government leaders that endorses the findings of a paper by Harvard economist Jeffrey Miron. Miron calculated that if marijuana was legalized, the government would save $7.7 billion annually in law enforcement costs, and it could bring in an additional $6.2 billion a year if pot was taxed at rates similar to alcohol and tobacco. That's $13.9 billion per year that could, and should, be earmarked to prevention campaigns and treatment.

In addition to the benefits of an influx of money, legalizing pot would lead to more effective prevention campaigns. Marijuana users would no longer be stigmatized as criminals, which would allow society to accept their drug use for what it is: for some, a choice, like having a drink in the evening; for others — including many teenagers — a response to their environment or social and psychological problems. For still others, it is a symptom of an illness that needs treating. In a recent year, more than 47 percent of all drug arrests in this country were for marijuana offenses. People shouldn't be arrested for smoking pot or even for dealing small amounts. They should be educated and, if problems develop, immediately treated so their problems don't escalate. If marijuana was legal, related problems, including addiction, could be addressed as health issues, not moral or criminal ones. Teenagers and others might be more willing to talk about their interest in or experience using. People with problems might seek help earlier. However, people who are arrested for drug use are likely to descend into more use. When people — especially children — enter the criminal justice system, the risk factors for drug abuse and addiction increase exponentially. Think about it: Take a child who does what so many kids do these days: he's with his friend, someone hands him a joint, and he tries it. Now he's broken the law. If his use escalates and he winds up in the criminal justice system, he's entered one of the highest risk groups for addiction. Previous offenders are more likely to use drugs. They're isolated from their families and neighborhoods, which increases their risk. They're under great stress, which increases their risk. They're stigmatized and their self-esteem is battered. If they're expelled from school or lose a job, their prospects are fewer. This recipe creates not only more drug use, but more dangerous use.

"In ninth grade I was caught smoking weed with some friends," a boy wrote. "I was suspended and sent to juvie [juvenile detention]. When I came back to school, I was put in a special class, the one for fuck-ups. The friends I'd been hanging out with before didn't do drugs much. We smoked a bit of weed when we weren't doing school or sports, but my new cohorts were the stoners, using shrooms, ecstasy, speed, Oxies, what have you. They thought they were the awesomist. The big thing then was to hide flasks of booze in their boots.

"As you may well imagine, my parents were pissed off at their young juvenile delinquent. My dad especially was on my case. I was his perfect son, the heir apparent, and I'd become the great disappointment. You'd think he never tried pot when he was a kid. You can imagine that I felt pretty shitty. I was the pariah at home, the pariah at family gatherings, the pariah at church, the pariah at school. I was treated like a loser and so I became a loser. I didn't have many options. The one place where I wasn't a pariah was when I was with the other fuck-ups. I started getting high with them — drinking, tripping, snorting. We were always high. There was the choir, the debate team, and our cadre: the Stoners. We'd trip at school and sell drugs. We all were selling, but naturally I was the one who was busted."

The letter continues for another page and then ends: "Now I'm 24. The prodigal son is now the less prodigal inmate. Here I languish."

Marijuana should be legalized. There should be a trial period during with the changes it brings are monitored. It should be taxed and controlled like alcohol. It should be regulated, and regulations should be modified as needed. There should be strictly enforced rules that limit advertising and promotion of marijuana to children. Indeed, given the potential extreme harm that marijuana can cause adolescents and young adults, it should remain illegal for anyone to sell to kids. Laws about underage using won't stop many kids from smoking; laws about alcohol don't stop kids from drinking. But underage pot smoking — and underage drinking, for that matter — should be addressed by positive intervention, including evidence-based education campaigns and early screening and treatment, not prosecution.

In many states, adults who supply alcohol to kids at parties and allow drinking at their homes are legally liable. They can be charged with crimes and can be held responsible if a child gets high at their house and then gets into a car accident. As much as possible, kids need to be protected, and grownups should be prohibited from aiding and abetting kids' self-destructive behavior. If they do, they should be held responsible. That shouldn't change with legalization.

A few people may still make bathtub gin, but it's rare, because it's easier to find alcohol at a nearby store. Currently, many kids wind up in emergency rooms after unintentionally smoking pot laced with speed, hallucinogens, lead (added to increase its weight), and other substances. Legalization would protect users from unscrupulous dealers and the crime that is often associated with illegal drug transactions.

The most convincing argument for me is that as long as pot remains a legal issue, we fail to address the most important problems related to marijuana smoking and, in fact, to other drug use. The drug's legal status fills prisons; makes drug use go underground; encourages a black market that's characterized by crime, including murder; and criminalizes innocent children — but it doesn't stop them from getting high. We know that criminalization doesn't work. It's time to try a new approach.

Legalizing Other Drugs?

I don't advocate legalizing other drugs. However, as the drug war ends, we should study alternative ways to treat the addicted — and to save their lives. In Vancouver, at a supervised injection site called Insite, IV drug users are given not only clean needles but a safe place to shoot up and stay while they're high. (Needle exchanges themselves are controversial in the United States, even though they've been shown to reduce drug use, crime, and the transmission of blood-borne illnesses.) Insite is set in a converted storefront in a neighborhood known for its street addicts and crime. Addicts shoot up in booths with clean needles and other gear supplied by the clinic. They're encouraged to stay in a "chill-out" room where there's coffee, couches, and a TV. They have the option of receiving medical advice and care, and there's a gentle push toward treatment.

The program is funded and run by the British Columbia Ministry of Health Services. A series of studies has shown that Insite is effective at getting addicts into treatment, lowering crime in the neighborhood, and reducing the number of overdoses and illnesses from IV drug use.

It would be rational to study options such as safe injection sites, but in the U.S. there's great resistance to any policy that's based on acceptance of drug use. Shortly after Insite opened, John Waters, President Bush's drug czar, denounced the program, calling it immoral and "state-sponsored suicide." This contradicts the findings that led to a landmark ruling by the Canada Supreme Court in 2011. Insite had faced opposition from the conservative government, but the court ruled that the clinic could remain open. BBC News reported that the court found that in the clinic's eight-year history, "Insite has been proven to save lives with no discernible negative impact on the public safety and health objectives of Canada."

There are needle-exchange programs in the United States that offer pared-down versions of Insite's program. A number of National Institutes of Health studies have shown that providing clean syringes to drug users is an effective way to curb the spread of HIV and hepatitis C, and such programs don't increase the numbers of drug users. Significantly, they've also been shown to help retain addicts in treatment.

Meanwhile, in the Netherlands, policies about drug use are focused on "preventing drug use and reducing the risks to users and those around them. Toleration (exemption from prosecution) is the main thrust of Dutch policy," as explained by the country's Ministry of Health. In the Netherlands, drug policies are different for soft and hard drugs. Pot and alcohol are soft drugs. Marijuana isn't legal, but there are official guidelines that state that possession of the drug for personal use won't be prosecuted. The country has a program in place that administers buprenorphine or methadone to heroin users. The Netherlands is famous for its coffee shops where patrons can get small quantities of marijuana and hashish along with an espresso. Numerous studies have shown drops in crime and, according to UCLA's Dr. Weiss, "no higher abuse, no higher dependence." Indeed, the *New York Times* reported that in spite of easy access to pot, "the Dutch are far less likely than Americans or many other Europeans to use marijuana" — only about 5 percent of the Dutch use pot, according to the U.N. Office on Drugs and Crime. Still, the easy accessibility of marijuana in cafés, at least for nonresidents, may end. In mid-2012 the current conservative government sought to prohibit the sale of pot in cafés, at least to nonresidents. The *Times* reports that the reason has nothing to do with health or crime issues, but — parking. For instance, in the southern city of Maastricht, "hundreds of drug tourists drive in daily from elsewhere in Europe to purchase marijuana, creating an infuriating traffic nuisance."

A more extreme approach to drug policy can be found in Portugal, where the government decriminalized the possession and use of all drugs — not only marijuana but heroin, cocaine, and the rest. Drugs are still illegal, but users caught with small quantities aren't sent to jail. Instead, they face a panel consisting of a psychologist, social worker, and legal adviser, who recommend appropriate treatment.

"At the time, critics in the poor, socially conservative and largely Catholic nation said decriminalizing drug possession would open the country to 'drug tourists' and exacerbate Portugal's drug problem," reported Maia Szalavitz in *Time*. "However, a study commissioned by the Cato Institute suggested otherwise." The study found that five years after personal possession was decriminalized, illegal drug use among teens declined, rates of new HIV infections had dropped, and the number of people seeking treatment for drug addiction more than doubled. Prior to the change in drug policy, Portugal had one of the highest rates of drug use in Europe; afterward, it had one of the lowest. In 2006, five years after implementing decriminalization policies, Portugal reportedly had a lifetime cannabis use in people over age fifteen of 10 percent — the lowest in the European Union. Drug-related crime there has been cut, and drug-related court cases dropped 66 percent. A significant finding that shouldn't be ignored: Since decriminalization, the number of regular users held steady — a fact that shows that decriminalization brought no surge in drug use.

Now the Global Commission on Drug Policy is looking at Portugal as a model and calling for national governments to "depenalize" if not legalize drug possession and sales. The commission suggests following strategies similar to the ones being tried in Portugal: stop the arrest and imprisonment of drug users and, in some cases, even the prosecution of smalltime drug dealers "whose arrest does nothing to dent the flow of illegal drugs." Whether or not Portugal's model is applicable to the United States, alternatives to the current archaic and harmful treatment must be explored.

Hope

We must end the War on Drugs and focus our efforts on the prevention and treatment of addiction. Doing so would save money, lower crime, and increase productivity. And we'll prevent more suffering than anyone can imagine.

When you're in the throes of active addiction, whether it's your own or that of someone you love, it's impossible to imagine that things can get better, but they can. People can get and stay clean, and their lives can improve in ways they never thought possible.

I've noted that, at least for now, addiction isn't curable. By definition, a chronic illness can't be cured. However, addiction treatment can lead to physiological and psychological changes that border on cure. Some recovering addicts should never be around others who drink or use, but some can become inured to the minefield of triggers that occur in social situations. It's possible to relapse at any time, but after treatment, sometimes multiple treatments, many people never do. Are they cured? A genetic predisposition remains. Neurological damage may remain too. Though they've been defused, triggers may lie dormant. Intense stress or the sight of one's drug of choice or a combination of the two may wake it up. Most experts maintain that many addicts remain vulnerable. But as we've seen, over time, preventing relapse gets easier for most people — time sober predicts more time sober, partly because of physical and psychological healing and partly because lives rebuild, and addicts have increasing incentive to keep doing the work associated with recovery. Indeed, to continue the positive trajectory, some people need ongoing treatment, whether in outpatient groups or therapy. Some need to stay on medication, though the drugs and dosages may be modified. Many addicts regularly attend AA meetings. Those with co-occurring illnesses must continue to have them treated. After treatment, some people may need to remain segregated in sober-living communities or halfway houses.

There are no guarantees, of course, but often the work that gets and keeps people sober makes them more resilient, wiser, and — yes — better, because they're no longer controlled by drugs or by destructive habits and behaviors associated with their drug use. They still live with the threat of relapse. But addicts who are effectively treated can successfully weather the ups and downs of life without relying on drugs. They can do what they couldn't do when they were using. They can make choices. The fear of calamity recedes. You would never choose to suffer the pain of addiction. You would never want someone you love to suffer this terrible disease. But surviving addiction changes addicts and their loved ones forever. They have a new appreciation for one another, and for life itself.

Epilogue

CLEAN ACKNOWLEDGES THE FAILURES of the current approaches to preventing drug use and treating addiction but celebrates new ones — approaches that, if they're adopted, can lead to fewer people using drugs and a far better prognosis for addicts who seek treatment. I describe practices that work but aren't widely used, either because people don't know about them or because they aren't accessible. I identify promising prevention strategies and treatments currently under development. But I also express great frustration in the fact that progress has been slowed by the stigmatization of addiction, the poor coordination of disparate efforts to improve things, a lack of resources, and resistance in a thoroughly entrenched system.

But recently there's been a development that could dramatically change the status quo.

As I reported, the War on Drugs and the war on cancer, both started in 1971, have had opposite effects on their respective diseases. The War on Drugs has worsened the problem it was meant to solve. But the war on cancer, while far from won, has been an unmitigated success when measured by the countless lives it has saved.

The war on cancer didn't begin in policymakers' offices but in the halls of the American Cancer Society, an organization founded in 1913. It's impossible to overstate the impact of the ACS on American health over the past century. The organization has supported the research that led to nearly every major cancer treatment breakthrough. It was a driving force behind studies that proved the link between cancer and smoking. It demonstrated the effectiveness of the Pap test and mammography and pioneered the development of lifesaving treatments that have lowered the death rates of breast cancer, leukemia, lung cancer, and more. According to its website, the American Cancer Society has invested $3.6 billion in research and supported the investigations of forty-six scientists who later went on to win Nobel Prizes for their work. The ACS has done more to educate the public and prevent cancer than any other entity, while also managing to destigmatize the disease. And it's lobbied for policies that have led to, for example, the Surgeon General's report linking smoking and cancer and increased government support for cancer research. The ACS contributes more than $1 billion annually to prevent and cure cancer.

The American Cancer Society was also the hidden force behind the Nixon administration's declaration of war on cancer. It lobbied for the passage of the National Cancer Act, which since then has directed billions of NIH dollars to cancer research, much of it through the National Cancer Institute, which has also been supported by the ACS. By working with myriad partners around the world (coordinating and funding research, supporting local and national prevention efforts), it remains at the vanguard of the ongoing effort to eradicate the disease. Nearly twelve million cancer survivors are alive today. Three hundred and fifty lives are saved every day, lives that otherwise would have been lost to cancer.

About the same number of people who die each day of drug addiction.

Half a decade ago, I called for the formation of the American Addiction Society, modeled after the American Cancer Society. Its purpose would mirror the ACS's: to support all efforts to prevent drug use and treat the addicted; to educate about addiction and end the stigmatization of drug users; to influence public policy; to unite and coordinate organizations throughout the United States devoted to fighting problems caused by drugs; and to guide and support research into effective prevention and treatment programs and implement those that prove to be effective.

In the summer of 2012, I met Gary Mendell, Brian's father. He had been working to found a national organization to prevent and treat substance abuse. Earlier that summer, he had stepped down as CEO of his hotel company (he remains chairman) and founded a nonprofit organization. He retained behavioral economists, behavioral psychologists, and leading experts in substance-abuse prevention and treatment to help hone the organization's vision and business plan. He has assembled a board of directors, board of advisers, and scientific board, which together include researchers, business leaders, policymakers, and representatives from the health-care industry. Tom McLellan has assumed the role of chairman of the organization's scientific board. (I am on the advisory board.)

Earlier, I noted that the squeaky wheel gets the grease, and as America's number one preventable health problem, substance-use disorders must become the squeakiest wheel of all. I am hopeful that Mendell's new organization will make this happen. It has already identified evidence-based prevention and treatment programs, and it will, Mendell says, adopt them nationwide with training, support, efficiency, and fidelity. He will also support cutting-edge research into the development and implementation of new prevention and treatment strategies. The organization will follow the American Cancer Society's model and support research, education, and prevention. The influx of attention and money into the field will draw a new generation of researchers and treatment professionals. The organization will work with experts to improve and implement assessment tools so drug problems can be detected and treated early. It will coordinate with other organizations devoted to fighting addiction. It will advocate for changes in public policy. And Mendell's organization will, he says, work with Tom McLellan's TRI on its development of a consumer guide to outpatient and inpatient treatment programs that offer evidence-based practices — something he and Brian never had.

Because of the tireless work of researchers, treatment professionals, and those working in schools, communities, and city-, county-, and state-based organizations to prevent drug use — and now because of the potential impact of a national organization devoted to prevention and treatment — there's reason to be optimistic about the prospects for dramatic change. It's reasonable to envision a time not too far away when fewer people will try and use drugs, when more addicts will be effectively treated. And in the long term? We just might end addiction. There's hope because of all of those who say to those who have died: We won't forget you and with you in our minds we will work to end this disease.

The Clean Paradigm
in Twelve Steps

IN THIS BOOK I DESCRIBE a new way to prevent drug use and treat addiction. Here I summarize how we can do that, in a series of steps—indeed, twelve of them.

Twelve steps? Obviously I'm borrowing the organizing principle behind the original Twelve Steps, which have been the main option for people seeking help with drug abuse and addiction since the 1930s. As I've explained, Twelve Step programs have helped countless addicts to get and stay clean. So why are new steps needed? First, the traditional steps don't address prevention, but successful prevention would avert addiction and reduce the health, legal, social, and personal problems that harm or destroy millions of lives. Moreover, as I've shown, only a fraction of those who need help ever make it into a Twelve Step program, and of those who do and "keep coming back," as the program exhorts them, only a minority stay sober. "There are millions of people who fervently believed that the twelve-step process saved their lives," David Brooks wrote in the New York Times in June 2010. "Yet the majority, even a vast majority, of the people who enroll in the program do not succeed in it."

The following steps, a distillation of the research that's described in *Clean,* can help addicts who are uninterested in the Twelve Steps or for whom the Twelve Steps haven't worked. At the same time, the new steps are compatible with the traditional ones, so they can also help people who are in the Program. That is, these new steps are relevant for anyone, no matter their background, age, gender, drug or drugs of choice, and religious beliefs, or lack of them.

Step 1: *Reject the view that America's drug problem is unsolvable, and that addicts can't be successfully treated.* Traditional approaches have failed, but research has led to breakthroughs in prevention and treatment, and offers help for every addict, and for our nation.

Step 2: *Understand that drugs don't cause addiction, life does.* That is, people become addicted because of genetic factors, the age they begin using, their environment and mental health, and stress. Effective prevention and treatment are tied to a recognition of why people use and abuse drugs.

Step 3: *Lessen the likelihood that children will abuse drugs by helping them navigate the challenges they face.* Ninety percent of addicts begin using as teenagers. Help kids grow up healthy.

Step 4: *Get help as soon as drugs become a problem.* The traditional approach to treatment insisted that addicts needed to hit bottom before they could stop using, but that's an archaic, misguided, and dangerous philosophy. Do not wait for an addict to hit bottom. If drug abuse isn't being treated, it usually gets worse.

Step 5: *Understand that addicts aren't bad people—they're ill.* For too long addicts have been judged as selfish hedonists out for a good time no matter the harm they cause to themselves or others. But bad behavior that appears to be a choice is a symptom of this chronic and progressive brain disease.

Step 6: *Try AA, but remember that it's only one of many available treatments.* If it doesn't help or isn't enough of a help, seek other options. Don't blame the patient when AA (or any other treatment) fails.

Step 7: *Go to a doctor—one trained in addiction medicine.* And get a second opinion.

Step 8: *Choose evidence-based treatments—that is, ones that science has shown to be effective in treating this disease.* Reject programs based on tough love, pseudoscience, contrition, and punishment.

Step 9: *Addicts' bodies must be detoxified, but that's not all it takes to treat addiction.* Purging drugs from an addict's system is the essential first stage of treatment in many cases, but it's not enough to prevent most addicts from relapsing. Follow detox with primary treatment.

Step 10: *Treat dual diagnosis.* A majority of addicts have one or more psychological disorders that occur along with their addiction. In most cases, if both aren't treated, neither will be.

Step 11: *Do all you can to prevent relapse, but don't consider it a sign of defeat.* Relapses can be fatal, but they're often a part of recovery from the chronic disease of addiction. If relapse occurs, address it immediately and adjust treatment accordingly.

Step 12: *End the war on drugs and treat addiction for what it is—not a criminal problem, but a health crisis.* As a nation, we must fight the right war: not against drugs but against addiction.

Afterword

It's been a year since the first edition of *Clean* was published. In that time, an estimated 127,000 people who suffered the disease of addiction have died because they never got the treatment they needed.

The horror continues unabated. In fact, it's worsened in some communities, where misused prescription medications, synthetic marijuana, heroin, and Molly (MDMA), a form of ecstasy, have raised the number of overdose deaths. The letters still flood in. Like this one:

My daughter is in the ICU due to a heroin overdose. She will not be one of the survivors. Her body is barely functioning; she has no brain activity. In the next 24 hours I will have to let her go. As a parent of an addict, I've already lost her once to the drug. Now I have to face the final goodbye. Her brother [and] sister are on their way to say goodbye to her physical shell. My heart is shattered.

Four days later, the mom responded to a note I'd sent:

David, she passed away Tuesday morning.

The heartbreak is unrelenting, but there has been progress, and I remain hopeful that we're moving toward a time when fewer people will become addicted and die from the disease. Tom McLellan points out that 2014 is the one hundredth anniversary of the Harrison Act, which took addiction out of the hands of physicians and put it in the hands of the criminal-justice system. This shift contributed to the current climate; as I've described, addiction has been treated as a problem of criminality, morals, and character. But a confluence of forces is beginning to reverse a century of harm, so that this disease will once again be faced as the health challenge it is.

There's still troubling resistance to the understanding that addiction is a disease, not a moral failing. I saw this in some of the responses to this book. "It's simple," one man wrote, echoing the reactions of many. "People make choices in their lives. They make good or bad choices. Their choices are informed by their consciences or lack thereof." But as more people are educated about the science of addiction, more are coming around. Clearly the Obama administration and many legislators have been listening to addiction scientists, because their rhetoric increasingly reflects the medical community's classification of addiction as a disease. The message is also being reinforced as the Affordable Care Act is being implemented. The act requires insurance plans to fully cover addiction treatment; health insurance covers disease, not bad behavior. And insurance plans, with an eye on the bottom line, will treat addiction like other diseases and demand accountability from practitioners and treatment programs. They won't pay for unscientific programs that blame addicts and punish them and demand their contrition. Programs will have to adapt and offer evidence-based treatments practiced by qualified professionals, or they'll go out of business.

There are still other encouraging steps forward. Scientists, including many of those I've written about in *Clean,* are progressing in their research into improved prevention and treatment strategies. Though they're still too scarce, more treatment programs are offering evidence-based treatment, including once-shunned addiction medications like methadone, buprenorphine, and Vivitrol.

I witnessed another significant change as I traveled around the country speaking at community events. I've seen a building grassroots movement. The public outcry by people and families afflicted with addiction is getting louder. They will no longer tolerate the silence. They refuse to hide in the shadows. They are organizing in communities around the nation, circulating petitions, lobbying their legislators. For example, parents who've lost their children to drugs have founded organizations that have succeeded in pushing "911 Good Samaritan" laws through legislatures in several states. These laws protect people who call 911 if they are with someone who is overdosing, so the callers themselves won't be afraid of arrest or criminal charges. In an op-ed I wrote for the *New York Times,* I reported the story of a father who told me about his only child, who overdosed on a combination of OxyContin and Jack Daniel's. The boy's friends put him in an ice-filled bathtub, a misguided intervention they had seen on TV. He died. None of the teens called 911 because they were afraid they would be arrested, and they probably would have been. This boy was one of many thousands whose lives might have been saved if someone had called for help.

Only a dozen states have laws shielding a person who calls 911 from arrest and prosecution for drug use or possession, underage alcohol use, and similar crimes. These are commonsense laws. No one should be arrested for saving a life.

Other groups are campaigning to make the drug naloxone (marketed as Narcan) widely available to addicts and their families. Narcan, which can be administered by injection or in a nasal spray, can reverse an opiate overdose. Coalitions of citizens are also educating their communities when new threats strike: an epidemic of ODs on Xanax and heroin, for example; kids getting sick because of synthetic marijuana; high school students overdosing on cough syrup; on college campuses, "Skittles parties" where kids swallow whatever pills they draw from a bowl without knowing what they're taking. People are holding teach-athons and organizing neighborhood- and school-based prevention programs. They're lobbying independent and public schools to increase support for mental health services, and are beginning to identify candidates for public office who are committed to working with them to improve addiction prevention and treatment in their communities.

We are also, at long last, ending some components of the War on Drugs. When I think about this catastrophic policy, I recall a Hunter S. Thompson–esque road trip I embarked on when I was nineteen, a college freshman. Motivated by the promise of quick cash and adventure, I got in my car and drove from Berkeley to San Diego with a few kilos of marijuana in the trunk. It was an uneventful drive south. I delivered the weed to a friend of a friend, slept on his couch, and headed home.

On the return trip, however, I was stopped by a highway patrol officer outside the city of Salinas. The officer called for backup, and more police arrived. They thoroughly searched the car, even looking under the spare tire and unscrewing a flashlight. They found nothing, because there was nothing to be found. I look back with abject horror at how much my life since then would have been different if I'd been stopped on my way to — rather than from — my one and only drug deal.

At that time, had I been convicted of drug possession and dealing, I would likely have spent at least two decades in prison. Instead of going to college, starting a family, and building a career, I would have been in a cell. Upon release, I'd have had a criminal record. That, and my interrupted education, would have made me far less employable. While incarcerated, I would probably have learned how to navigate prison, but not life outside it. My youthful transgression would have all but destroyed my life. Would justice have been served? Would society have benefited? Would America have been safer?

It was a significant step forward when, in mid-2013, U.S. Attorney General Eric Holder issued a directive to federal prosecutors that ended federal mandatory sentencing for minor drug crimes. Mandatory minimums have led to the incarceration of hundreds of thousands of Americans convicted of such crimes, including many that were far less serious than mine. Those laws, Holder said, would be replaced by a set of guidelines designed to decrease imprisonment rates for "low-level, nonviolent drug offenders who have no ties to large-scale organizations, gangs or cartels." New provisions would direct some violators to drug treatment. Another advance came when, after Colorado and Washington legalized marijuana, the Obama administration announced that it would not challenge those states' laws. Finally, the Office of National Drug Control Policy's 2013 budget includes $25 billion, more money than ever before, for prevention of drug use and treatment for addiction.

Despite these positive changes, however, critical policy shifts are still to be made; the War on Drugs is far from over. Though there are some improvements in the 2013 federal budget, $15 billion of the $25 billion is earmarked for the same wartime tactics, including interdiction, law enforcement, and eradication programs, that for decades have failed to lower the supply of drugs and the number of deaths from addiction. There has been no indication that the mandatory-sentencing prohibition will be retroactive, which means that hundreds of thousands of citizens, including a disproportionate number of African Americans, will languish in prison for minor drug crimes. There has been no serious consideration of some harm-reduction strategies, including the safe injection sites for IV drug users that I describe in *Clean,* which have shown promise in other nations. And people are still being arrested and locked up for no crime other than being ill. The drug war must be ended and a new war declared: a war on the disease of addiction.

As I've explained, it wasn't by choice that I became immersed in this field a decade ago. I was dragged in when my son became addicted and was on a trajectory that was leading to his death. He just turned thirty-one and celebrated five years clean. After many near misses, my son is alive. He's lucky. I'm lucky. He underwent (and continues) intensive evidence-based treatment developed and practiced by doctors trained in addiction medicine. They saved the life of my son, just as they will save the lives of countless others' sons and daughters.

October 2013

Appendix: Just Say *Know*

IN A SURVEY COMMISSIONED by the Partnership at Drugfree.org, teenagers were asked what would dissuade them from using drugs. Essentially they said: The truth.

The internal and external factors that drive drug use are the most salient forces in users' lives, and so the most important prevention strategy is to address them. But even that isn't enough. If kids (and others) are to make informed choices about drugs, they need to have facts about them. They need to know what they're risking in order to get high.

Kids already know that drugs make people feel great. They should know why: the facts I explained earlier about the flood of dopamine, the full-blast go system, and the sidelined prefrontal cortex that would, if it were fully developed, moderate impulsivity and the desire for pleasure but also regulate the flow of chemicals. The chemistry of addiction explains why drugs in general make us feel so good, and also why they can be so dangerous. But kids aren't deciding whether or not to do drugs in general; they're deciding specifically whether to smoke, drink, take cocaine, or use other drugs.

Some drugs they'll encounter are perennially obtainable, while others come and go depending on social trends, availability, and cost (supply and demand operates in the black market too). Here, I'll describe the most prevalent drugs and their effects, starting with the most ubiquitous drug of all.

Alcohol

One hundred and thirty-one million people drink, nearly half of Americans. Most of us drink casually without negative consequences.

You hear (or say) it all the time: "I need a drink." Why? Alcohol can calm people when they're stressed. Some people feel energized, at least for a while. Some people lose their inhibitions, which can feel liberating. Alcohol can also make people feel morose and depressed. It can lead to reckless behavior. It can cause illness, brain damage, and death.

ER visits and hospital admissions for alcohol overdose, alcohol-caused maladies, and alcohol-related car and other accidents are up 29 percent over the past decade. In 2005, the CDC estimated that 35,000 people a year died from cirrhosis of the liver and other diseases linked to drinking, and at least 40,000 died from car crashes and other accidents caused by excessive alcohol use. Of those teens who reported alcohol use, a majority (62 percent) said they had had their first alcoholic drink by age fifteen, and a fourth had been younger than twelve.

The fact is, most people drink moderately. A martini. A couple of beers. Wine with dinner. And for most people, moderate drinking is harmless. (The effects of alcohol vary according to the individual's gender, body size, amount of body fat, amount of alcohol consumed, and other factors.) However, the brains of heavy drinkers and those with malfunctioning stop systems — that is, those predisposed to addiction — can change quickly, and the addiction cycle begins.

When a person has a drink, ethanol, a form of alcohol, reaches the brain and all the organs of the body within ninety seconds. Ten percent of the ethanol is eliminated (through sweat, breath, etc.), and the liver begins working to metabolize the rest; alcohol is toxic, and the body tries to get rid of it as quickly as possible. On average, the liver metabolizes a half an ounce of ethanol in an hour. When there's more alcohol in the body than the liver can break down, the concentration of alcohol in the bloodstream increases.

Alcohol slows brain function in two ways. It primarily affects the neurotransmitter GABA, the one that inhibits, or controls, neural activity, and glutamate, which acts as the brain's general-purpose excitatory neurotransmitter. Alcohol decreases function, particularly in areas of the brain involved in memory formation, decision-making, and impulse control. By preventing glutamate from doing its work, ethanol slows reaction times, impairs memory, dampens motor skills, and can cause slurred speech, nausea, emotional volatility, loss of coordination, and visual distortions. Like other drugs, alcohol increases the flow of dopamine. The dopamine flow may cause an initial sense of euphoria, but that soon dissipates. When it does, it can cause feelings of depression. Alcohol activates serotonin receptors, disrupting the neurotransmitter system that helps regulate mood and sleep, and it damages a part of neurons in the cerebellum, a structure involved in motor skills, which is why drinking causes people to lose coordination. Elsewhere in the body, alcohol is toxic in the liver, kidney, and nervous system, though it affects every organ in the drinker's body and can damage a developing fetus. Alcohol slows breathing and heart rate, sometimes to the point that coma — even death — results.

From 10 to 15 percent of people who try alcohol will become alcoholics. Alcohol actually damages more neurotransmitter systems than many other drugs — dopamine, serotonin, glutamate, and GABA. The earlier a child begins drinking, the more likely he'll abuse alcohol.

Some people think it takes decades for alcohol to damage the brain, but teens are vulnerable to immediate harm, some of which may be irreversible. At the University of California at San Diego, researchers looked at twelve- to fourteen-year-olds before they used any alcohol or drugs and then followed them as they began drinking. Some became binge drinkers. The researchers scanned binge drinkers' brains and compared them to the brains of kids who drank moderately. They also tested their thinking and memory.

Binge drinking is especially prevalent — and deadly — among teenagers. Nearly a quarter of those over twelve — almost sixty million people — binge drink. More than 40 percent of college students do. This number contrasts starkly with the number of parents who think their children binge drink; according to one study, only 3 percent thought their teens had indulged in binge drinking in the past month.

Adolescents who binge drink are often motivated to do it by all the reasons they try other drugs, but there are also factors unique to their biology that drive them to alcohol. One is that teenage bodies are better able to tolerate the negative immediate effects of drinking, such as nausea, which makes them likelier to drink more—feeling more of a buzz in the short term but increasing their likelihood for addiction and other health problems in the long term.

In some schools, bingeing has become a perverse rite of passage. Kids have died at parties at which they drink twenty-one shots to celebrate their twenty-first birthdays.

These events have also given rise to an epidemic of date rape. For college-age youths between eighteen and twenty-four, there were almost a hundred thousand cases of alcohol-related sexual assault or date rape reported. (Alcohol is sometimes combined with date-rape drugs.)

Like binge drinking, car accidents are especially prevalent—and deadly—among teens. And both are the result of the peculiar way alcohol interacts with teenage biology. In the case of car crashes, alcohol impairs reaction time and judgment, exaggerating the deficits of the adolescent brain, which hasn't yet developed the ability to control impulses and assess risks (such as the risk of getting in a car driven by someone who's drunk a six-pack in an hour). Alcohol is involved in car crashes that account for more than one in three teenage deaths.

Not all the havoc alcohol causes is as dramatic as a car wreck. The drug produces a calm, drowsy effect and is a depressant (even if it can initially feel like it's countering depression). Alcohol seems to have the same depressant effect in younger people as it does in adults, and alcohol use has been associated with half of teenage suicides. Indeed, increased teen drinking may be to blame for the rising rates of teenage suicide since 1950.

After first stimulating the production of dopamine, serotonin, and another neurotransmitter—norepinephrine—alcohol lowers the levels of these substances in the brain, which can explain its depressive aspects. In addition, it can cause depression by inhibiting the neurological system that regulates moods. Alcohol contributes to depression in other ways too. Its toxicity makes people feel physically ill, and abusing it can induce guilt. Also, alcohol is used disproportionately by people who are already depressed. An article on WebMD reports, "Nearly a third of those with major depression also have an alcohol problem, according to one major study conducted by the National Institute on Alcohol Abuse and Alcoholism. Research shows that children who are depressed are more prone to develop alcohol problems once they reach adolescence. Teens who've had an episode of major depression are twice as likely as those who aren't depressed to start drinking alcohol." "The problem," says the Menninger Clinic's Dr. Flack, "is that a beer or two can appear to relieve depression for a little while, but by the time you have your eighth beer you feel suicidal, angry, or out of control and more depressed."

Long-term heavy drinking can cause a number of physical problems, particularly liver disease. Alcohol abuse is the most common cause of liver disease in North America. It can also cause or contribute to pancreatitis, epilepsy, and heart disease. Using it increases the risk of developing cardiovascular disease and some forms of cancer. It can damage the nervous system and cause impotence. Fetal alcohol spectrum disorders occur in babies born to mothers addicted to alcohol, and the disorders affect 40,000 newborns a year in the United States. As I said earlier, withdrawal from alcohol can cause seizures, including ones that are fatal.

Marijuana

According to a 2011 study, daily marijuana use among high-school seniors is currently at its highest level in thirty years. In a survey conducted in 2008, 42 percent of teens twelve to seventeen years old said they could buy marijuana in a day or less; 23 percent said they could buy weed in an hour or less. Marijuana smokers now include people from just about every demographic. *Marie Claire* magazine ran a story about "stiletto stoners," professional women who wind down after work with a joint instead of a martini. "They've got killer careers and enviable social lives. They're also major potheads." Use is up, and so are health problems attributed to pot smoking. In a recent year, nearly four hundred thousand of the nation's two million drug-related ER visits involved marijuana.

There's widespread misinformation about all drugs, but pot is the most misunderstood. Some say it's evil; others maintain that it's harmless. Warnings about the dangers of marijuana are confusing, because they belie the experience of many people who enjoy smoking, whether occasionally or frequently, and feel that there's no downside. Those users defend it as natural, harmless, and safe, or at least safer than alcohol. They claim it isn't addictive. They laugh at the idea that marijuana is a gateway drug that leads to hard drugs. Many teenagers have told me that almost everyone they know smokes, including stellar students. (Many get high on "edibles" — a menu of pot-laced delicacies that include the classic marijuana brownies plus gourmet ice cream, scones, BBQ sauce, and, from one of many cookbooks, Ganja Granny's Smoked Mac 'N' Cheese.)

The first thing to say about marijuana is that many people use it without any obvious negative impacts on their lives. *Obvious* is the operative term here — there are negative impacts that may be subtle or may not become relevant for years. But those who preach that marijuana will kill you, make you crazy, or make you shoot heroin are wrong — usually. That said, it must also be noted that those who claim marijuana is harmless are wrong too. Here are the facts:

In a number of studies, long-term marijuana users have reported poor outcomes on a variety of life satisfaction and achievement measures, including educational attainment. Fewer smokers than nonsmokers complete college, and smokers are far more likely than nonsmokers to earn yearly incomes of less than $30,000. Also, the IQs of heavy users who began smoking pot as teenagers are an average of eight points lower than IQs of nonsmokers. Marijuana users are more likely to suffer from depression than others, but, as Ty S. Schepis, assistant professor of psychology at Texas State University, clarifies, "It's unknown if pot causes depression; it may be that depressed people smoke pot."

Pot may cause something called amotivational syndrome. The THC in marijuana binds to the brain's cannabinoid receptors, many of which are in the prefrontal cortex. The drug docks on the receptors and blocks the mechanism that normally would inhibit the release of dopamine and other neurotransmitters. Dopamine flows, activating parts of the neurological system that make you feel relaxed and calm. By stunting communication between brain regions, it impairs the cognitive process — high-level thinking. One effect of all this is what researchers describe as amotivational syndrome, a "diminished or absent drive to engage in typically rewarding activities," as the National Institute on Drug Abuse defines it. In *Jackie Brown*, the Quentin Tarantino movie, Samuel L. Jackson's character tells his girlfriend, "You smoke too much of that shit.

That shit's gonna rob you of your ambition, girl." She answers, "Not if your ambition is to get stoned and watch TV." A recent meta-study of a body of research into amotivational syndrome found consistent evidence of "impaired motivation" as a symptom of chronic pot smoking. Ultimately, the research about whether pot drains motivation isn't conclusive — motivation is difficult to quantify and measure, especially over decades. The fact is that many of us know pot smokers who seem as motivated as anyone. However, it's also true that many long-term pot smokers describe impaired motivation that affected, and in some cases defined, their lives. Says Dr. Richard N. Rosenthal, chairman of psychiatry at St. Luke's–Roosevelt Hospital in Manhattan and professor of clinical psychiatry at Columbia University: "The people who become chronic users don't have the same lives and the same achievements as people who don't use chronically."

The existence of amotivational syndrome may be arguable, but there's no arguing with the research that proves that pot affects brain structure, cognitive functioning, and memory. In the main text of *Clean* I reported research that shows the changes marijuana causes in the brains of adolescents. Susan Tapert's research has shown the dramatic diminution in the white matter. What does it matter if the white matter is changed, especially if the changes are subtle? Tapert's and others' tests have shown that the fact that messages between brain regions don't flow as efficiently has significant repercussions. Retarded communication between these regions explains functional deficits found in marijuana smokers. It explains the fact that marijuana has been shown to impair attention, judgment, coordination and balance, learning skills, reaction time, and the ability to organize and integrate complex information, and it compromises memory.

For her studies, Dr. Tapert and her colleagues recruited children as young as twelve years old. In one of her studies, a control group of nonusers (they consistently tested negative for drugs) was compared to a group of heavy pot smokers. The researchers examined the differences and changes in brain tissue and determined how the changes correlated with cognitive abilities, specifically their learning and memory. In another study, they worked with twelve-year-olds who had never smoked pot and followed them. Over the course of the study, some of them began smoking. The researchers measured the differences in functioning before and after they started using. Dr. Vicki Nejtek, referring to Tapert's and others' research, concludes, "There seems to be a reduction in brain cell activity which appears to correlate with some memory loss and a reduced ability to concentrate. When combined with a loss of concentration, even the slightest memory loss amounts to a significant loss in decision-making during complex tasks."

There's already a large body of evidence that shows that when people are high, they can't concentrate well, don't learn well, can't remember well, and have slowed reaction times. Tapert's studies help explain why. She looked at the effects of marijuana when users weren't stoned and after they'd stopped smoking for some time. The studies all showed "consistent differences" in marijuana users compared to nonusers, Tapert says. A presentation of her research at the American Academy of Pediatrics, "Neuroimaging Marijuana Use and Its Effects on Cognitive Function," showed that chronic, heavy marijuana use during adolescence is associated with poorer performance on thinking tasks, including slower psychomotor speed and poorer complex-attention, verbal-memory, and planning abilities.

Tapert's colleague Krista Lisdahl Medina said that some findings suggest that former pot smokers did better on some tests, which may indicate partial recovery of verbal-memory functioning, but she added that complex-attention skills continued to be affected. "Not only are their thinking abilities worse, their brain activation to cognitive tasks is abnormal," she explains. "The tasks are fairly easy, such as remembering the location of objects, and they may be able to complete the tasks, but what we saw is that adolescent marijuana users are using more of their parietal and frontal cortices to complete the tasks. Their brain is working harder than it should." She notes, "We find that the adolescent marijuana users use larger portions of their brain to complete the same task as non-smokers. As teens mature, they tend to use smaller, more focused neural circuitry — we believe using marijuana heavily disrupts this maturation. Short term, they appear less efficient and accurate on cognitive tests. This is especially true for more difficult tasks that need to be sustained over time and require a lot of effort. Given this, when current marijuana users or recently abstinent users are in school or on the job they are likely working slower, learning less, and performing at a lower level than they would if they were not heavy users. Because they have to work harder, they may be more likely to quit tasks that are challenging. We are currently following teens over time to see if sustained abstinence (e.g., greater than six months) results in complete recovery, or if long-lasting effects can be measured even after teens stay abstinent."

MARIJUANA CAN IMPEDE MATURATION

Most people who use drugs begin in high school, which is the worst possible time for them to be using, for many reasons. In the past, it was generally accepted as fact that the human brain is more or less fixed after a person is twelve or so, but scientists now understand that the brain continues to develop, and, after the first few years of life, human neurobiology is most plastic — able to adapt and change — during adolescence and into one's early twenties. Drugs — including marijuana — can wreak havoc on developing brains precisely at the time they're supposed to be maturing. According to Dr. Schepis, "This is a period of strong change in the brain. We're very concerned that marijuana alters the ways in which adolescent brains normally mature, particularly among heavy users."

"And the younger, the more impact it seems to have," says Dr. Jacobus. Younger smokers — twelve, thirteen, fourteen — "consistently have a poorer outcome in the long term compared to those who start when they're older." The impact isn't limited to cognitive functions like memory. It's inseparable from the psychological and emotional development that occurs during adolescence.

"An eighteen-year-old who walks into my office and asks for help with his addiction who's been using since he was twelve years old is twelve years old," Fred Holmes says. "That's when his social-skill development stopped working, because he started using opiates or other drugs to figure out problems he should have figured out in appropriate ways."

Pot (like other drugs) can prevent people from having to feel, so as teenagers, pot smokers never feel or learn how to deal with those feelings. Kids who are alienated may be drawn to pot, but pot may alienate them further. (This is ironic, because initially it can feel as if drugs make it easier to have relationships.) Even if users aren't clinically depressed, marijuana can induce depressive feelings, which may cause them to isolate more. In a real way, adolescents can miss much of their teenage years and early twenties if they spend them in a haze of pot smoke. "Adolescents are making the transition from childhood to adulthood," Robert Schwebel wrote in *Saying No Is Not Enough.* "Teenagers with drug problems will not be prepared for adult roles. . . . They will chronologically mature while remaining emotional adolescents."

MARIJUANA CAN CAUSE OR WORSEN DEPRESSION, ANXIETY, AND OTHER PSYCHOLOGICAL DISORDERS. IT CAN EVEN TRIGGER MENTAL ILLNESS.

Though some people use pot to ameliorate depression and anxiety, there's evidence that it can cause or trigger those very conditions and make them worse — both common depression and anxiety and the more serious versions that qualify as psychological disorders. And though some advocates of marijuana dismiss the claim that the drug can cause people to become psychotic or schizophrenic, there's a growing body of evidence that it can trigger depression and bipolar disorder and trigger or exacerbate a range of emotional and behavioral disorders. One out of five adolescents has one or more of these.

Several studies show a relationship between teenage marijuana use and later psychosis. Once again, it's impossible to know if pot caused the psychosis or if people who later develop psychosis are for some reason drawn to smoke pot. Some researchers believe that the drug "turns on" and worsens preexisting disorders. They've observed that marijuana use can worsen the course of illness in patients with schizophrenia and some other mental illnesses and it can produce a brief psychotic reaction in some users (it usually fades when the drug wears off, but it doesn't always). In addition to the documented links between marijuana use and schizophrenia, anxiety, and depression, associations between marijuana use and suicidal thoughts and attempts and personality disorders are being investigated.

"We know that some kids become psychotic from smoking pot," according to Dr. Matthew Large of the University of New South Wales, whose study showed that the onset of mental illness was hastened by three years among marijuana users compared to kids who hadn't used. There's no proof that marijuana *caused* the mental illness, of course, and Large's study showed that the highest-risk kids are those with a family history of psychosis or some psychotic symptom, but they aren't the only ones whose pot smoking triggers mental illness. Kids struggling in school or experiencing stress at home are also highly vulnerable, Large said. "There's probably something in marijuana that triggers schizophrenia," he told Reuters. "What that is isn't clear yet, but there's a connection." It's important to emphasize that this is rare, but it's also important to emphasize that it happens — using is a risk. To protect the vulnerable from this, some proponents of marijuana use would agree that kids with mental illness, behavioral disorders, learning disabilities, or similar problems shouldn't smoke, but they're missing an essential point. When people say that pot's fine, they can't also caution, "It's fine if you don't have mental illness" — most children who begin using don't know if they have mental illnesses. Their parents probably don't know either. Every kid who starts using thinks it's not a big deal and it'll never be a problem.

Beyond the cause-and-effect relationship between pot and mental illness, it's clear that many people with psychological disorders use pot and other drugs to escape from the confusion and pain associated with mental illness and whatever else is happening inside and outside their heads. It's accurate to say that people attempt to self-medicate and escape psychic and physical pain with marijuana (and other drugs). But when symptoms are hidden, they aren't noticed, and they can't be diagnosed and treated. Often delaying treatment, especially among teenagers, dramatically worsens mental disorders. When I visited Hazelden Adolescent Center, I was informed that 90 percent of patients from fifteen to nineteen years of age who were pot smokers (and some, but not all, used other drugs) had been diagnosed with co-occurring psychological disorders.

MARIJUANA *ISN'T* A GATEWAY DRUG — AND IT IS

Okay, marijuana isn't always a gateway drug, of course, but no honest person would argue that any twelve-year-old starts out with a needle and heroin or a line of meth. Pot was certainly a gateway drug for me. When I accepted the first joint, I crossed a line. Before that, I was certain I'd never use drugs. Suddenly the gate was open. I liked being high and wanted to be higher. Marijuana didn't make me paranoid or crazy, it just made me feel good, so I became less fearful of other drugs. I overcame whatever it was that had stopped me from using before that — conscience, fear of getting caught, fear of what drugs might do. I hung out with a new crowd of kids, ones who got stoned. Before long, in addition to joints, people were offering me pills and lines of coke.

My experience is anything but unique. For example, a study of over three hundred fraternal and identical twins found that a subject who had used marijuana before the age of seventeen had a higher rate of other drug use and drug problems later on than his twin who hadn't used before he turned seventeen.

MARIJUANA *CAN* BE ADDICTIVE

One of the major myths about marijuana is that it isn't addictive, but it can be. This doesn't mean that everyone who tries pot will become addicted, of course, but that's also true of cocaine and many other drugs. Regardless of whether it's a physical or psychological addiction (it's almost certainly both), more adults and adolescents are now admitted to treatment for primary marijuana addictions than for primary addictions to heroin, cocaine, and hallucinogens, according to the Substance Abuse and Mental Health Services Administration. By the time most people arrive in treatment, they've experienced some or all of the conditions that define addiction. Indeed, marijuana addiction has most of the hallmarks of other addictions. The simplest measure of dependency on a drug is that people have difficulty controlling their use and some can't stop even when it interferes with their lives. In scans and other tests, the brains of people who are addicted generally appear different than "normal" brains, and there are physical anomalies found in the brains of heavy marijuana users. Another quality of addictive drugs is that users can build up a tolerance to them, so more is required to achieve the same effect. This is true of marijuana. Addictions also cause withdrawal symptoms. People trying to quit marijuana report irritability, sleeping difficulties, craving, and anxiety. They show increased aggression on psychological tests.

It's estimated that 5 percent of people who use marijuana will become dependent on it. The number goes up among those who start using in their teens, and among daily users. But it's true that the odds of becoming addicted to pot are lower than the odds of becoming addicted to alcohol and other drugs.

MARIJUANA *CAN* KILL

Some people defend marijuana by claiming that it's never killed anyone, whereas the truly dangerous drugs, including alcohol, have taken countless lives. It's a misleading assertion, because it doesn't take into consideration the likelihood that pot has caused or contributed to fatal accidents. Research shows that "behavioral and cognitive skills related to driving performance [are] impaired in a dose-dependent fashion with increasing THC blood levels," according to the summation of a meta-analysis of approximately sixty studies of marijuana and driving. A thorough recent study, published in the *British Medical Journal,* reviewed nine studies of more than 49,000 people involved in accidents on public roads involving one or more motor vehicles, including cars, trucks, buses, and motorcycles. Marijuana use was confirmed by blood tests or self-reporting. Researchers found drivers who had used marijuana within three hours of beginning to drive had nearly *double the risk* of causing a collision, especially a fatal one. Mark Asbridge, associate professor in the Department of Community Health and Epidemiology at Dalhousie University in Halifax, Nova Scotia, where the study was conducted, told TheFix.com, "Cannabis affects drivers' spatial sense, potentially causing them to follow cars too closely or swerve in and out of lanes. This differs from the main effect alcohol has on drivers: slower reaction times." It was no surprise, but younger people (below thirty-five) were more likely that older ones to be in fatal accidents.

As I've said, an essential fact about any drug, including marijuana, is that a person doesn't have to be an abuser or addict to have negative, even catastrophic, consequences. One-time use can lead to accidents or other dangerous events. Meanwhile, in a survey in 2012, 19 percent of teen drivers reported driving under the influence of pot, while 36 percent of the teens surveyed said that they were confident the drug had no effect on their abilities behind the wheel.

Hard Drugs

Across all ages and most demographics, abuse of prescription pills is America's fastest-growing drug problem, with skyrocketing teenage use. Cocaine, date-rape drugs like roofies, opiates that range from OxyContin to heroin, ecstasy, psychedelics like LSD, paint thinner, synthetic pot, methamphetamine, DXM, Adderall . . . each drug has particular properties that cause different highs, and each carries specific risks. Here's some basic information, and there's more to be found online, on the NIDA website and elsewhere. (An entertaining explanation of the interaction of various drugs on the brain can be found at Mouse Party, created by the University of Utah's Genetic Science Learning Center.)

More than 3.7 million teenagers regularly — more than twice a month — use prescription and over-the-counter pharmaceuticals to get high. According to the White House Office of National Drug Control Policy, the number of people seeking care for abuse of prescription painkillers rose 400 percent from 1998 to 2008. People entering treatment for benzodiazepine addiction (these include Valium, Xanax, and Klonopin) tripled between 1998 and 2008. A study issued by the Centers for Disease Control in 2012 showed a doubling of fatal poisonings among American children from 2000 to 2009. Prescription-drug abuse was largely to blame.

In America, two million people either abuse or are dependent on opiates or opioid pain medications like OxyContin, the most widely abused prescription painkiller. Oxy tablets are crushed and then snorted, smoked, or injected. Like other opiates, including Vicodin, codeine, hydrocodone, Roxicodone, fentanyl, and morphine, OxyContin is related to heroin — and misuse of them all often leads to heroin. Ty S. Schepis, of Texas State University, explains, "A sixteen-year-old's looking in his parents' medicine cabinet. It's unlikely he's going to find a bag of meth or cocaine, but there's a bottle with ten Percocets that his parents have around from when Mom or Dad had surgery. They're curious and try it. *Whoa, that was fun.* They try it again. They run through the ten pills. Need to get some more. They raid a friend's parents' medicine cabinet. They're trying to buy them at school." Then they learn that heroin provides a similar high for a fraction of the cost. The jump from prescription drugs to heroin is partly why heroin use has increased sharply in many parts of the country. In 2010, 359,000 Americans age twelve and older were addicted to heroin. A father wrote from Texas, saying that his son, addicted to prescription drugs, was a regular in emergency rooms — from January to June 2009, he was in the ER thirty times — "more often than not leaving with a prescription for a narcotic in hand. Two weeks ago he visited a hospital and got a prescription for Valium. The next night, the same emergency room prescribed him with Percocet and a narcotic cough medicine. He returned home, went to sleep, and never woke up again."

Heroin and other narcotics are agonists, drugs that mimic a chemical in the body. Heroin, OxyContin, and other opiates can cause breathing to slow and eventually stop. Most deaths from heroin ODs are caused by respiratory failure. The drug can also cause heart attacks. Heroin withdrawal is characterized by physical pain, anxiety, insomnia, diarrhea, vomiting, and hot and cold flashes. Many of the deaths from heroin or other opiates occur in opiate neophytes or addicts with high tolerance to the drug who detox and then relapse and take doses they're no longer able to tolerate. Dr. Flack saw a patient who was taking 800 milligrams of methadone a day — "enough to kill eight to ten people," he said. He got clean and relapsed on a similarly high dosage when he no longer had the tolerance.

Cocaine, methamphetamine, and other amphetamines (forms of speed) act directly on the dopamine system, causing a spray of the chemical as if from a fire hose. More babies are born exposed to meth than to heroin and cocaine combined. Meth is tied to higher numbers of incidents of child abuse and spousal abuse. Whereas a decade ago a majority of meth was made in mom-and-pop labs in garages or trailers, there are now superlabs — huge state-of-the-art factories producing more than a ton of crystal a week — in Malaysia, Mexico, and elsewhere. There were more than 350,000 meth users in America in 2010. Worldwide, there are twenty-five million users.

Meth causes an intense and long-lasting rush, but it is also one of the most toxic and addictive drugs. Animal research going back more than twenty years shows that high doses of methamphetamine damage nerve-cell endings and this leads to long-lasting memory and cognitive deficits. Meth can lead to anorexia, mood disturbances, violent behavior, anxiety, confusion, paranoia, delusions, convulsions, and insomnia. Meth use and withdrawal often include severe depression and high levels of anxiety. The drug increases breathing rates, body temperature, and blood pressure and can cause strokes and heart attacks (cardiovascular collapse). When San Francisco cardiologist Charles Morris was director of the cardiac catheterization lab at St. Luke's Hospital, he often performed angiograms on meth patients who came in for chest pain or heart failure. "What I saw were extremely damaged hearts, often end-stage cardiomyopathies — they're in heart failure that will relentlessly progress toward death," Morris says.

The number of cocaine-related emergency-room visits, including cocaine-induced cardiac arrests, has doubled over the past five years. Normally after dopamine is released and triggers its rewards in the neurological system, it recirculates, whereas meth causes it to seep through cell walls. Cocaine blocks the transporters, leaving the drug trapped where it repeatedly stimulates the receptors. In autopsies, cocaine users are found to have fewer dopamine receptors than normal and lower gray-matter density in regions of the brain associated with memory, attention, and learning. When a person takes cocaine, he's twenty-four times more likely than normal to have a heart attack within an hour. At St. Luke's and California Pacific Medical Center, Dr. Morris has seen addicts with "blown-out aortas" — aortic dissections — caused by cocaine.

Prescription stimulants such as Adderall and Ritalin, used to help people with ADHD focus, can energize those without the disorder. The drugs have become common on college campuses and, more recently, in high schools, where students take them to study better, do better on tests, stay up all night writing research papers — and to party. Abuse of these drugs is up an estimated 92 percent over the past decade. They can cause symptoms of psychosis and delirium, paranoia, depression, and, because they elevate blood pressure and cause heart palpitations, like other stimulants they can cause strokes or heart attacks. About 10 percent of people who use them become addicted.

About 695,000 people use ecstasy. Like other drugs, ecstasy stimulates the flow of dopamine, but it also affects serotonin, the neurotransmitter responsible for mood, sleep, perception, and appetite. Many ecstasy tablets are "dirty," meaning they're laced with other drugs, sometimes methamphetamine. *Science Daily* reported on studies that showed long-term ecstasy use causes the hippocampus region of the brain to shrink an average of 10 percent. As the authors of the study pointed out, "hippocampal atrophy is a hallmark for diseases of progressive cognitive impairment in older patients, such as Alzheimer's disease." Overdose can cause seizures and heart or kidney failure.

Like ecstasy, Rohypnol (roofies) and GHB are so-called party drugs. The latter two are also known as date-rape drugs, because victims who are slipped them (they dissolve in liquid) pass out and — after they're raped — often don't remember what happened. When prescribed (outside the United States; the drug isn't approved in this country), Rohypnol is used to treat anxiety disorders. GHB, or gamma-hydroxybutyrate, is a central nervous system depressant. Its primary ingredients are used as floor strippers and drain cleaners. Rarely, users of these drugs fall into comas, and some die.

More than a hundred thousand people use PCP, ketamine, and DXM (dextromethorphan, which is in over-the-counter medications); they're classed together because they're dissociative drugs — they cause delusions, hallucinations, and anxiety, plus impair motor functions. They increase heart rate and blood pressure and decrease respiration and can cause psychosis, convulsions, and a fever so high that it can lead to death. Use of PCP has dissociative effects that can also lead to psychosis. Ketamine has similar effects. The drug is an anesthetic that's used by veterinarians as an animal tranquilizer, and it affects memory, attention, and learning. It can cause high blood pressure and depression, and it can slow breathing to the point that it becomes fatal.

About a million people use LSD and other hallucinogens (such as psilocybin mushrooms and mescaline) each year. LSD also affects serotonin, binding to serotonin receptors, both inhibiting and exciting a part of the brain that sends neurons to sensory areas of the brain, which is why the drug causes hallucinations, distortions in perception, and dramatic mood swings. These drugs also raise body temperature and increase heart rate and blood pressure.

Often people don't take drugs singly but combine them. Most drug overdoses involve the use of more than one drug. The Drug Abuse Warning Network reported an average of 2.7 drugs involved in every fatal overdose. When drugs are combined, the potential for brain damage, heart attack, stroke, and overdose increases. The U.S. National Household Drug Survey estimated that around five million people use alcohol and cocaine together each month. When cocaine is combined with alcohol, a chemical called cocaethylene results; it's toxic to the liver and can cause heart attacks. Another dangerous combination of drugs is heroin and cocaine in what's known as a speedball; it can cause heart attacks and respiratory failure. Generally, using two or more drugs together doesn't simply double or triple the odds of causing damage; it raises the risk exponentially.

There are always new drug trends. In 2012, a study published in *Pediatrics* reported forty-five hundred calls to poison control centers between 2010 to 2011 related to K2, Spice, and other "synthetic pot," which can cause seizures, panic attacks, and psychosis. These synthetics became illegal in 2012, but soon after, there were new formulations available on the streets based on knock-off molecules that weren't illegal.

Inhalants aren't new, but now more than two million people, mostly teenagers, use them — glue, paint thinner, gasoline, nail polish remover, and aerosols. They can permanently damage the nervous system and cause heart failure. Another trendy drug is what's known as bath salts, a combination of the toxic chemicals mephedrone and methylenedioxypyrovalerone, and it's led to seizures, violence, suicide, and lethal overdose.

"Lean" or "purple drank" is a relatively new way kids use opiates. They mix medications that contain codeine — principally promethazine VC — with soda and candy. Robitussin DXM is also used to make lean. There are increasing reports of children, many high-school kids but also middle-schoolers, showing up in emergency rooms after Robotripping — drinking Robitussin or other cough syrups that contain DXM. A bottle of the syrup can get kids high, but it can also make them psychotic. Those who don't use drugs can't conceive of a child voluntarily drinking cough syrup or taking cold medication — or sniffing nail polish remover. But as Luke explained, though he'd regularly get high on ecstasy, cocaine, and pot, his need for drugs was such that, as he said, "If I didn't have anything, I'd take gasoline out of the lawnmower and huff that."

Acknowledgments

I AM GRATEFUL TO ALL of those who allowed me into their lives and shared their stories, and to the many researchers, doctors, therapists, social workers, nurses, staff members of treatment centers and prevention programs, and others who educated me about addiction. I am indebted to Amelia Arria, Fran Benton, Anne Besser, Peter Boeschenstein, Melissa Burton, Diana Clark, Anna David, Lennard Davis, Michael L. Dennis, Laura Duran, Eileen Dwyer, Christopher J. Evans, Marica Ferri, Jim Flack, Susan E. Foster, Gannt Galloway, Kevin Gogin, Luke Gsell, Mark Gsell, Father John Hardin, Ulrike Heberlein, Fred Holmes, Keith Humphreys, Joanna Jacobus, Paulina Kalaj, Rebecca Keithahn, Kathleen Kelly, Patrick Kennedy, Beau Kilmer, Matthew Large, Joseph Lee, Sharon Levy, Walter Ling, Roberta Lojak, Bertha Madras, Gabor Maté, Michael McCann, Krista Lisdahl Medina, John Mendelson, Rudolph Moos, Vicki Nejtek, Jeannie Obert, Charles O'Brien, David Olds, Jan Osborn, Michael Pantalon, Steve Pasierb, Shannon Pearce, Jacqueline Periman, Helen M. Pettinati, Steve Randall, John Roll, Barbara Rothbaum, Ty S. Schepis, Joe Schrank, Marvin Seppala, Cheryl Shine, Michael D. Slater, Kali Spencer, Josh Spitalnick, Jim Steinhagen, Susan Tapert, Martha Lee Taylor, J. Scott Tonigan, and Ken C. Winters.

I particularly want to acknowledge the immeasurable contributions of Steve Shoptaw, Rick Rawson, and Tom McLellan, who generously shared their vast knowledge and experience, patiently indulged my endless queries, and vetted portions of the book. I'm also thankful to Tom for sharing his personal story. In addition to the other scientists

I've listed, I thank Nora Volkow, head of the National Institute on Drug Abuse, a tireless advocate for the addicted, and her colleagues at NIDA, including Ruben Baler, Kevin Conway, Joseph Frascella, Dave McCann, Stephanie Older, Lisa Onken, Eve Reider, Elizabeth Robertson, David Shurtleff, and Susan Weiss.

Others who helped on various aspects of *Clean* include Lori Glazer, Megan Wilson, Carla Gray, Ben Hyman, Lois Wasoff, Sanj Kharbanda, and Larry Cooper at Houghton Mifflin Harcourt; Ron Bernstein, Molly Atlas, Margaret Southard, and Michael Griffo at ICM; Ling Ma, who fact-checked the manuscript; Tracy Roe, who copyedited it; Melissa Lotfy and Alex Camlin, who designed the book inside and out.

Gary Mendell's contributions to *Clean* were invaluable. I'm in awe of Gary and the way he has undertaken to build an organization that can—that *will*—help turn the tide on addiction. I'm grateful to him, Janet Mendell, and Greg Mendell.

As it was in *Beautiful Boy,* the elegant touch of Eamon Dolan, my editor, can be seen on every page of *Clean.* Eamon guided this book from its inception. He's the editor every writer dreams of working with.

It's impossible to adequately express my thanks to Amanda Urban for her guidance, advocacy, wisdom, and caring.

I'm grateful to two sources quoted in *Clean* who are also dear friends, Charles Morris and Kyle Redford. (I'm also grateful to their spouses, Jamie and Andrea.) Peggy Knickerbocker is testament to the profundity of the Twelve Steps. Thanks to her and Robert Fisher for edifying conversations about recovery, and for their friendship. I thank my many other friends for their support, encouragement, and advice. Finally, I thank my parents, Joan and Sumner Sheff, and the rest of my family: Debra, Mark, Jenny, Becca, Bear, Nancy, Steve, Mark, and the newest addition, Jette. Don Barbour provided invaluable research from medical journals. Susan Barbour vetted portions of the manuscript. Lucy Briggs provided stellar research assistance. Nic Sheff conducted the interview with Anna David. Indeed, there would be no book without Nic, Jasper, and Daisy Sheff, and without my remarkable wife, Karen Barbour.

Notes

Quotations that are not specifically sourced in the notes come from interviews with the author.

PREFACE

xv *Almost 80 percent of America's children:* National Center on Addiction and Substance Abuse, "Adolescent Substance Use: America's #1 Public Health Problem," May 21, 2012. The number excludes cigarettes. Partnership at DrugFree.org, "2011 Partnership Attitude Tracking Study," May 2, 2012; "Teen Alcohol and Illicit Drug Use and Abuse Starts Earlier Than You Might Think," *Science Daily,* April 2012, http://www.sciencedaily.com/releases/2012/04/120402162601.htm.

xvi *more than twenty million people:* Substance Abuse and Mental Health Services Administration, *Results from the 2011 National Survey on Drug Use and Health: Summary of National Findings,* NSDUH Series H-44, HHS Publication No. (SMA) 12-4713 (Rockville, MD: Substance Abuse and Mental Health Services Administration, 2012). The number is 20.6 million. Per the study, "Of these, 2.6 million were classified with dependence or abuse of both alcohol and illicit drugs, 3.9 million had dependence or abuse of illicit drugs but not alcohol, and 14.1 million had dependence or abuse of alcohol but not illicit drugs."

doubling of drug-related deaths: Lisa Girion, Scott Glover, and Doug Smith, "Drug Deaths Now Outnumber Traffic Fatalities in U.S., Data Shows," *Los Angeles Times,* September 17, 2011; National Institute on Drug Abuse, "Medical Consequences of Drug Abuse," http://www.drugabuse.gov/related-topics/medical-consequences-drug-abuse, last accessed October 2012.

365 Americans: National Center on Addiction and Substance Abuse at Columbia University (CASA), "Addiction Medicine: Closing the Gap Between Science and Practice," June 2012.

Approximately 135,000 deaths: Ibid.

xvi *septicemia, and on and on:* If cigarettes were included, the number would be 560,000 deaths a year; CASA, "Addiction Medicine: Closing the Gap."

Approximately one in twelve: The number hovers around 10 percent. In 2012, it was one in twelve — 20.6 million out of 253 million people. Substance Abuse and Mental Health Services Administration, *Results from the 2010 National Survey on Drug Use and Health: Summary of National Findings*, NSDUH Series H-41, HHS Publication No. (SMA) 11-4658 (Rockville, MD: Substance Abuse and Mental Health Services Administration, 2011).

Addiction is more prevalent: According to the American Cancer Society's "Cancer Basics," in 2008, twelve million people were diagnosed with cancer. Americans have fewer than a million strokes a year, and slightly more than a million Americans have HIV, according to the Centers for Disease Control. The Alzheimer's Association reported in 2012 that 5.4 million Americans had Alzheimer's disease.

ER visits: Drug Abuse Warning Network, "The Dawn Report," revised May 2011. Available at http://www.drugabuse.gov/publications/drugfacts/drug-related-hospital-emergency-room-visits references.

In 2010, 85 percent: of the 2.3 million inmates in U.S. prisons, 65 percent meet the criteria for substance abuse dependence and addiction. Another 20 percent were under the influence at the time of their offense, stole money to buy drugs, violated drug laws, etc. National Center on Addiction and Substance Abuse, "Behind Bars II: Substance Abuse and America's Prison Population," February 2010, http://www.casacolumbia.org/articlefiles/575-report2010behindbars2.pdf.

xvii *Almost 80 percent:* CASA, "Addiction Medicine: Closing the Gap." A child who is arrested three or more times is five and a half times more likely than others to have an addiction. Of the 10- to 17-year-olds in the U.S. juvenile justice system, 78.4 percent are "substance involved."

From one-half to three-quarters: Ibid.

At least 60 percent of homeless people: National Coalition for the Homeless, "Substance Abuse and Homelessness," July 2009, http://www.nationalhomeless.org/factsheets/addiction.html.

$400 billion a year: "What Are the Costs of Drug Abuse to Society?," DrugAbuse.gov, http://archives.drugabuse.gov/NIDA_Notes/NNVol19N2/Tearoff.html; Center for Behavioral Health Statistics and Quality, "2010 National Survey on Drug Use," detailed tables; Office of National Drug Control Policy, "The Economic Costs of Drug Abuse in the United States, 1992–2002," available at www.ncjrs.gov/ondcppubs/publications/pdf/economic_costs.pdf; National Drug Intelligence Center, "The Economic Impact of Illicit Drug Use on American Society," http://www.justice.gov/archive/ndic/pubs44/44731/44731p.pdf; J. Rehm et al., "Global Burden of Disease and Injury and Economic Cost Attributable to Alcohol Use and Alcohol-Use Disorders," *Lancet* 373 (2009): 2223–33. Illicit drug use alone costs the United States almost $200 billion a year.

In this competition: In 2012, the American Society of Interventional Pain Physicians reported that the U.S. consumes 80 percent of the world's opiate painkillers. The U.S. placed first out of seventeen countries in a World Health Organization survey of illegal drug use. The survey showed that Americans were four times more likely to have used cocaine than citizens of the next closest country. The U.S. was number one for pot smoking, at 41 percent. China had a negligible .03 percent, Japan 1.5 percent, and Germany 17.5 percent. And the future is grim too: American teenagers also lead the world's teenagers in drug use. According to a recent University of Michigan Monitoring the Future study, the U.S. ranks first in the proportion of students using hallucinogens, ecstasy, amphetamines. Only France and Monaco had higher rates of marijuana use, at 24 percent and 21 percent, respectively. The average across all the European countries was 7 percent, or less than half the rate of the U.S. See European Monitoring Centre for Drugs and Drug Addiction EMCDDA 2012 Country Overviews, http://www.emcdda.europa.eu/; "Greg Laden, "Stoned Nation: International Study of Drug Use Places US in the Lead," *ScienceBlogs,* June 30, 2008, http://scienceblogs .com/gregladen/2008/06/30/stoned-nation-international-st/.

"We knew K.": Unless I have explicit permission, I don't use the names of those I've corresponded with.

xx   *more than $1 trillion:* I'm using a conservative figure. The estimates range from $1 trillion to $2½ trillion; the sum depends on what's tallied. The low-end number is frequently quoted. It's based on an average of $25 billion a year spent for forty years. (The 2013 National Drug Control Budget is $25.6.) However, this number accounts for federal spending only, and it does not take into account secondary and tertiary costs of the War on Drugs. A high-end figure of $ 2½ trillion, which includes criminal justice and other costs, was reported in *Time* magazine (Claire Suddath, "The War on Drugs," *Time,* March 25, 2009).

1. THIS IS YOUR BRAIN ON DRUGS

11   *"kissing the creator":* http://www.drugs-forum.com/forum/showthread.php?t=1233# ixzzlaj6AAzWD.

2. THIS IS OUR COUNTRY ON DRUGS

12   *seven million people a year:* Substance Abuse and Mental Health Services Administration, *Results from the 2010 National Survey on Drug Use and Health: Summary of National Findings,* NSDUH Series H-41, HHS Publication No. (SMA) 11-4658 (Rockville, MD: Substance Abuse and Mental Health Services Administration, 2011).

Lifetime marijuana use: Partnership at DrugFree.org, "2011 Partnership Attitude Tracking Study," May 2, 2012, http://www.drugfree.org/tag/partnership-attitude -tracking-study.

Daily marijuana use: L. D. Johnston et al., *Monitoring the Future: National Survey Results on Drug Use, 1975–2011: Volume II, College Students and Adults Ages 19–50* (Ann Arbor: Institute for Social Research, University of Michigan, 2012).

More than 40 percent: Substance Abuse and Mental Health Services Administration, *Results from the 2010 National Survey.*

Binge drinking is defined: Ibid.

More people died from overdoses: Centers for Disease Control, "Vital Signs Report," July 2012, http://www.cdc.gov/vitalsigns/.

median age of initial drug use: "Teen Alcohol and Illicit Drug Use and Abuse Starts Earlier Than You Might Think," *Science Daily,* April 2, 2012, http://www.sciencedaily .com/releases/2012/04/120402162601.htm.

before the age of eighteen: National Center on Addiction and Substance Abuse (CASA), "Adolescent Substance Abuse: America's #1 Public Health Problem," June 2011, http:// www.casacolumbia.org/upload/2011/20110629adolescentsubstanceuse.pdf.

13   *"a growing belief":* Partnership for a Drug-Free America, "2009 Partnership Atti-

tude Tracking Study," released March 2, 2010, http://www.drugfree.org/wp-content/uploads/2011/04/FULL-REPORT-PATS-2009-3-2-10.pdf.

a precipitous drop: Ibid.

expect that their children will try: National Center on Addiction and Substance Abuse at Columbia University, *National Survey of American Attitudes on Substance Abuse XII: Teens and Parents,* August 2007, www.google.com/url?sa=t&rct=j&q=&esrc=s&source=web&cd=1&ved=0CCIQFjAA&url=http%3A%2F%2Fwww.casacolumbia.org%2Fdownload.aspx%3Fpath%3D%2FUploadedFiles%2Fvilf5lvw.pdf&ei=ZQuAUMnjL8PU0gHH_4HIDA&usg=AFQjCNG55WKPN5BMDCBpdMxTWPA4ZpoQqg&sig2.

14 *"full-fledged junkies, addicted to pills, or tweakers":* Junkies are heroin addicts. Tweakers are addicted to methamphetamine.

15 *Ninety percent of people who need help:* According to the National Survey on Drug Use and Health, in 2007, 23.2 million people (9.4 percent of the U.S. population) twelve and older needed treatment for drug problems. Almost 21 million of them, or 10 percent (8.4 percent of the population twelve and older), didn't get it.

17 *relapse within the first year:* A. Thomas McLellan et al., "Drug Dependence, a Chronic Medical Illness: Implications for Treatment, Insurance, and Outcomes Evaluation," *Journal of the American Medical Association* 284 (2000): 1689–95; H. Xie et al., "The 10-Year Course of Remission, Abstinence, and Recovery in Dual Diagnosis," *Journal of Substance Abuse Treatment* 39 (2010): 132–40.

"Seventy to eighty percent drop out": Quoted in Sharon Waxman, "Stars Check In, Stars Check Out," *New York Times,* June 17, 2007.

18 *"My makeup wasn't smeared":* Kati Marton, *Hidden Power: Presidential Marriages That Shaped Our Recent History* (New York: G. K. Hall and Company, 2002), 211.

"stupid," "weak": Hazelden Foundation, *Results from the Fall 2008 National Study of Public Attitudes Toward Addiction* (Center City, MN: Center for Public Advocacy, 2008), www.hazelden.org/web/public/.../2008publicsurvey.pdf.

"a total abdication of reason": Peg O'Connor, "In the Cave: Philosophy and Addiction," *New York Times,* January 2, 2012.

19 *In 2006, alcohol and other drugs:* National Center on Addiction and Substance Abuse at Columbia University, "Behind Bars II: Substance Abuse and America's Prison Population," February 2010, http://www.casacolumbia.org/articlefiles/575-report2010behindbars2.pdf.

One-third of the songs: Brian A. Primack et al., "Content Analysis of Tobacco, Alcohol, and Other Drugs in Popular Music," *Archives of Pediatric and Adolescent Medicine* 162 (2008): 169–75.

20 *"The average adolescent is exposed":* Tara Parker-Pope, "Under the Influence of . . . Music?" *New York Times* blog *Well,* February 5, 2008.

A study of sixteen thousand teenagers: Reiner Hanewinkel et al., "Alcohol Consumption in Movies and Adolescent Binge Drinking in 6 European Countries," *Pediatrics,* March 5, 2012, doi: 10.1542/peds.2011-2809.

"nothing but voluntary madness": The Roman philosopher Lucius Annaeus Seneca said this in the first century; see Robert Andrews, *The Concise Columbia Dictionary of Quotations* (New York: Columbia University Press, 1989).

21 *"Muslims and Mormons":* Malcolm Gladwell, "Drinking Games," *New Yorker,* February 15, 2010.

"alcohol seemed to exacerbate": David F. Musto and Eric D. Wish, "Historical Perspectives," in *Lowinson and Ruiz's Substance Abuse: A Comprehensive Textbook*, eds. Pedro Ruiz and Eric C. Strain, 5th ed. (Philadelphia: Lippincott Williams and Wilkins, 2011). *"the magical drug"*: David Bakan, *Sigmund Freud and the Jewish Mystical Tradition* (Mineola, NY: Dover Publications, 2004).

22 *"bohemians, gamblers"*: Paul Vallely, "Drug That Spans the Ages: The History of Cocaine," *Independent*, March 2, 2006.
"medieval plagues": Maia Szalavitz, "Cracked Up," Salon.com, May 11, 1999.
Fallu concluded: Jean-Sébastien Fallu et al., "The Influence of Close Friends on Adolescent Substance Use: Does Popularity Matter?," in A. Ittel et al., eds., *Jahrbuch Jugendforschung* (Wiesbaden: VS Verlag, 2011).

23 *"The media function as a kind of 'super-peer'"*: http://books.google.com/books/about /Children_adolescents_and_the_media.html?id=wpooAAAAYAAJ.

24 *trouble getting insurance:* Addicts told me they were unable to get health insurance, and some tried but were unable to get life insurance.

3. EVERYBODY DOES IT

29 *"I had never smoked pot"*: Seth Mnookin, "Harvard and Heroin," Salon.com, August 27, 1999.
"The presence of peers": Tara Parker-Pope, "Teenagers, Friends and Bad Decisions," *New York Times* blog *Well*, February 3, 2011.

32 *Most parents assumed:* Partnership for a Drug-Free America, 2007 Partnership Attitude Tracking Study, http://www.drugfree.org/wp-content/uploads/2011/04/PATS -Teens-2007-Full-Report.pdf.

33 *a study conducted across Europe:* "Young People Are Intentionally Drinking and Taking Drugs for Better Sex, European Survey Finds," *ScienceDaily*, May 9, 2008, http:// www.sciencedaily.com/releases/2008/05/080508222420.htm.

36 *People living below the poverty line:* Beau Kilmer and Rosalie Liccardo Pacula, "Preventing Drug Use," in *Targeting Investments in Children: Fighting Poverty When Resources are Limited*, eds. Phillip B. Levine and David J. Zimmerman (Chicago: University of Chicago Press, 2010), 181–220.

37 *number one cause of poverty:* NPR/Kaiser/Kennedy School Poll, "Poverty in America," 2001, http://www.npr.org/programs/specials/poll/poverty/staticresults.html.
the greatest need for addiction treatment: http://www.samhsa.gov/data/2k10/173/ 173poverty.htm.
Overall, of the alcoholics studied: Ming-Chyi Huang et al., "Impact of Multiple Types of Childhood Trauma Exposure on Risk of Psychiatric Comorbidity Among Alcoholic Inpatients," *Alcoholism: Clinical and Experimental Research* 36 (2012): 598–606.
"Addiction is always an attempt": In his book *In the Realm of Hungry Ghosts*, Gabor says that all addictions are related to trauma, including behavioral addictions such as gambling and sex; see Gabor Maté, *In The Realm of Hungry Ghosts: Close Encounters with Addiction* (Berkeley, CA: North Atlantic Books, 2010).

38 *"teenagers in single-parent households"*: Tara Parker-Pope, "Marijuana Use in High School," *New York Times* blog *Well*, March 10, 2011.
"Divorce can be deceptive": Barbara Dafoe Whitehead, "Dan Quayle Was Right," *Atlantic*, April 1993.

teens with divorced parents: http://rehabcenters.com/resources/effects-of-divorce-on
-teen-drug-use/.

39 *If one parent is a heavy drinker:* Melanie Chalder et al., "Drinking and Motivations to
Drink Among Adolescent Children of Parents with Alcohol Problems," *Alcohol and
Alcoholism* 41 (2006): 107–13.
children of alcoholics: American Academy of Child and Adolescent Psychiatry, "Facts
for Families: Children of Alcoholics," December 2011, http://www.aacap.org/cs/root/
facts_for_families/facts_for_families.
respond to stress by drinking: "Stress Drives Alcoholics' Children to Drink, Study Suggests," *Science Daily,* September 24, 2011, http://www.sciencedaily.com/releases/2011/
09/110920075518.htm.

40 *studies of twins:* Dr. Volkow explained, "When you study identical twins (who have
the exact genetic background but more or less different life experiences) a researcher
can ask: what is the likelihood that, if one brother or sister becomes addicted to a psychoactive substance, the other brother or sister will also be affected? If genes were the
only determinant risk factor, one would expect a 100% concordance. But in fact, the
concordance in substance use disorders among identical twins is much lower, closer
to about 50%, which shows that many other, non-genetic factors (like socioeconomic
status, deviant peers, drug availability) also play important contributing roles in substance abuse and addiction."

41 *"Academic failure":* National Center on Addiction and Substance Abuse at Columbia University, "Substance Abuse and Learning Disabilities," September 2000, http://
www.google.com/url?sa=t&rct=j&q=&esrc=s&source=web&cd=2&ved=0CCoQFjA
B&url=http%3A%2F%2Fwww.casacolumbia.org%2Fdownload.aspx%3Fpath%3D%
2FUploadedFiles%2Fzgayicmc.pdf&ei=aB-AUL6uAoH68gSstIDIDg&usg=AFQjCN
FartQdYOQwEIWO5Qbb4Jvhx5lthQ&sig.
"seeming like they don't care": Kyle Redford is a friend of the author.
kids with ADHD: Sophie Terbush, "Kids with ADHD More Likely to Use Drugs,
Analysis Finds," *USA Today,* April 24, 2011; Steve Lee et al., "Prospective Association of Childhood Attention-Deficit/Hyperactivity Disorder (ADHD) and Substance
Use and Abuse/Dependence: A Meta-analytic Review," *Clinical Psychology Review* 31
(2011): 328–41.
mental-health problems: Substance Abuse and Mental Health Services Administration, *Results from the 2010 National Survey on Drug Use and Health: Summary of
National Findings,* NSDUH Series H-41, HHS Publication No. (SMA) 11-4658 (Rockville, MD: Substance Abuse and Mental Health Services Administration, 2011.
Anxiety disorders: National Institute of Mental Health, "The Numbers Count: Mental
Disorders in America," http://www.nimh.nih.gov/health/publications/the-numbers
-count-mental-disorders-in-america/index.shtml; last reviewed October 12, 2012.
affected by depression: Centers for Disease Control and Prevention, "An Estimated 1
in 10 U.S. Adults Report Depression," http://www.cdc.gov/features/dsdepression/, last
updated March 31, 2011.

42 *an estimated two million kids:* Substance Abuse and Mental Health Services Administration, *Results from the 2010 National Survey.*
anxiety or mood disorder: "Understanding the Facts: Substance Abuse," Anxiety and
Depression Association of America, 2010–2012, http://www.adaa.org/about-adaa/
press-room/facts-statistics.
conditions such as schizophrenia: Theresa H. M. Moore et al., "Cannabis Use and Risk

of Psychotic or Affective Mental Health Outcomes: A Systematic Review," *Lancet* 370 (2007): 319–28.

4. HELPING KIDS GROW UP

44 *"little influence"*: Partnership for a Drug-Free America, "2007 Partnership Attitude Tracking Study," released June 11, 2008, http://www.drugfree.org/wp-content/uploads/2011/04/PATS-parents-2007-Full-Report-FINAL.pdf.

45 *nine out of ten people who become addicted:* National Center on Addiction and Substance Abuse (CASA), "Adolescent Substance Abuse: America's #1 Public Health Problem," June 2011, http://www.casacolumbia.org/templates/NewsRoom.aspx?articleid=631&zoneid=51.

"Even if the onset of psychosis were inevitable": David Freeman, "Psychosis Triggered by Smoking Pot? Marijuana Study Says Yes," CBS News, February 8, 2011. Even marijuana alone has been shown to turn on mental illnesses in some adolescents. A study by Dr. Large showed that people over eighteen who had used marijuana had twice the risk of mental illness as the general population, but kids under fifteen had five times the risk.

48 *California Nurse-Family Partnership branch:* The national office of the Nurse-Family Partnership arranged for me to spend an afternoon with a nurse in California. I agreed to use pseudonyms for all participants and to obscure the location.

52 *those who've gone through the program:* David L. Olds, "Prenatal and Infancy Home Visiting by Nurses: From Randomized Trials to Community Replication," *Prevention Science* 3 (2002): 153–72; D. L. Olds et al., "Long-Term Effects of Home Visitation on Maternal Life Course and Child Abuse and Neglect: Fifteen-Year Follow-Up of a Randomized Trial," *Journal of the American Medical Association* 278 (1997): 637–43; David Olds et al., "Enduring Effects of Prenatal and Infancy Home Visiting by Nurses on Children," *Archives of Pediatric and Adolescent Med* 164 (2010): 412–18.

"Preventing Drug Abuse Among Children and Adolescents": http://www.drugabuse.gov/sites/default/files/redbook_0.pdf.

53 *dinner with their families:* National Center on Addiction and Substance Abuse, "The Importance of Family Dinners VII," released September 2011.

54 *helped the kids with their homework:* Substance Abuse and Mental Health Services Administration, *Results from the 2010 National Survey on Drug Use and Health: Summary of National Findings*, NSDUH Series H-41, HHS Publication No. (SMA) 11-4658 (Rockville, MD: Substance Abuse and Mental Health Services Administration, 2011).

56 *"parental disapproval of substance use"*: National Center on Addiction and Substance Abuse, "Adolescent Substance Abuse."

57 *three to ten times more THC:* Jeanne Meserve and Mike M. Ahlers., "Marijuana Potency Surpasses 10 Percent, U.S. says," CNN.com, May 14, 2009, http://edition.cnn.com/2009/HEALTH/05/14/marijuana.potency/.

58 *"Drugs shield children"*: Robert Schwebel, *Saying No Is Not Enough* (New York: New Market Press, 1998).

if their parents told them honestly: http://www.hazelden.org/web/public/four_generations_overcoming_addiction.page.

59 *Meditation, yoga, journaling:* Some other strategies are listed on the Mayo Clinic website: http://www.mayoclinic.com/health/relaxation-technique/SR00007.

increased flow of dopamine: Panayotis K. Thanos et al., "Chronic Forced Exercise During Adolescence Decreases Cocaine Conditioned Place Preference in Lewis Rats," *Behavioral Brain Research* 215 (2010): 77–82.

who reported exercising daily: Karen McNulty Walsh, "New Findings Imply Exercise in Adolescence May Help Prevent Drug Abuse," *Brookhaven National Laboratory News,* August 4, 2010. There are many theories about why exercise helps. It may stimulate a reward pathway in the brain that leaves people less responsive to drugs. It may lower drug use because exercise acts as a mild antidepressant and relieves stress. Another theory is that people who get natural highs — endorphin rushes — from exercise may be less interested in alternative highs. Still another theory holds that exercise improves the way the brain processes dopamine. All that said, it's obvious that exercise isn't enough protection for many people; there are countless examples of athletes succumbing to drugs.

62 *most U.S. middle schools:* Chris Ringwalt et al., "The Prevalence of Evidence-Based Drug Use Prevention Curricula in U.S. Middle Schools in 2008," *Prevention Science* 12 (2011): 63–69.

DARE not only doesn't lower drug use: Numerous studies have shown this. The U.S. General Accounting Office, the National Academy of Sciences, and the National Institutes of Health have all released reports about the ineffectiveness of DARE. The U.S. Department of Education prohibits schools from spending federal money on DARE.

the DARE website: http://www.dare.com/home/about_dare.asp.

66 *Life Skills Training does have significant:* "Long-Term Effectiveness of School-Based Drug Prevention Programs Prove Successful." *Addiction Treatment,* May 25, 2012, http://www.addictiontreatmentmagazine.com/addiction-news/school-drug-prevention -programs/.

69 *4-H Clubs:* Richard Lerner et al., "The Positive Development of Youth: Report of the Findings of the First Eight Years of the 4-H Study of Positive Youth Development," Institute for Applied Research in Youth Development, Tufts University, 2012.

70 *study of Communities That Care:* J. David Hawkins et al., "Results of a Type 2 Translational Research Trial to Prevent Adolescent Drug Use and Delinquency: A Test of Communities That Care," *Archives of Pediatrics and Adolescent Medicine* 163 (2009): 789–98.

the ads had made it more *likely:* Ryan Grim, "A White House Drug Deal Gone Bad," Slate.com, September 7, 2006, http://www.slate.com/articles/health_and_science/science/2006/09/a_white_house_drug_deal_gone_bad.html.

"may have promoted perceptions": U.S. Government Accountability Office, "Contractor's National Evaluation Did Not Find that the Youth Anti-Drug Media Campaign Was Effective in Reducing Youth Drug Use," August 25, 2006, http://www.gao.gov/products/GAO-06-818.

72 *Truth Campaign ads:* Kevin C. Davis et al., "The Impact of National Smoking Prevention Campaigns on Tobacco-Related Beliefs, Intentions to Smoke and Smoking Initiation: Results from a Longitudinal Survey of Youth in the United States," *International Journal of Environmental Research and Public Health* 6 (2009): 722–40.

Slater's research into Above the Influence: Michael D. Slater, "Assessing Media Campaigns Linking Marijuana Non-Use with Autonomy and Aspirations: 'Be Under Your own Influence' and ONDCP's 'Above the Influence,'" *Prevention Science* 12 (2011): 12–22.

In 2001, a Partnership ad campaign: See "Brief History," http://www.drugfree.org/brief-history.

annual media budget: Andrew McMains, "Anti-Drug Campaign Takes Funding Hit," *Adweek,* December 21, 2011.

5. USE BECOMES ABUSE, AND ABUSE BECOMES ADDICTION

77 *as it did for Ian Sullivan:* Sullivan is a pseudonym. He requested that one be used because of his "professional, social, and family circumstances."

80 *"poses a huge problem":* Maia Szalavitz, "*DSM-5* Could Categorize 40% of College Students as Alcoholics," Time.com, May 14, 2012.

"we can treat them earlier": Ian Urbina, "Addiction Diagnosis May Rise Under Guideline Changes," *New York Times,* May 11, 2012.

81 *more than 13,000 babies:* "About 3.4 of every 1,000 infants born in a hospital in 2009 suffered from a type of drug withdrawal commonly seen in the babies of pregnant women who abuse narcotic pain medications," according to a study published in the *Journal of the American Medical Association* (Liz Szabo, "Number of Painkiller-Addicted Newborns Triples in 10 Years," *USA Today,* May 1, 2012).

82 *More than 60 percent of those who try heroin:* National Epidemiological Survey on Alcohol and Related Conditions (NESARC), U.S. Department of Health and Human Services, December 2006.

Kids who are abusing: "How to Spot Drug and Alcohol Use: Is Your Teen Using? Signs and Symptoms of Substance Abuse," Parent Toolkit, Partnership at Drugfree.org.

84 *the efficacy of testing:* There's a debate about the effectiveness of testing in schools. A study published in 2007 in the *Journal of Adolescent Health* found that student athletes who participated in randomized drug testing had overall rates of drug use similar to students who didn't take part in the program; see Linn Goldberg et al., "Outcomes of a Prospective Trial of Student-Athlete Drug Testing: The Student Athlete Testing Using Random Notification (SATURN) Study," *Journal of Adolescent Health* 41 (2007): 421–29. Other studies have shown moderately lower rates of use. Testing in schools is complicated, however. "Just as it's hard for parents to get it right," Dr. Sharon Levy points out, "it's hard for schools to get it right." Workplace drug testing is controversial too. It's been shown to be an effective deterrent in some professions. A study showed that drug testing truck drivers resulted in a 9 to 10 percent reduction in accident fatalities. Another study of construction companies by Cornell University showed that after implementing drug testing, companies had a 51 percent reduction in injury rates. Airline pilots, routinely drug tested, have low rates of use that may or may not be related to the fact that they know they'll be tested, and stoned pilots are automatically grounded.

85 *NIDAMED, at the NIDA website:* http://www.drugabuse.gov/nmassist/.

86 *SBIRT can be "remarkably effective":* Bertha K. Madreas et al., "Screening, Brief Interventions, Referral to Treatment (SBIRT) for Illicit Drug and Alcohol Use at Multiple Healthcare Sites: Comparison at Intake and 6 Months Later," *Drug and Alcohol Dependence* 99 (2009): 280–95.

"No one knew": Anna David, executive editor of TheFix.com, was interviewed by Nic Sheff, my son. Nic knows David from his job writing a column for that webzine.

6. ADDICTS AREN'T WEAK, SELFISH, OR AMORAL — THEY'RE ILL

91 *the brains of binge drinkers:* Michelle Trudeau, "Teen Drinking May Cause Irreversible Brain Damage," NPR, January 25, 2010.

"Taken together, the studies suggest": "Young Addicts 'Risk Damage Similar to Alzheimer's,'" *Scotsman,* June 22, 2005.

meth causes structural changes: Stephen Kish, a researcher at the University of Toronto's Medical Center, is one of the scientists who discovered neurologic damage in the brains of meth users.

93 *"We know the myelin sheath":* John Burnett, "What If Marijuana Were Legal? Possible Outcomes," NPR, April 20, 2009.

95 *fifty cocaine addicts and their siblings:* Karen D. Ersche et al., "Abnormal Brain Structure Implicated in Stimulant Drug Addiction," *Science* 335 (2012): 601–4.

brain scans showed that both siblings: Jon Hamilton, "Addicts' Brains May Be Wired at Birth for Less Self-Control." National Public Radio, February 3, 2012.

96 *studies of adopted children:* Kenneth Kendler et al., "Genetic and Familial Environmental Influences on the Risk for Drug Abuse," *Archives of General Psychiatry* 69 (July 2012): 690–97.

"Some people have a genetic predisposition": Michael Lemonick, "How We Get Addicted," *Time,* July 5, 2007.

97 *"These allergic types":* Alcoholics Anonymous, Big Book Online, http://www.aa.org/bigbookonline/.

101 *very small fraction actually quit on their own:* Alan I. Leshner, "Exploring Myths About Drug Abuse," http://archives.drugabuse.gov/Published_Articles/Myths.html.

102 *"It's a brain problem":* Alexis Geier Horan, "ASAM Releases New Definition of Addiction," American Society of Addiction Medicine, August 15, 2011.

7. DON'T DENY ADDICTION, DON'T ENABLE IT, AND DON'T WAIT FOR AN ADDICT TO HIT BOTTOM — HE COULD DIE

105 *The Alcoholics Anonymous Twelve Steps:* Bill Wilson, *Twelve Steps and Twelve Traditions* (New York: Alcoholics Anonymous Publishing Inc., 1953).

109 *"Who isn't?":* Wendy Kaminer, "Chances Are You're Codependent Too," *New York Times Book Review,* February 11, 1990.

8. INTERVENTION

114 *Joan and Richard Laurel:* The Laurels asked that all names and identifying features in their story be changed.

121 *Maia Szalavitz cited a 1999 study:* Maia Szalavitz, "When the Cure Is Not Worth the Cost," *New York Times,* April 11, 2007.

122 *get kickbacks from interventionists:* I've been told about interventionists receiving kickbacks, but I've also heard about doctors, therapists, counselors, and sober-living house directors receiving kickbacks from programs they refer to. "It's rife," said Joe Schrank, the owner of Loft 107, a sober-living house in Brooklyn. Schrank said,

"Since we don't play that game, I don't get any big checks at the end of the year like some people do. At the most I may get a box of pears and a [Christmas] card."

9. FINDING TREATMENT

129 *Brian Mendell:* Brian Mendell's story was reported by his father, Gary Mendell, in a series of tape-recorded interviews. Gary supplied copies of medical records, e-mails, letters, and other documentation. I also interviewed Greg Mendell, Brian's brother.

135 *"I've made a very close personal analysis":* William C. Moyers, "Crusader to Critic," *Beyond Addiction,* July 3, 2012, http://www.hazelden.org/web/public/100703ba.page? printable=true&showlogo=true&callprint=true .

137 *only 6 percent of primary care physicians:* National Center on Addiction and Substance Abuse, "Missed Opportunity: The CASA National Survey of Primary Care Physicians and Patients on Substance Abuse," April 2000, www.casacolumbia.org.

138 *evidence indicating that a physician has adequate training:* American Society of Addiction Medicine, "How to Identify a Physician Recognized for Expertness in the Diagnosis and Treatment of Addiction and Substance-related Health Conditions," http://www.asam.org/advocacy/find-a-policy-statement/view-policy-statement/public-policy-statements/2011/12/16/how-to-identify-a-physician-recognized-for-expertness-in-the-diagnosis-and-treatment-of-addiction-and-substance-related-health-conditions; last reviewed January 15, 2010.
     ASAM maintains a list: The ASAM website is at www.asam.org. Click on "Find a Physician Near You."
     ABAM website: http://www.abam.net/find-a-doctor.
     I wrote about her daughter Ashley: Roberta and Ashley Lojak's story appeared in the book *Addiction: Why Can't They Just Stop.* I interviewed Roberta for the book that accompanied the HBO documentary series.

139 *Medicaid and Medicare coverage:* "Eliminating Disparities in Medicare and Medicaid for Addiction Treatment," *American Society of Addiction Medicine:* April 2004. Web.

10. DETOX

142 *"abstain . . . suddenly and entirely":* Benjamin Rush, *Medical Inquiries and Observations* (Philadelphia: Johnson and Warner, 1809).

11. BEGINNING TREATMENT

152 *histories of suicidal thoughts or attempts:* P. A. Harrison and S. E. Asche, "Comparison of Substance Abuse Treatment Outcomes for Inpatients and Outpatients," *Journal of Substance Abuse Treatment* 17 (1999): 207–20.
     "somewhat" better outcomes: R. H. Moos, J. W. Finney, and B. S. Moos, "Inpatient Substance Abuse Care and the Outcome of Subsequent Community Residential and Outpatient Care," *Addiction* 95 (2000): 833–46.

153 *"outpatients, regardless of level of psychiatric severity":* H. M. Pettinati et al., "Inpatient

vs. Outpatient Treatment for Substance Dependence Revisited," *Psychiatry Quarterly* 64 (1993): 173–82.

156 *After ninety days, however:* National Institute on Drug Abuse, "Drug Abuse Treatment Outcome Studies," March 2008, http://www.drugabuse.gov/.
Yale University researchers concluded: Michael A. Lemonick, "How We Get Addicted," *Time,* July 5, 2007.

157 *A SAMHSA website has three types of directories:* http://www.dpt.samhsa.gov/ treatment/treatmentindex.aspx.
$34 billion industry: Catherine New. "The Real Tab for Rehab: Inside the Addiction Treatment Biz," *Daily Finance,* June 3, 2011.
"the most trustworthy accreditation": http://www.carf.org/advancedProviderSearch .aspx; http://www.qualitycheck.org/consumer/searchQCR.aspx.

159 *National Registry of Evidence-Based Programs and Practices:* http://www.nrepp .samhsa.gov/.

162 *Another on the list of ASAM guidelines:* American Society of Addiction Medicine, "How to Identify a Physician Recognized for Expertness in the Diagnosis and Treatment of Addiction and Substance-related Health Conditions," http://www.asam.org/ advocacy/find-a-policy-statement/view-policy-statement/public-policy-statements/ 2011/12/16/how-to-identify-a-physician-recognized-for-expertness-in-the-diagnosis -and-treatment-of-addiction-and-substance-related-health-conditions; last reviewed January 15, 2010.

162 *in California there's actually a statute:* http://sooo.senate.ca.gov/sites/sooo.senate .ca.gov/files/Rogue%20Rehab%209_4_12.pdf.

163 *"employing tactics of intimidation and humiliation":* National Mental Health Association, "Mental Health Treatment for Youth in the Juvenile Justice System," 2004, https://www.nttac.org/views/docs/jabg/mhcurriculum/mh_mht.pdf.
"not only ineffective, but harmful": Bruce Selcraig, "Camp Fear," *Mother Jones* (November/December 2000).

164 *When visiting one rehab:* This event occurred at a rehab I was allowed to enter only under the condition that I didn't reveal its location or its therapists' and patients' names. I've received numerous letters from addicts and family members who describe similar occurrences.

165 *kicked out of Promises:* Paul Pringle, "The Trouble with Rehab, Malibu Style," *Los Angeles Times,* October 9, 2007.

167 *average cost of a day in a hospital:* http://www.beckershospitalreview.com/lists/average-cost-per-inpatient-day-across-50-states-in-2010.html.
For cancer patients: http://www.hcup-us.ahrq.gov/reports/statbriefs/sb125.jsp.
There are online directories: www.clinicaltrials.gov.

12. PRIMARY TREATMENT

180 *I'll call her Ruth:* I was asked to use pseudonyms for Matrix's therapist and clients.

187 *patients who earned vouchers:* Alan J. Budney et al., "Adding Voucher-Based Incentives to Coping Skills and Motivational Enhancement Improves Outcomes During Treatment for Marijuana Dependence," *Journal of Consulting and Clinical Psychology* 68 (2000): 1051–61.

194 *"Anyone who is instrumental":* Center for Substance Abuse Treatment, "Substance

Abuse Treatment and Family Therapy: A Treatment Improvement Protocol," 2004, http://www.ncbi.nlm.nih.gov/books/NBK64265/.

13. TREATING DRUG PROBLEMS WITH DRUGS

198 *fastest-growing category of abused substances:* Office of National Drug Control Policy, "Epidemic: Responding to America's Prescription Drug Abuse Crisis," 2011, http://www.whitehouse.gov/sites/default/files/ondcp/policy-and-research/rx_abuse_plan.pdf.

201 *group's therapist, Kenneth:* Once again, the participants in this therapy group aren't called by their real names.

204 *Suboxone at Hazelden:* Maia Szalavitz. "Hazelden Introduces Antiaddiction Medications into Recovery for First Time," *Time,* Nov 5, 2012, http://healthland.time.com/2012/11/05/hazelden-introduces-antiaddiction-medications-in-recovery-for-first-time/.

205 *"Anonymous1234":* http://www.prescriptiondrug-info.com/Discuss/Difference-between-Suboxne-and-methadone-189168.htm.

14. WHERE DOES AA FIT IN?

207 *"In the wake of my spiritual experience":* Beverly Conyers, *Everything Changes: Help for Families of Newly Recovering Addicts* (Center City, MN: Hazelden Publishing, 2009).

208 *"It seemed to me, in the mind's eye":* Brendan I. Koerner, "Secret of AA: After 75 Years, We Don't Know How It Works," *Wired,* June 23, 2010.

209 *members shared stories:* Christopher Cavanaugh, *AA to Z: An Addictionary of the 12-Step Culture* (New York: Random House, 1998).

210 *"Some 1.2 million people":* Koerner, "Secret of AA."

"I believe, along with many other people": David Sheff, "Interview: M. Scott Peck," *Playboy* (March 1992): 44.

"After years of despair": Alcoholics Anonymous, "This Is A.A.: An Introduction to the A.A. Recovery Program" (Alcoholics Anonymous World Services Inc., 1984), online at http://www.aa.org/catalog.cfm?origpage=198&product=4.

212 *"I'm Rick and I'm an alcoholic-addict":* In AA meetings, participants identify themselves by first names only. I follow that protocol here.

213 *"'Alcoholics Anonymous is a fellowship'":* Alcoholics Anonymous, "A.A. Preamble" (Alcoholics Anonymous, A.A. Grapevine, Inc., 2002), online at http://www.aa.org/en_pdfs/smf-92_en.pdf.

"'We admitted we were powerless'": Alcoholics Anonymous, "The Twelve Steps and Twelve Traditions," online at http://www.aa.org/1212/.

215 *"If it had been a Christian-based book":* Michelle Boorstein, "AA Original Manuscript Reveals Profound Debate over Religion," *Washington Post,* September 22, 2010.

Wilson emphasized in speeches: Bill Wilson, "National Clergy Conference on Alcoholism," National Catholic Council on Addictions, *Blue Book,* Volume 12, 1960.

"Alcoholics Anonymous is a religious program": Susan Cheever, *My Name Is Bill* (New York: Simon and Schuster, 2005).

217 *"To its credit, AA insists":* Clancy Martin, "The Drunk's Club," *Harper's Magazine* (January 2011): 28–38.

218 *They can take credit:* Blaming the patient is not exclusive to drug-treatment centers.

A study showed that most therapists blame treatment failures on their clients' lack of motivation or commitment rather than on themselves. However, the fact that it's consistent with the broader field of psychology doesn't make it less insidious.

221 *In 2011, Susan Cheever:* Susan Cheever, "The Column That Ignited a National Furor: Is It Time to Take the Anonymous out of A.A.?," TheFix.com, April 7, 2011, http://www.thefix.com/content/breaking-rule-anonymity-aa.

"It seems crazy": David Colman, "Challenging the Second 'A' in A.A.," *New York Times,* May 6, 2011.

222 *"If we slip":* Adi Jaffe, "Is Anonymity the Final Shame Frontier in Addiction?" *Psychology Today,* June 17, 2010.

"That attitude in itself": Daniel Goleman, "Breaking Bad Habits: New Therapy Focuses on the Relapse," *New York Times,* December 27, 1988.

224 *"wrong to deprive any alcoholic":* http://www.aa.org/pdf/products/p-11_aamembersMedDrug.pdf.

225 *"Everyone said the same thing":* Martin, "The Drunk's Club."

227 *sound evidence-based practice:* In the EBT-based Matrix outpatient program in Los Angeles, patients count sober time differently. After a relapse, rather than saying he is one day sober, a patient will say, "Of the past ninety days, I've been sober eighty-nine." "If a person with an addiction problem relapses, it doesn't hold the same sense of defeat and shame," according to Matrix's Jeanne Obert. In Matrix, patients keep calendars on which they place blue dots for sober days and red ones for days they slipped. A calendar filled with blue dots is an accomplishment to be proud of, but one with a few red dots may not seem like a catastrophe. AA's system of rewarding sober time works for some people, but Matrix's model is a sound alternative that saves a relapsing addict from the overwhelming anxiety of going back to square one.

227 *AA's own surveys:* Alcoholics Anonymous, "2011 Membership Survey," Alcoholics Anonymous World Services Inc., 2011.

an internal report: Bankole A. Johnson, "We're Addicted to Rehab; It Doesn't Even Work," *Washington Post,* August 8, 2010.

"merely dabbled": Rudolf H. Moos and Bernice S. Moos, "Participation in Treatment and Alcoholics Anonymous: A 16-Year Follow-up of Initially Untreated Individuals," *Journal of Clinical Psychology* 62 (2006): 735–50.

studies conducted by Marica Ferri: Nicholas Bakalar, "Review Sees No Advantage in 12-Step Programs," *New York Times,* July 25, 2006.

229 *one of the alernatives:* I've heard from people for whom a program called Rational Recovery, an alternative to AA and other Twelve-Step groups, was useful.

230 *40 percent of those who try AA:* Hal Arkowitz and Scott O. Lilienfeld, "Does Alcoholics Anonymous Work?," *Scientific American,* March 29, 2011.

"We do not think": Alcoholics Anonymous, "This Is A.A."

15. TREATING DUAL DIAGNOSIS

242 *"serious" mental illness:* Substance Abuse and Mental Health Services Administration, *Results from the 2010 National Survey on Drug Use and Health: Summary of National Findings,* NSDUH Series H-41, HHS Publication No. (SMA) 11-4658 (Rockville, MD: Substance Abuse and Mental Health Services Administration, 2011).

fifteen million children and teens: American Academy of Child and Adolescent Psychiatry, "AACAP Workforce Fact Sheet," 2010, http://www.aacap.org/cs/root/legislative_action/aacap_workforce_fact_sheet.

have episodes of mental illness: Substance Abuse and Mental Health Services Administration, *Results from the 2010 National Survey.*

46 percent of schizophrenics: Dartmouth-Hitchcock Behavioral Healthcare, Dual Diagnosis Fact Sheet.

50 percent of those with mental disorders: Darrel Regier et al., "Comorbidity of Mental Disorders with Alcohol and Other Drug Abuse," *Journal of the American Medical Association* 264 (1990): 2511–18.

243 *Dr. Volkow at NIDA:* Nora Volkow, "Addiction and Co-Occurring Mental Disorders," National Institutes of Health, February 2007, http://www.drugabuse.gov/news-events/nida-notes/2007/02/addiction-co-occurring-mental-disorders.

244 *relapsed at least once:* H. Xie et al., "The 10-Year Course of Remission, Abstinence, and Recovery in Dual Diagnosis," *Journal of Substance Abuse Treatment* (2010): 132–40.

246 *recommended by psychiatrists and researchers:* My sources cited these programs as of the initial publication of *Clean* in April 2013, and some of their recommendations may no longer be current. As I've written above, patients must consult doctors before choosing any treatment program.

16. RELAPSE PREVENTION

251 *Steven Garfield:* At his request, the names and some details in Steven's story have been changed.

254 *ecstasy at least twenty-five times:* Tamra B. Orr, *Ecstasy* (New York: Rosen Publishing, 2008).

it appeared to be normal: Alan I. Leshner, "Treatment: Effects on the Brain and Body," National Methamphetamine Drug Conference, Office of National Drug Control Policy, https://www.ncjrs.gov/ondcppubs/publications/drugfact/methconf/plenary2.html.

growth in the damaged dopamine receptors: "The Meth Epidemic: How Meth Destroys the Body," *Frontline*; Patrick Zickler, "Methamphetamine Abuse Linked to Impaired Cognitive and Motor Skills Despite Recovery of Dopamine Transporters," *NIDA Notes* (April 2002).

258 *The speaker, Clark:* As always, I have changed the names of participants in the meeting and residents of the program.

261 *Scott and Dennis:* Hazelden.org, "Drs. Michael Dennis and Christy Scott Earn Hazelden's Dan Anderson Research Award," December 12, 2011, http://www.hazelden.org/web/public/dennisscott2011dara.page.

17. THE FUTURE OF PREVENTION AND TREATMENT

275 *"Addiction treatment is largely disconnected":* National Center on Addiction and Substance Abuse at Columbia University, "Addiction Medicine: Closing the Gap Between Science and Practice," June 2012, http://www.casacolumbia.org/templates/PressReleases.aspx?articleid=680&zoneid=95.

12,500 oncologists: http://www.advisory.com/Research/Oncology-Roundtable/Oncology-Rounds/2011/06/Estimating-the-Demand-for-Oncology-Physicians.

20,000 cardiologists: http://www.nejm.org/doi/full/10.1056/NEJMp038201.

"It's not a very good vaccine": Roni Caryn Rabin, "Cocaine Vaccine Is Developed, but It Does Not Keep Users from Wanting the Drug," *New York Times,* October 6, 2009.

278 *Yale researchers:* http://www.yaledailynews.com/news/2011/oct/25/brain-scan-pre dicts-addiction/?print.

"Addiction is a medical condition": Michael D. Lemonick, "How We Get Addicted," *Time,* July 5, 2007.

18. FIGHTING THE RIGHT WAR

284 *"America's public enemy":* Martin A. Lee, *Smoke Signals: A Social History of Marijuana* (New York: Simon and Schuster, 2012).

285 *$25 billion:* Office of National Drug Control Policy, "The National Drug Control Budget: FY 2013 Funding Highlights," http://www.whitehouse.gov/ondcp/ the-national-drug-control-budget-fy-2013-funding-highlights.

U.S. jail and prison population: National Center on Addiction and Substance Abuse at Columbia University, "Behind Bars II: Substance Abuse and America's Prison Population," February 2010, http://www.casacolumbia.org/articlefiles/575-report2010be-hindbars2.pdf.

286 *"This increase":* Veronique de Rugy, "'Prison Math' and the War on Drugs," *National Review,* June 9, 2011.

are parents: See http://bjs.ojp.usdoj.gov/index.cfm?ty=pbdetail&iid=2230 and http:// www.ojp.usdoj.gov/newsroom/pressreleases/2008/bjs08101.htm.

"Although the pain": Patricia Allard and Judith Greene, Justice Strategies, "Children on the Outside: Voicing the Pain and Human Costs of Parental Incarceration: Justice Strategies Report," January 2011, http://www.justicestrategies.org/publications/2011/ children-outside-voicing-pain-and-human-costs-parental-incarceration.

blacks are arrested: Human Rights Watch, "Decades of Disparity: Drug Arrests and Race in the United States," 2009, http://www.countthecosts.org/sites/default/files/ Decades%20of%20Disparity.pdf.

287 *"costs of the drug war":* http://online.wsj.com/article/SB1000142405270230439270457 6377514098776094.html.

"our nation's drug policies": Drug Policy Alliance, "About the Drug Policy Alliance," http://www.drugpolicy.org/.

"Without meaning to": http://www.forbes.com/sites/artcarden/2012/04/19/lets-be -blunt-its-time-to-end-the-drug-war/.

"war on drugs, while well-intentioned": http://www.huffingtonpost.com/2012/07/09/ chris-christie-drugs-war-on-drugs_n_1659687.html.

greatest cause of prison population growth: http://www.nytimes.com/2011/06/17/ opinion/17carter.html.

it was a failure: Angus Reid Public Opinion poll, "Americans Decry War on Drugs, Support Legalizing Marijuana," June 6, 2012, http://www.angus-reid.com/polls/45091/ americans-decry-war-on-drugs-support-legalizing-marijuana/.

"I will also ask": Richard Nixon, "Annual Message to the Congress on the State of the Union," January 22, 1971; posted online by Gerhard Peters and John T. Woolley at http://www.presidency.ucsb.edu/.

289 *"death rates plunged":* Amanda Gardner, "Cancer Death Rates Continue to Drop," *USA Today,* January 5, 2012.

290 *National Cancer Institute's 2011 budget:* National Cancer Institute, U.S. Department of Health and Human Services, "2011 Fact Book," 2011, http://obf.cancer.gov/financial/attachments/11Factbk.pdf.

just over $1 billion: National Institute on Drug Abuse, "Fiscal Year 2011 Budget Information: Congressional Justification for National Institute on Drug Abuse," 2011, http://www.drugabuse.gov/about-nida/legislative-activities/budget-information/fiscal-year-2011-budget-information.

Americans with AIDS: Centers for Disease Control and Prevention, "HIV in the United States: At a Glance," March 14, 2012, http://www.cdc.gov/hiv/resources/factsheets/us.htm.

total spent on AIDS research: NIH Office of AIDS Research, "2011 Congressional Budget Justification," 2011, http://www.oar.nih.gov/budget/pdf/2010_0129_CJ2011.pdf.

291 *"reduced costs of crime":* Susan L. Ettner et al., "Benefit-Cost in the California Treatment Outcome Project: Does Substance Abuse Treatment 'Pay for Itself'?," *Health Services Research* 41 (2006): 192–213.

292 *"In the early 1980s":* Vicki Browder, "The Squeaky Wheel Gets the Grease," *EMBO Reports* 6 (2005): 1014–17.

293 *"Typically, a segregated illness":* Sally Chew, "Why Obama's Deputy Drug Czar Ditched DC," TheFix.com, June 9, 2011.

294 *Thirty-two states:* The most recent figure reported is from 2005; http://www.asam.org/advocacy/find-a-policy-statement/view-policy-statement/public-policy-statements/2011/12/15/repeal-of-the-uniform-accident-and-sickness-policy-provision-law-%28uppl%29.

296 *the felony re-arrest rate:* Linda Truitt et al., "Evaluating Drug Courts in Kansas City, Missouri, and Pensacola, Florida: Final Reports for Phase I and Phase II," National Institute of Justice, March 2002, http://www.abtassociates.com/reports/ES-eval_treatment.pdf.

"Seventy-five percent": National Association of Drug Court Professionals, "Drug Courts Work," http://www.nadcp.org/nadcp-home/.

297 *support legalization:* "Half in U.S. Support Legalizing Marijuana Use: Poll," Reuters, October 18, 2011.

"periodic pain": Josh Harkinson, How to Get a Pot Card (Without Really Trying)," *Mother Jones,* October 11, 2010.

298 *"What I think is horrible":* "Former Surgeon General Calls for Marijuana Legalization," CNN, October 18, 2010.

"because they are illegal": Marsha Rosenbaum, "Kids, Drugs, and Drug Education: A Harm Reduction Approach," National Council on Crime and Delinquency, 1996, http://www.drugtext.org/Education-and-Prevention/kids-drugs-and-drug-education-a-harm-reduction-approach.html.

299 *inaccurate and dangerous message:* Beau Kilmer et al., "Altered States? Assessing How Marijuana Legalization in California Could Influence Marijuana Consumption and Public Budgets," Rand Corporation, 2010, http://www.rand.org/pubs/occasional_papers/2010/RAND_OP315.pdf.

spike in marijuana use: Kilmer, "Altered States."

Miron calculated: Jeffrey A. Miron, "The Budgetary Implications of Marijuana Prohibition," Marijuana Policy Project, June 2005, http://www.prohibitioncosts.org/mironreport/.

300 *marijuana offenses:* Joe Klein, "Why Legalizing Marijuana Makes Sense," *Time,* April 2, 2009.

302 *Insite is effective:* "Vancouver's Insite Drug Injection Clinic Will Stay Open," CBC News, September 30, 2011.

303 *"state-sponsored suicide":* Jeremy Hainsworth, "Worldwide Interest as Canada Drug Program in Court," Associated Press, May 11, 2011.

"Insite has been proven": See http://www.bbc.co.uk/news/world-us-canada-15130282.

help retain addicts in treatment: U.S. Department of Health and Human Services, "Research Shows Needle Exchange Programs Reduce HIV Infections Without Increasing Drug Use," 1998, http://archive.hhs.gov/news/press/1998pres/980420a.html.

"Dutch are far less likely than Americans": David Jolly, "Law Could Hamper Drug Tourism in the Netherlands," *New York Times,* April 2, 2012.

304 *"Portugal's drug problem":* Maia Szalavitz, "Drugs in Portugal: Did Decriminalization Work?," *Time,* April 26, 2009.

Portugal reportedly had: Barry Hatton, "Portugal's Drug Policy Pays Off; US Eyes Lessons," Associated Press, December 27, 2010.

"whose arrest does nothing": Eduardo Porter, "Numbers Tell of Failure in Drug War," *New York Times,* July 3, 2012.

EPILOGUE

308 *The ACS contributes:* American Cancer Society, "About the American Cancer Society: Our History," http://www.cancer.org.

APPENDIX: JUST SAY *KNOW*

314 *the truth:* "This is an insight we've garnered from years of qualitative research with our teen audience," says Caryn Pace, who runs the National Youth Anti-Drug Media Campaign for the Partnership at Drugfree.org.

315 *Of those teens:* Partnership at DrugFree.org, "2010 Partnership Attitude Tracking Study," 2011, http://www.drugfree.org/the-partnership-at-drugfree-org.

316 *will become alcoholics:* Benjamin R. Nordstrom and Herbert D. Kleber, "Clinical and Societal Implications of Drug Legalization," in *Lowinson and Ruiz's Substance Abuse: A Comprehensive Textbook,* eds. Pedro Ruiz and Eric C. Strain, 5th ed. (Philadelphia: Lippincott Williams and Wilkins, 2011).

Binge drinking is especially prevalent: Substance Abuse and Mental Health Services Administration, *Results from the 2010 National Survey on Drug Use and Health: Summary of National Findings,* NSDUH Series H-41, HHS Publication No. (SMA) 11-4658 (Rockville, MD: Substance Abuse and Mental Health Services Administration, 2011).

317 *For college-age youths:* National Institute on Alcohol Abuse and Alcoholism, "College Drinking," National Institutes on Health, http://www.niaaa.nih.gov/alcohol-health/special-populations-co-occurring-disorders/college-drinking.

teenage deaths: Centers for Disease Control and Prevention, "Mortality Among Teenagers Aged 12–19 Years: United States, 1999–2006," NCHS Data Brief, May 2010, http://www.cdc.gov/nchs/data/databriefs/db37.htm.

rates of teenage suicide: Committee on Adolescence, "Suicide and Suicide Attempts in Adolescents," *Pediatrics* 105 (2000): 871–74.

318 *episode of major depression:* "Alcohol and Depression," WebMD.com, last accessed October 17, 2005; http://www.webmd.com/depression/alcohol-and-depression.

Fetal alcohol spectrum disorders: Substance Abuse and Mental Health Services Administration, "The FASD Center," July 27, 2012; Centers for Disease Control and Prevention, "Facts about FASDs," September 22, 2011.

daily marijuana use: National Institute on Drug Abuse, *Monitoring the Future: National Survey Results on Drug Use, 1975–2011. Volume I: Secondary School Students* (Ann Arbor: Institute for Social Research, 2011); National Institute on Drug Abuse, *Marijuana Use Continues to Rise Among U.S. Teens, While Alcohol Use Hits Historic Lows* (Ann Arbor: Institute for Social Research, University of Michigan, 2011).

they could buy marijuana: National Center on Addiction and Substance Abuse, *National Survey of American Attitudes on Substance Abuse XIII: Teens and Parents* (New York: Columbia University, 2008).

"major potheads": Yael Kohen, "Stiletto Stoners," *Marie Claire*, October 1, 2009.

drug-related ER visits: Substance Abuse and Mental Health Services Administration, Center for Behavioral Health Statistics and Quality, *Drug Abuse Warning Network: Detailed Tables: National Estimates, Drug-Related Emergency Department Visits for 2004–2009* (Rockville, MD: Substance Abuse and Mental Health Services Administration, 2011).

319 *Fewer smokers than nonsmokers complete college:* National Institute on Drug Abuse, "How Does Marijuana Use Affect School, Work, and Social Life?," September 2010.

IQs of heavy users: http://well.blogs.nytimes.com/2012/08/27/early-marijuana-use-linked-to-i-q-loss/.

320 *"chronic users":* Sarah Kershaw and Rebecca Cathcart, "Marijuana Is Gateway Drug for Two Debates," *New York Times*, July 17, 2009.

321 *"brain activation to cognitive tasks":* Dawn Fuller, "Research Finds That Marijuana Use Takes Toll on Adolescent Brain Function," *University of Cincinnati News*, October 13, 2008.

323 *"transition from childhood":* Ibid.

one out of five adolescents: Office of Adolescent Health, "Mental Health," http://www.hhs.gov/ash/oah/adolescent-health-topics/mental-health/, last accessed October 17, 2012.

324 *"triggers schizophrenia":* Nancy Lapid, "Smoking Pot May Hasten Onset of Mental Illness," Reuters, February 7, 2011.

325 *fraternal and identical twins:* M. T. Lynskey et al., "Escalation of Drug Use in Early-Onset Cannabis Users vs. Co-Twin Controls," *Journal of the American Medical Association* 289 (2003): 427–33.

primary marijuana addictions: Substance Abuse and Mental Health Services Administration, *Results from the 2010 National Survey.*

326 *The number goes up:* "Is Marijuana Addictive?" National Institute on Drug Abuse, July 2012, http://www.drugabuse.gov/publications/research-reports/marijuana-abuse.

Marijuana use was confirmed: Mark Asbridge et al., "Acute Cannabis Consumption and Motor Vehicle Collision Risk: Systematic Review of Observational Studies and Meta-Analysis," *British Medical Journal* 344 (2012).

"Cannabis affects drivers' spatial sense": McCarton Ackerman, "Pot Use Doubles Car Crash Risk," TheFix.com, February 10, 2012.

326 *confident the drug had no effect:* Michelle Healy, "Teen Drivers and Marijuana: A 'Dangerous Trend,'" *USA Today*, February 23, 2012.

327 *the NIDA website:* http://www.drugabuse.gov/drugs-abuse.

at Mouse Party: http://learn.genetics.utah.edu/content/addiction/drugs/mouse.html.

rose 400 percent: United States Office of National Drug Control Policy, *Epidemic: Re-*

sponding to America's Prescription Drug Abuse Crisis (Washington, DC: Executive Office of the President of the United States, 2011).

doubling of fatal poisonings: Jeffrey Young, "Prescription Drug Abuse Drives Huge Spike in Poisoning Deaths Among Children: Report," Huffington Post, April 16, 2012.

328 359,000 Americans: Substance Abuse and Mental Health Services Administration, Results from the 2010 National Survey.

350,000 meth users: Ibid.

329 cocaine-related emergency-room visits: Drug Abuse Warning Network (DAWN) report, "National Estimates of Drug-Related Emergency Department Visits," 2005, http://www.samhsa.gov/data/2k10/DAWN/ED2007/DAWN2k7ED.htm.

have a heart attack: "Cocaine Increases Heart Attack Risk," BBC News, June 1, 1999.

330 "hippocampal atrophy": "Long-Term Users of Ecstasy Risk Structural Brain Damage, Study Suggests," Science Daily, April 15, 2011.

use LSD and other hallucinogens: Substance Abuse and Mental Health Services Administration, Results from the 2010 National Survey.

331 alcohol and cocaine together: Jamie Doward, "Warning of Extra Heart Dangers from Mixing Cocaine and Alcohol," Guardian, November 7, 2009.

"synthetic pot": Joanna Cohen et al., "Clinical Presentation of Intoxication Due to Synthetic Cannabinoids," Pediatrics 129 (2012): e1064–67.

Index